SLEEPING WELL

The Sourcebook for Sleep and Sleep Disorders

Michael J. Thorpy, M.D., and
Jan Yager, Ph.D.

ILLINOIS PRAIRIE DISTRICT LIBRARY

☑® Checkmark Books®

An imprint of Facts On File, Inc.

Sleeping Well: The Sourcebook for Sleep and Sleep Disorders

Checkmark Books
An imprint of Facts On File, Inc.
132 West 31st Street
New York NY 10001

Library of Congress Cataloging-in-Publication Data

Thorpy, Michael J.
    Sleeping Well: the sourcebook for sleep and sleep disorders / by Michael J. Thorpy and Jan Yager
        p. cm.
Includes bibliographical references and index.
ISBN 0-8160-4090-7 (pbk. : alk. paper)
1. Sleep disorders—Popular works. 2. Sleep—Popular works. I. Yager, Jan, 1948—
II. Title

RC547 T47 2001
616.8†498—dc21   2001028323

The electroencephalographic characteristics of the human sleep stages chart is reprinted, with permission, from Peter Hauri's *Current Concepts: The Sleep Disorders*. Kalamazoo, Michigan: The Upjohn Company, 1982.
    The chart "When to Seek Help," created by Dr. Michael J. Thorpy, is reprinted with permission.

Checkmark Books are available at special discounts when purchased in bulk quantities for businesses, associations, institutions or sales promotions. Please call our Special Sales Department in New York at (212) 967-8800 or (800) 322-8755.

You can find Facts On File on the World Wide Web at http://www.factsonfile.com

Text design by Evelyn Horovicz
Cover design by Cathy Rincon

Printed in the United States of America

MP FOF 10 9 8 7 6 5 4 3 2 1

This book is printed on acid-free paper.

CONTENTS

LIST OF CHARTS AND ILLUSTRATIONS

IMPORTANT NOTE AND DISCLAIMER

This book is not intended to take the place of medical advice from your medical professional or psychological or psychiatric advice from your therapist. Readers are advised to consult a physician, psychologist, psychiatrist or other qualified health or psychological professional regarding treatment of their sleep, health or psychological problems. Neither the publisher nor the authors take any responsibility for any possible consequences from any treatment, action or application of medicine or preparation by any person reading or following the information in this book.

Before you make any changes in your sleep or health care regimens, or take any medications described in this book, make sure you consult a licensed physician. While this book provides general information on sleep strategies and disorders, since every person is unique, it is not intended to be a substitute for appropriate medical or psychological diagnosis or treatment. If you are having a sleep-related concern or a persistent problem, consult your physician or a physician or qualified health care professional at one of the accredited sleep disorders centers listed at the website of the American Academy of Sleep Medicine (AASM), which continually updates its list of accredited sleep disorders centers (http://www.aasm-net.org).

Throughout this book, you will find street addresses for associations or organizations, phone numbers, fax numbers, e-mail addresses, or websites. Since this information may change at any time, including even the name of an association or even the existence of a website on the Internet, neither the publisher nor the authors take any responsibility for the accuracy of any listings.

FOREWORD

Please note: Although the rest of *Sleeping Well* reads as one voice (except for Chapter 10, by Drs. Spielman and Glovinsky) for the purpose of this foreword we are writing individually about our unique backgrounds and approaches to the subject of sleep and sleep disorders.

When I first became interested in the area of sleep medicine, sleep was still little understood by the medical profession. There was no training in medical school on the subject of sleep disorders and thus I, as every other physician, had no formal training in this area. My primary interest was in neurology, and particularly the subject of neuroendocrinology, the study of how the brain produces hormones. Neuroendocrinology was in its beginning stages, and there were also very few training programs in the subject, but I managed to find a fellowship program at Montefiore Medical Center in New York. This program focused on the study of hormone production over a 24-hour period and involved the study of humans in a time isolation facility. It was there that I realized that circadian patterns of sleep and wakefulness had a profound control over hormone production, and my interest in sleep began. I assisted in the study of hormone production and sleep patterns of patients who were isolated from any knowledge of the time of day for periods of up to six months.

In 1977, Montefiore became the first sleep disorders center to be accredited in the United States, and I began to see patients with a variety of sleep problems. During the next two years, I became more engrossed in the clinical aspects of sleep medicine. I found an area of medicine that was little known, not only by physicians, but also the public, and discovered that many wonderful, strange and even dangerous things could happen during sleep. The most interesting question of all, and one that is still unanswered is, "Why do we need sleep?" In 1982 I was appointed the director of the Sleep-Wake Disorders Center at Montefiore Medical Center, a position I still hold.

In the 20 years I've been in sleep medicine, I've had the rewarding experience of helping thousands of men and women with sleep-related problems. I have helped cure hundreds of men and women who were snoring so loudly their partner could no longer share the marital bed, and those who needed help developing sleep patterns so they could sleep through the night and no longer be fatigued and exhausted during the day at home or on the job. I helped a young woman whose sleep terrors were so bad that she was unable to stay overnight with friends and was even embarrassed to spend the night in a hotel in case she would scream in the middle of the night. And I helped a man whose restless legs syndrome was so bad that he did not have a single night without pain in his legs for over 40 years. When relieved of the pain, he thought that it was a miracle. I've lost track of all the men and women with narcolepsy whom I've helped become more awake during the daytime, but I haven't forgotten the words they share when they call to thank me for helping them become more functional and active, such as "I have a new life" and "I feel younger and more energetic."

I also feel grateful for having the opportunity to save the lives of so many men with such severe sleep apnea that they could have died in their sleep. In addition to treating patients, I have found pleasure in being able to advise patients on their misconceptions about sleep; for example, many patients with insomnia feel that they will never be able to sleep again naturally if they start taking sleeping pills. However, if someone can sleep with the help of sleeping pills, he or she can sleep without them, and getting a patient to sleep well without medication is the ultimate aim.

Here are a few other examples of the countless patients with sleep-related problems whom I have helped over the years:

Jed, who was 62 years of age, enjoyed watching television in the evening but found that he was unable to stay awake after 8 P.M., when his favorite programs were shown. He would fall asleep in his chair, in front of the television, until he was awakened by his wife and told to go to bed. Although he fell asleep easily in the evening, he was unable to remain asleep at night and would lie in bed awake for hours after 3 A.M. trying to get back to sleep. He was referred to a sleep disorders center where he was diagnosed as having the advanced sleep phase syndrome. He was placed on a strict schedule of delaying his sleep by 15 minutes each day, becoming exposed to very bright light in the evening, and taking 3 mg of melatonin at bedtime. After two weeks, he was able to stay awake until 11 P.M. and slept until 6 A.M., a major improvement over his previous sleep pattern.

Michelle was 31 years of age and a physician. After a lecture I gave at a local hospital on sleep disorders, she came up to me and confided that she had been banging her head in bed since she was an infant. It was something that she had never told anyone about as she was embarrassed by the activity. In fact, she had purposefully avoided making any close relationships with the opposite sex because of the headbanging. I saw her as a patient and recommended some behavioral manipulations such as lining her bed with pillows, as it has been shown that close contact with the body provides a stimulation that reduces the tendency for rhythmical body movements. In addition, she started a benzodiazepine medication to help her sleep better and reduce the frequency of the movements. Although the activity did not cease completely, her movements became more controllable and less worrisome.

My daughter called me one day to say that her 26-year-old high school teacher was unable to stay awake long enough to mark their assignments that week. She had not been sleeping well and felt tired and sleepy all day long. She had seen her physician about the problem and was being investigated for insomnia. Interestingly, that week my wife and I had been to a parent-teacher meeting with that teacher, and during our two-minute meeting, something emotional came up and she flushed, faltered in her speech, and her head drooped. I thought it strange at the time but did not think anything else about it until my daughter mentioned the sleepiness. I thought to myself that it could be narcolepsy and had my daughter ask her teacher to make an appointment to see me. I saw the teacher as a patient and studies confirmed that rather than having insomnia, she had narcolepsy. Treatment with the medication Provigil (modafinil) led to significant improvement in her alertness during the day, and I am pleased to report that after that she was able to keep alert to mark her student assignments.

—Michael Thorpy, M.D.

. . . . . .

Dr. Thorpy and I began our collaboration back in 1987, when we began working together on the first edition of *The Encyclopedia of Sleep and Sleep Disorders,* published by Facts On File in 1991. At the request of our publisher, we recently completed the revision of the second edition of *The Encyclopedia of Sleep and Sleep Disorders* (Facts On File, 2001).

When we began work on this book, of course I brought to this project all the knowledge about sleep and sleep disorders I had gained through my collaboration with Dr. Thorpy over the last decade. But I also brought to the project my own training in related health care fields. I did a year of graduate work in psychiatric art therapy, including internships at an psychiatric hospital and a home for abused children. I also had a predoctoral fellowship from the National Science Foundation in medical sociology through Mt. Sinai Medical College and the City University of New York Graduate School, where I obtained my Ph.D. in sociology in 1983. Medical sociology was one of my three areas of specialization for my sociology doctorate. Other credits include my authorship of more than a dozen books, including an extensive study of friendship that evolved out of my sociology dissertation on friendship, entitled *Friendshifts®: The Power of Friendship and How It Shapes Our Lives,* as well as an annotated guide on where to get help in 52 areas of concern, including health, titled *The Help Book.* I have also researched and published health articles on such topics as lupus, pregnancy, childbearing and food labeling, that have appeared in *Woman's Day, McCall's, Newsday* and other publications.

In addition to working with Dr. Thorpy on these two sleep books, I have been researching an article on Sleep and Your Career. For that research, I interviewed sleep experts Joyce Walsleben, Ph.D., Dr. Amy Wolfson, Dr. Alan Jasper, Dr. Dennis Harris, Dr. Deelip Chatterjee, Dr.

Karen Wolfe, Dr. Bill Anthony (who, with his wife, Camille, maintains the www.napping.com website), as well as Pat Agostino, an emergency room nurse and freelance writer, and Andrea Herman from the Better Sleep Council. Also helpful were Gwen A. Henson, Laura Gilbert, Bob Abbott, Karen Allen, Terri Raab, Vicki Gladden, Linda Olson, Caryl Frawley, Jim Blassingame, Richard Laermer, Will Veitch and John Antonio Negroni. I also want to acknowledge the help of Marcia C. Stein of the National Sleep Foundation as well as numerous other publicists and information officers including Erin Hill, Ken Davis, Vicki Garfinkel, Susan Kaplan, Andrea Papa, Nadine Woloshin, Marcia Goodrich, Rebecca Tessitore, Tom Durso, Barbara Wenner, Elaine Hamnett, Barbara Lewis, Judith Lederman and Ayoka Pond, all of whom were kind enough to respond to the query that I placed on the Internet research tool known as Profnet.com describing my sleep-related article research.

I also bring to *Sleeping Well* an expertise in time management as the author of two books on time management: *Creative Time Management* (Prentice Hall, 1984) and *Creative Time Management for the New Millennium* (Hannacroix Creek Books, 1999). At first, there may not seem to be a relationship between getting enough sleep and time management. But Stephanie Allmon, in her article "Wake-up Call Sounded on Need for More Sleep," published in *The Washington Times* (April 26, 2000, page A2), points out how Duane Slegel, clinical director of the Sleep Disorders Center of Texas, based in Dallas, relates the two. Allmon writes: "'The most important change people can make to get enough sleep at night is to be more efficient during the day,' Mr. Slegel said, 'One way to do this is to get more work done during normal working hours so you don't need to arrive early or stay late at your job,' he said."

Before Dr. Thorpy and I finished writing *Sleeping Well*, I had a frightening personal experience that subjectively reinforced just one example of the life-and-death value of the information that is shared in *Sleeping Well*. Like so many working parents, simultaneously juggling multiple responsibilities (for me, mother, wife, researcher, author, consultant and homemaker), I sometimes functioned on less sleep than I actually needed. When necessary, I compensated for that sleep deprivation by taking a 20-minute nap or getting more sleep the next night. This particular day, however, although tired in the late afternoon (around 4 P.M.), I ignored the warning signs of exhaustion.

I was fortunate that there were almost no cars on the road and that I was driving at or below the speed limit of 45 miles an hour because, in a split second, I fell asleep at the wheel. Fortunately, no one was hurt, but falling asleep at the wheel even once is a frightening experience. For me, it certainly was a crystal-clear wake-up call to the very real dangers of driving when exhausted. It taught me to listen to my instincts when I feel I am too tired to drive. The split second that it took to go from awake and alert to asleep at the wheel also showed me that this type of situation could truly happen to anyone, even someone like me who tries to be a careful driver, constantly aware of road conditions as well as any physical or mental condition related to driving, including the necessity of taking rest breaks or having clear driving directions if driving somewhere unfamiliar.

Since that horrific personal experience, I have been reading up on "drowsy driving," as it is called, and I have been astonished by just how many vehicle-related deaths and injuries are attributed to this widespread problem. The National Sleep Foundation's 2000 Omnibus Sleep in America survey found that 17% of people surveyed reported that in the previous year they had fallen asleep at the wheel and 51% reported driving a car or other vehicle while feeling drowsy. The National Sleep Foundation literature states that "fatigue contributes to more than 100,000 highway crashes, causing 71,000 injuries and 1,500 deaths each year in the United States alone." However, it is only in the last few years that "drowsy driving" is getting the attention that has been accorded an equally dangerous driving problem, namely drunk driving.

We want to thank Drs. Arthur Spielman and Paul Glovinsky for contributing their chapter on psychology and sleep. Finally, thanks to the staff at Facts On File, Inc., especially our dedicated editor on this book and on the second edition of *The Encyclopedia of Sleep and Sleep Disorders*, James Chambers, as well as his editorial assistant Regina Sampogna, Dorothy Cummings, Ben Jacobs, Pat McPartland, Kate Moore, Laurie Fishman, Megan Kennedy and the rest of the production, marketing and sales departments who helped us take this book from an idea to a published entity.

—Jan Yager, Ph.D.

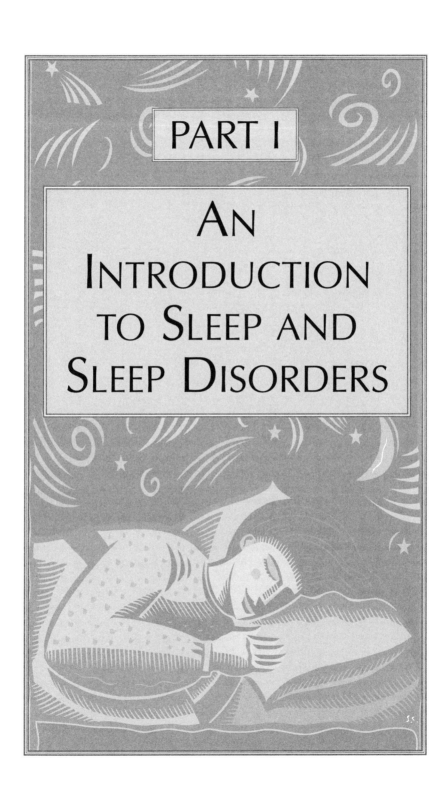

PART I

AN INTRODUCTION TO SLEEP AND SLEEP DISORDERS

CHAPTER 1
SLEEP: AN OVERVIEW

- A middle-aged man with obstructive sleep apnea snores so loudly that his wife has to move to another room in the house to sleep. The daytime sleepiness that accompanies his snoring and sleep apnea manifests itself whenever he is in a quiet situation—he falls asleep when he is reading or watching TV. Since at least twice he has fallen asleep while driving, his concerned wife now does most of the driving.
- The mother of a 10-month-old infant who does not yet sleep through the night, sleeping only five hours at a stretch, longs for a complete night of sleep. Sleep deprivation is taking an emotional toll on her as she begins each day exhausted and cranky.
- A 43-year-old investment banker, father of two school-age sons, falls asleep at the wheel while driving home on the highway. He is killed and his wife is injured.
- A teacher confides that she "loses sleep" over her supervisor's negative comments about her job performance.

Sleep—the hours separating one day from the next. On average, sleep comprises about eight hours of our day, or about one-third of our lives. If all goes well, we take sleep for granted. We wake up feeling alert and refreshed and remain alert throughout the day.

But, as the above examples indicate, when sleep is less than ideal because of physical or psychological reasons, the results can range from a mild case of exhaustion, like the sleep-deprived mother of the infant, to causing a disruption of the marital bed, as in the case of the man with sleep apnea and daytime sleepiness, or the extreme (but not uncommon) fatal consequence of when someone falls asleep at the wheel.

According to the National Sleep Foundation 2000 telephone survey of 1,154 men and women in the United States, the average number of hours of sleep during the workweek is 6 hours, 54 minutes, at least one hour fewer each night than the recommended 8 hours.

Few physiological conditions have received as much attention through the ages by poets, novelists, scholars and scientists as sleep. From Aristotle, Ovid and Shakespeare, to Dante and Frost, writers have been fascinated with sleep and its impact upon emotions, behavior and health. The cause and reason for sleep has been pondered by some of the world's greatest minds, including Hippocrates and Freud, who attempted explanations of the physiological basis of sleep and dreams.

As we increasingly become a 24/7 world, with supermarkets and some restaurants open 24 hours a day, an estimated one-fourth of the U.S. workforce, or more than 20 million workers, must deal with the night shift or shift work and the sleep-related problems that usually accompany that schedule. Similarly, as some school systems start the school day earlier and earlier, for children sleep has become more of a concern than ever before. Since sleep is a daily need, sleeping well tonight is no guarantee that you will sleep well every night. If you change, or environmental influences change, such as the addition of a newborn to the household, job stress, the noise caused by construction of a new building across the street, or even the development of a sleep disorder, your sleep may be disturbed; no one is ever totally devoid of any sleep disturbance all the time.

The sleep environment has also undergone a change: from communal sleeping rooms with beds of twigs, straw or skins, the bedroom has evolved in the 21st century into a private place with electronic equipment including computers, remote-controlled television, and video cassette recorders, thermostats controlling the temperature, and artificial lighting.

A rudimentary understanding of insomnia and sleepiness was known in ancient times, but specific sleep disorders, such as narcolepsy, began to be recognized only in the late 19th century. Explorations into the causes of sleepiness and insomnia have reached a peak in the last 50 years thanks to the development of sophisticated technology.

Although most sleep disorders have probably been present since humans evolved, modern society has produced several new disorders. Thomas Edison's electric light bulb has allowed the light of day to be extended into night so that shift work can now occur around the clock, but at the expense of a disruption of the circadian rhythm (or natural body clock) and sleep disturbance. Similarly, international travel by plane has enabled the rapid crossing of time zones, which also can lead to a disruption of circadian rhythms and sleep disturbance, commonly termed *jet lag*.

DEFINITION OF SLEEP

What is this condition known as sleep that we do for one-third of our lives? Sleep could be defined as a behavioral state characterized by rest, immobility, reduced perception of environmental stimuli and suspension of cognition and consciousness. Sleep occurs when the brain waves slow, and the erratic activity of many parts of the brain starts to coalesce into a coordinated, synchronized background rhythm. The heart rate slows, the muscles relax and the wakeful brain mentation calms to the point that a satisfying sense of contentment occurs as we mentally drift away from our environment into peaceful unconsciousness.

We usually refer to the main sleep episode at night as being either *nighttime* or *nocturnal sleep*. A nap is a sleep episode that is not the major sleep episode. However, for a shift worker who has to work at night and sleep during the day, the major sleep episode may occur during the day-time and not be related to nighttime.

The term *circadian* applies to rhythms that occur every 24 hours. The most obvious circadian rhythm is the sleep-wake cycle itself. However, there are circadian rhythms of many hormonal and biochemical factors such as the hormone cortisol or growth hormone.

How Much Sleep Is Enough Sleep?

For most of the population, $7^1/_2$ to 8 hours of sleep is sufficient. However, the need for sleep varies greatly, depending upon the age and the particular physiology of an individual. Infants will spend two-thirds of the day asleep, and the sleep need gradually reduces over a lifetime. In early adolescence, there is still a requirement for as much as 9 or 10 hours of sleep.

There is evidence that the elderly do require less sleep. The difference in the elderly is very small compared with the middle-aged population. Unfortunately, many elderly people cannot obtain adequate sleep at night due to physical conditions related to aging and consequently suffer from increasing tiredness and sleepiness during the daytime.

It is during our prepubertal years that sleep is best. That is when we have the smallest number of awakenings and the lowest amount of light sleep, and alertness during the day is optimal. However, from that age on, there is a gradual deterioration in the quality of the sleep at night, and we tend to become more tired and sleepy as we get older.

Are You Getting Enough Sleep?

Do *you* get enough sleep? Maybe you have a quick and definite "yes" or "no" answer to that question, or maybe you are unsure about yourself or about a spouse, child, friend or coworker. If you are in doubt about whether or not you or someone you know and care about, gets enough sleep, take the quiz on page 6.

How Much Sleep Are You Really Getting?

How many hours a night do you actually sleep? During the week? On weekends? Do you know when you go to sleep, how long you stay asleep, and when you wake up (throughout the workweek or school week) as well as on weekends or holidays? If you need to get a more accurate record of just how much you are sleeping throughout the week, then keep a sleep diary like the one below to track your sleep pattern. Use the sleep diary on page 6 to keep track of the time you go to sleep and wake up (the overall number of hours that you sleep) over a 7-day period. Make a photocopy of this master diary so you will always have a blank version available if you wish to create another sleep diary at a later date; this will also help you to avoid writing in the book (especially if it is a library book).

Are You Sleep-Deprived?

Ask yourself the following questions and answer "yes" or "no," keeping track of your answers:

Do you need to set an alarm in order to wake up in the morning?

Do you need a cup of coffee to "feel awake" in the morning?

Do you feel tired and fatigued upon awakening as well as exhausted in the morning?

Do you find that you catch yourself from drifting off or falling asleep at the wheel at any time during the day or evening when you are driving your car?

Do you fall asleep easily when traveling as a passenger in a bus, car, plane, train or subway?

Do you often doze when watching television or sitting quietly reading?

Do you find yourself needing a nap in the afternoon?

Do you find that you say to yourself at any time during the workweek, "I can't wait until the weekend so I can 'sleep in'"?

Do you find yourself falling asleep the instant your head hits the pillow?

If you answered "yes" *to more than one* of the above questions, you may be sleep deprived.

Sleep Diary

Name: _____   Date: _____

Complete this form for each day of the week. Add any additional comments to the side or on the back.

	Bedtime	Time to fall asleep	Number of awakenings	Wake time	Out-of-bed time	Comments
Monday						
Tuesday						
Wednesday						
Thursday						
Friday						
Saturday						
Sunday						

Why Do We Sleep?

Ironically, after all the research into sleep, we still do not know *why* we need to sleep. The cause-and-effect relationship between sleep and life is not as clear as it is between food and life or air and water and life. It is possible to go for an extended period of time without sleep, although it is not recommended. The world record is held by Randy Gardner who, in 1965, when he was a San Diego high school student, broke the *Guinness Book of World Records* record for the longest time awake: 264 hours or 11 days. He was monitored by the sleep researcher William Dement, who later wrote in his book *The Promise of Sleep*, "After recently reviewing the movies and audiotapes we recorded and the papers about Randy we published in scientific journals, I can say with absolute certainty that his staying awake for 264 hours did not cause any psychiatric problems whatsoever." However, Dement also notes that in 1965, the monitoring equipment was not as advanced as today; it is possible that "Randy may have been in the sleepwalking state some of the time."

Randy Gardner, however, is an exception to the rule; for most of us, even missing a few hours of the amount of sleep we usually need, or pulling an "all nighter" and missing an entire night, can have severe physical and mental consequences.

What Are the Benefits of Sleep and the Consequences of Sleepiness?

We may not know why we sleep, but we do see the benefits of sleep by looking at what happens when someone does not get enough sleep or goes without it for even one night. Too little sleep has a negative impact on mood; those who are sleep-deprived tend to be more agitated, depressed, cranky and pessimistic. Not getting enough sleep may also be the basis for stomach upset as well as heightened sensitivity to pain. Dr. David Dinges, who studied the impact of $4^1/_2$ hours sleep for one week on his subjects, found that partial sleep deprivation resulted in an increase in stress, muddled thinking, complaints about stomach ailments, greater sadness and a higher degree of mental and physical exhaustion.

An American Cancer Society study in the 1950s found that the amount of time spent sleeping might be one of the best predictors of how long we will live. Those adults who slept nine or ten hours or more*, and those who slept four or less hours, had higher mortality rates than those who slept about eight hours, who had the lowest mortality rates. (A nine-year follow-up study, as well as a repetition of the study by other researchers, found similar results.)

Besides promoting longevity, researchers have discovered that sleep is a better predictor than exposure to infection of whether or not someone

---

*Children, however, on average, need 9 to 10 hours of sleep a night.

will get a cold. During sleep, the immune system is reinforced. Another benefit of sleep is that hormones, such as cortisol, prolactin and the growth hormone, are discharged into the bloodstream.

Daytime fatigue, whether or not it is related to getting enough sleep the night before, is certainly a condition that also needs to be understood and addressed. One of the many tragic examples of this is the New Hampshire high school student who, in 1989, won a car for his recognition as "America's Safest Teen Driver" after competing in a national driver safety competition. The next year, however, that teen fell asleep at the wheel at 5 P.M. as he drove home from college. He drifted over the yellow line into oncoming traffic, killing himself as well as the 19-year-old driver of another car.

Other well-known tragedies that sleep researchers William C. Dement, James B. Maas and others suggest may be linked to daytime or nighttime sleepiness or exhaustion and severe sleep deprivation include the Challenger space shuttle explosion, the Exxon Valdez oil spill disaster and the Chernobyl nuclear reactor accident.

Sleepiness makes it harder for children and teens to learn at school and reduces worker productivity. The National Sleep Foundation's 2000 telephone survey of 1,154 adults in the United States found that these six skills were more difficult because of sleepiness, listed in order of descending frequency: concentrating (68%); handling stress (66%); solving problems (58%); decision making (58%); listening to coworkers (57%); and relating to coworkers (39%). Stated in an even more emphatic way, 61%, or more than six out of 10, said that sleepiness *diminished* their concentration, and more than 40% (four out of 10) said that the quality of their work suffers because of sleepiness.

EXPLAINING BASIC SLEEP TERMS

With the development of sleep medicine, many terms related to sleep and sleep disorders have been created. To adequately understand sleep and sleep disorders, it is useful to understand some of the basic terminology and concepts.

The Five Stages of Sleep

Before the birth of modern sleep research, in the early 1950s, it was commonly assumed that sleep was one long episode of six to nine hours when very little was going on except perhaps a dream or two. We now know that when we are asleep, the brain still produces electroencephalographic (EEG) waves although the waves are slower and distinctive from the awake state. While awake, the brain waves are beta waves, which are fast, and during a relaxed, eyes-closed state, the waves are alpha waves, which

HUMAN SLEEP STAGES

Awake—low voltage—random, fast

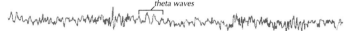

Drowsy—8 to 12 cps—alpha waves

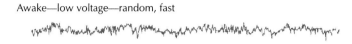

Stage 1—3 to 7 cps—theta waves

theta waves

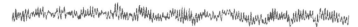

Stage 2—12 to 14 cps—sleep spindles and K complexes

sleep spindles   *K complex* ———

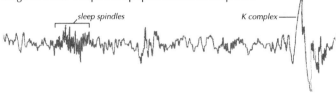

Delta sleep—1/2 to 2 cps—delta waves > 75 μV

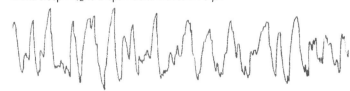

REM sleep—low voltage—random, fast with sawtooth waves

sawtooth waves

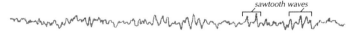

Source: Electroencephalographic characteristics of the human sleep stages. (From P. Hauri, *Current Concepts: The Sleep Disorders*. Kalamazoo, Mich.: The Upjohn Company, 1982; reprinted with permission).

are a little slower at 8 to 12 cycles per second. During sleep, the electroencephalographic waves are the much slower, and bigger amplitude delta and theta waves occur.

Although sleep may seem like a single state, physiology differs markedly during certain times of the major sleep episode since sleep is made up of various stages. As discussed below, it begins with stage one and progresses through stage four. These are the stages known as non-REM sleep, followed by the REM (rapid eye movements) stage, sometimes known as stage five sleep. The stages also are repeated several times throughout the night; we go through stages one through four, followed by a period of REM sleep, several times each night; a cycle that has a 90- to 100-minute duration. Each night, there are usually four or five sleep cycles occurring during the hours that we are sleeping.

Non-REM Sleep

Non-REM sleep is the type of sleep not associated with rapid eye movements (REMs); it includes four separate stages. Non-REM sleep consists of stage one, stage two, stage three and stage four sleep. All these stages lack REMs; hence these stages are grouped together as NREM or non-REM sleep. The body, including brain activity, rests during NREM sleep. (It is during REM sleep that the brain is active and dreaming occurs, but the body continues to rest even during REM sleep.)

Stage One (Theta Waves)

The lighter type of sleep is called stage one sleep. Stage one sleep is the transition between wakefulness and sleep, and it lasts about five minutes. If you awake out of stage one sleep, you often feel as though you have remained awake. However, stage one sleep is associated with changes in the brain wave pattern as your brain wave rhythms become slower, your muscles start to relax and your eye movements change to a slow rolling pattern (contrasted to the rapid eye movements seen during wakefulness). Usually, we only have about 4% to 5% of the night (total sleep time) spent in stage one sleep. But people with insomnia may have a greater percentage of lighter sleep. People who are sleep deprived can have less than 5% of stage one sleep because they go into deep sleep more quickly. In stage one sleep, there are no spindles, K-complexes or REMs.

Stage Two (Light Sleep—Sleep Spindles and K-Complexes)

Typically, we pass from stage one sleep into stage two sleep, which is a very specific sleep stage accounting for 45% to 50% of total sleep time. Stage two sleep has characteristic features associated with it, such as sleep spindle activity. Sleep spindles are fast brain wave rhythms that last up to $1^1/_2$ seconds, have a peculiar and specific spindle shape and can be detected using an EEG (electroencephalograph). In addition to sleep spindles, there is another unusual pattern that occurs in stage two sleep called the K-complex. The K-complex is an episodic large brain wave that stands out from the background pattern. This particular wave is only seen during stage two sleep, and is often seen in conjunction with the sleep spindles.

Usually, if we have been in stage two for several minutes and then awoken, we will have the sensation that we have been asleep.

Stage Three (Slow Wave Sleep)

As we get into deeper sleep stages, our muscles become more and more relaxed so there is little activity occurring in our muscles except what is required for breathing. Our brain wave activity starts to slow down and the brain waves become coordinated or synchronized into a large rhythmic pattern. This slow wave activity gives rise to *slow wave sleep,* the term used to describe both stage three and four sleep. The percentage of slow waves during a 10- or 15-second episode of sleep determines whether we are in stage three or stage four sleep.

Stage three sleep comprises 4% to 6% of total sleep time, and eye movement is typically absent during this stage. This stage is sometimes combined with stage four into NREM stages three and four because of the physiological similarities between the two stages.

Stage Four (Deepest Sleep)

Stage four sleep is scored when more than 50% of the epoch contains delta waves of the same frequency and amplitude as those seen in stage three sleep. This stage, the deepest of the four N-REM stages, is synonymous with slow wave sleep and usually comprises 12% to 15% of total sleep time. It is during this stage that sleep terrors or sleepwalking may occur. As noted above, it is sometimes combined with stage three into NREM stages three and four because the stages are so similar. Although rare, sleep spindles may occur during stage four sleep.

REM Sleep (Paradoxical Sleep When Dreaming Occurs)

One of the most dramatic forms of sleep is called rapid eye movement sleep, or REM sleep. REM sleep is so named because of the rapid eye movements that occur during this stage of sleep. There is also loss of muscle tone and a mixed frequency, low voltage EEG pattern with occasional bursts of "sawtooth" theta waves. Dreaming occurs during REM sleep.

Rapid eye movements are similar to looking quickly from side to side, or up or down, while we are asleep. In fact, the movements can be so much like the rapid eye movements when we are awake that this stage of sleep may be in some cases mistaken for wakefulness. In general, when we sleep at night our eye movements are nonexistent. Initially, there may be slow, rolling eye movements as our eyes go backward and forward under our eyelids. But when we get into deeper sleep, the eyes stop moving completely.

REM is actually the final stage of sleep, the stage when you dream. The first REM phase begins about 90 minutes after you begin sleeping. Several times each night, your sleep will follow this typical pattern: a deep NREM stage three or four sleep into a light stage two sleep before starting the first REM sleep.

The percentage of the night spent in each sleep stage differs according to age. Infants may have as much as 50% of the night spent in the REM sleep, preadolescent children may have more than 50% of slow wave sleep and the elderly may not have any slow wave sleep at all.

Physiological Changes During Sleep

A number of physiological changes are important during sleep. As mentioned above, the brain wave pattern, eye movements and muscle activity are three measures that are usually used for determining sleep stages. In addition, in measuring sleep we often record other physiological variables. These include the heart rhythm or EKG, and chest movements, abdominal movements or airflow through the nostrils and mouth, which can measure the pattern of breathing. The oxygen level is often measured in the blood; this is important in disorders where breathing is affected, when the oxygen level might fall. This measure of oxygen level is called the oxygen saturation.

Movements of the limbs are also often measured. There is a specific sleep disorder called periodic limb movement disorder in which the legs, and sometimes the arms, will have episodic jerks that occur every 20 to 40 seconds throughout sleep. Sensors for the detection of these movements are usually placed on the lower legs or arms. In addition, an individual may be videotaped during sleep to see if there are any abnormal behaviors that occur during sleep. All of the above measures are usually determined during sleep studies, also known as polysomnography.

SLEEP DISORDERS AND THE SLEEP INDUSTRY

Associated with the improved recognition and awareness of sleep disorders is the development of a whole industry around sleep. This industry provides information, diagnostic techniques and treatment of sleep disorders. Most popular magazines that deal with social or health issues have published stories on sleep disorders in recent years, and numerous popular books have been written on the topic. The National Sleep Foundation (NSF), established in 1990, conducts surveys, disseminates information on sleep and sleep disorders through its written publications as well as its website (http://www.sleepfoundation.org) and heightens public awareness of sleep through its annual National Sleep Awareness Week that takes place in March.

The medical profession has created professional associations for the practitioners of sleep medicine, such as the American Academy of Sleep Medicine (AASM). Textbooks and educational programs provide information on the current research and knowledge of sleep disorders. Professional examinations have been established, not only for clinicians, but also for the technologists involved in performing sleep testing, such as the Association of Polysomnographic Technologists (APT). Freestanding and hospital-based sleep disorders centers have been created extensively throughout the United States and much of the world. Diagnostic equipment companies and medical supply companies provide treatment means such as continuous positive air pressure device (CPAP) machines, for the treatment of sleep apnea. Clearly, sleep has become a big business.

Fortunately, patients and the general public have benefited from all these advances in sleep medicine. Patients are now being diagnosed much more quickly and are receiving more specific and more effective treatments. These advances and treatment issues are discussed further in Chapters 2–10 and in the A-to-Z entries of *Sleeping Well*. The general public is beginning to gain a better understanding of this everyday yet mysterious occurrence that we call sleep.

Still, there are many misconceptions and biases about sleep, particularly when it comes to the use of medications in the treatment of sleep disorders. For example, some sleep researchers believe that sleeping pills may be harmful because of their potential for addiction, whereas others believe that they can be beneficial in reconditioning a person back to good sleep habits.

The medical texts describe more than 80 different sleep disorders. For many of these disorders, such as obstructive sleep apnea syndrome or restless legs syndrome, a recipe-like approach emphasizing diagnosis and specific treatments is useful. However, for numerous sleep disorders, such as insomnia, chronic fatigue syndrome, or headbanging, effective treatment is very dependent upon the skill and expertise of the clinician.

Dealing with sleep disorders is still very much an art, as well as a science. Furthermore, because the range of sleep disorders is so large, and every patient is unique, it usually takes considerable clinical experience for a medical practitioner or other qualified health care professional, such as a psychologist with training in sleep disorders, to feel comfortable in dealing with patients who may have a sleep disorder.

There are several sleep disorders that have captured the public's attention, namely, insomnia, sleep apnea, narcolepsy and jet lag. These disorders are commonly discussed in the media at the expense of the other 75 or so other sleep disorders. Chapters 3 through 8 of *Sleeping Well* provide an overview to these common sleep disorders as well as several additional sleep disorders (shift-work sleep disorder, sleepwalking, sleep terrors, REM-sleep behavior disorder, headbanging, sleep-related eating disorder, restless legs syndrome). In Part II, the A-to-Z entries, you will be able to find basic information and suggested treatments for a wider range of sleep disorders, among them advanced sleep phase syndrome, alcohol-dependent sleep disorder, altitude insomnia, confusional arousals, limit-setting sleep disorder and much more, including definitions of terms and descriptions of sleep medications and treatments.

Of all the sleep disorders, sleep apnea is the sleep ailment that has received the most attention and concern from the medical profession. Sleep apnea can be associated with sudden death during sleep at night and typically is associated with the very common symptom of snoring. It also produces tiredness and fatigue during the daytime.

Although sleep apnea affects up to 24% of males on a chronic basis and has the potential of being a fatal ailment, insomnia (the inability to get to sleep or to remain asleep) is far more common. According to a 2000 National Sleep Foundation Sleep in America Poll, 58% of the adults surveyed reported having insomnia a few nights per week or more within the year prior to the survey.

In the last several years, the neurological disorder of narcolepsy has received a lot of attention. Narcolepsy is a disorder or excessive sleepiness that during daytime episodes of sleep is often accompanied by dreams and the sensation of an inability to move the body (sleep paralysis) upon awakening. Part of the reason for the increased attention to narcolepsy is the availability of new medication and treatments. Also, recent research has demonstrated a better understanding of the cause of narcolepsy. This knowledge is having a major impact upon our understanding of the brain's control of sleep and wakefulness.

With the increasing frequency of international travel, jet lag, especially as it relates to business travel, has received a lot of interest, as has the somewhat similar shift-work sleep disorder. Shift-work sleep disorder affects workers who work the night shift, such as 11 P.M. to 7 A.M., and who typically have a disturbed sleep-wake pattern. These disorders are usually transient and can affect anyone regardless of whether they have any ill health.

Although there are a large number of sleep disorders, most do not occur at every phase of the lifespan. For example, there are disorders that affect only infants, and some that only affect the elderly. Chapter 9 discusses the disorders that typically occur at different stages in life. Gender also plays a part, and women develop sleep disorders that differ in their prevalence from males; sleep disorders may be related to menstruation, pregnancy or menopause. Women are more likely to suffer from difficulty in sleeping than men. Women fall asleep less quickly and have more awakenings, but have an increase in slow wave sleep that does not reduce with age as quickly as it does in men. Insomnia is more common in women; snoring and sleep apnea are less common. However, after menopause some women start to snore more, and sleep apnea becomes more prevalent. These differences in sleep features are thought to be related to differences in sex steroids.

In Chapter 2, before the discussion of specific sleep disorders in Chapters 3 through 8, you will learn information that is relevant to everyone, namely, how to increase the likelihood that you will get a good night's sleep by promoting optimal sleep hygiene.

INCREASING YOUR CHANCES OF GETTING A GOOD NIGHT'S SLEEP

PROMOTING SLEEP HYGIENE

Sleep specialists use the term *sleep hygiene* to apply to those everyday activities that can be beneficial to promoting continuous and effective sleep. Sleep hygiene revolves around the timing and quantity of sleep as well as practices that are performed during the day or evening that may be counterproductive to good sleep. These are common behaviors that may have little consequence to someone who has no difficulty in sleep, but for someone who is suffering from a sleep disturbance—not only those suffering from insomnia, but also people who may have sleep apnea, narcolepsy or some other type of sleep disorder—they may become paramount.

Unfortunately, a lot of these basic sleep hygiene recommendations are not taught to our children, otherwise we would probably see fewer sleep problems occurring in older age groups. Good sleep practices should be taught at an early age. Parents need to be aware of the importance of promoting exemplary sleep habits so that they can institute exemplary practices in their children.

Regularity Is Key

Probably the most helpful information that anyone who has a sleep problem should understand is that maintaining a regular bedtime and having a regular time of awakening is of vital importance in reducing the severity of a sleep disorder. The amount of time you spend in bed is also crucial. In general, much of our population tends to cut itself short of sleep. The insufficient amount of sleep at night results in tiredness and sleepiness during the daytime. Another large portion of the population spends an excessive amount of time in bed, with resulting complaints of inability to sleep at night, or frequent awakenings at night.

Sleep as a Conditioned Response

We become conditioned to the environment and the circumstances around going to bed at night. Good sleepers usually do not think about how their sleep is going to be on any particular night. They may look at their watch, see a specific time that they usually go to bed and, although they may be wide awake and alert and conversing at that time, once in bed, they fall asleep rapidly, without difficulty. They are also able to sleep soundly until their time of awakening the next morning.

This ability to change from near full alertness to sound sleep is promoted by a set of conditioned responses. These responses are affected by going into a bedroom where we are exposed to an environment that we use for sleeping. The practices around going to bed, such as changing into nightwear, going to the bathroom and turning out the bedroom light, all have a positive effect on our sleep. People who have significant sleep disturbances often lose these typical conditioned responses and their night-to-night behavior can be quite variable.

Ideally, we should avoid any mental stimulation for the hour or so before going to bed at night. Many people will read a book, have a hot bath, do some light exercise or rest prior to getting into bed. All of these practices are generally helpful in any particular individual. However, if somebody has a sleep disturbance and suffers from a disorder such as insomnia, then spending time awake in the bedroom and doing wakeful activities may be counterproductive to the development of good sleep. The bedroom should be viewed as the place for sleep at night, not a place for wakeful activities other than sexual activity.

Beds and the Sleep Environment

Although the bedding industry would have everyone believe that a bad bed is the primary cause of most sleep disturbances, there is little scientific evidence to support this. Certainly, if a bed is uncomfortable and causes pain or discomfort, it is likely to interfere with our sleep. However, it is important to recognize the fact that people who sleep in different cultures, such as those who sleep on the ground on hard mats, can sleep as well as someone sleeping in a comfortable, high-quality, expensive mattress set.

There are some, however, who have reported improved sleep because of a specific mattress. Sleep research pioneer William C. Dement, in *The Promise of Sleep*, writes about the two times in 30 years that he thought the mattress made a difference in providing him with the best nights of sleep he ever had. First was the time he slept at the famed Beverly Hilton Hotel and found it was "like sleeping on a cloud" and second was the time he stayed at a bed-and-breakfast in Pasco, Washington, "operated by a patient with narcolepsy." "Once again," he writes, "I had a magical night" because of the mattress he slept on. (If you want to read guidelines on mattress selection, provided by Andrea Hermann of the Better Sleep Council, see Appendix 1.)

When we stay at a hotel, or sleep in a different environment, a change in the sleeping surface may be important. However, other factors, such as the stress of being in a new environment, may be as important in causing us to sleep less soundly.

Stress

The part that stress plays in the development of sleep problems varies greatly. There is no question that there are people under high stress who sleep very well at night without difficulty. If you have sleep difficulties, it is very easy to ascribe stress as the primary cause, and certainly at times this may be correct. Changes in levels of stress are more important than chronic ongoing stress. Everybody has experienced a sleepless night related to some increase in anxiety or worries. In general, it is better to do something restful, such as reading, to reduce an increased anxiety level before going to sleep at night. (For additional comments about the relationship between stress and sleep, see Chapter 10, "The Interplay Between Psychology and Sleep," by psychologists and sleep experts Arthur J. Spielman, Ph.D., and Paul B. Glovinsky, Ph.D.)

Light

In recent years there has been evidence about the importance of light exposure in controlling the day-to-day pattern of sleep and wakefulness. Light follows very definite pathways within the brain that affect the sleep centers. Bright light during the waking portion of the day is very helpful in maintaining our circadian pattern of sleep and wakefulness. Light is often used as a means for adjusting the timing of sleep and can be useful for people who suffer from jet lag, shift work or other sleep disorders where the timing of sleep within the 24-hour day is altered.

In general, bright light immediately before going to bed at night tends to delay our sleep to a later time. Bright light immediately upon awakening in the morning is more likely to cause our sleep pattern to advance, so that we tend to fall asleep earlier in the evening.

Exercise

There is ample evidence to indicate that exercise is beneficial for sleep. Exercise, particularly in the late afternoon or early evening, is more helpful to improving sleep patterns than exercise that occurs immediately before bedtime, or upon awakening in the morning. If exercise is taken late at night, generally it should be relaxing exercise, such as yoga, which may be conducive to sleep. More energetic exercise, such as playing a game of squash, should be avoided.

Exercise is important, not only in promoting good sleep habits, but also in controlling body weight. Sleep apnea, a common sleep disorder particularly in middle-aged males, is greatly affected by body weight; exercise may be helpful in allowing a person to maintain an ideal body weight.

Patients with sleep apnea should make exercise a regular part of their daily routine.

Noise

Much has been written about the effect of noise upon sleep. In general, loud noise can disrupt sleep and cause frequent awakenings at night. However, there are countless people who sleep next to airports, with planes taking off and landing at night, or who sleep near railroad tracks or highways, who sleep extremely well and without difficulty.

Some people are very susceptible to noise, and this will prevent them from being able to get back to sleep. For most patients who have insomnia, noise is not the cause of their sleep disturbance, although they may think that this is the reason that they cannot sleep. In general, patients who are awake will become aware of any noise in the environment, and if they focus and dwell on that noise, it may become a cause of their inability to fall back to sleep.

Certain curtains have been marketed as being important for keeping out sound from the bedroom. However, these curtains are not necessary for most people who have a sleep disturbance. If we travel to a different environment, such as staying in a hotel, however, strange noises may be disturbing. The soundproofing of hotel rooms is much more important than in a home bedroom. We tend to become conditioned to noise in a familiar environment to the point that it does not bother us. However, sometimes we can become so focused on the noise in an unfamiliar environment that until it is excluded, we may have difficulty in being able to return to sleep.

Food

Hunger can also be a factor in disturbing our sleep at night. Ideally, we do not want to go to bed hungry and therefore a light snack before going to bed can be useful for some people. Large meals generally are disruptive to sleep, and a change in dietary intake may also be disruptive. For example, someone who is not used to a new spicy cuisine may find that it disturbs his or her sleep. The cause of the sleep disturbance is not specifically the spicy food, as individuals who eat that type of food every day do not sleep any worse than the average person does.

Large meals before sleep may be disruptive and can be particularly detrimental for someone who suffers from loud snoring or a tendency for sleep apnea. A large meal before sleep at night may promote indigestion with acid coming back into the mouth. This acid reflux can be inhaled, causing gasping, coughing and choking. Dietary factors are also very important for the overweight individual who needs to lose weight in order to reduce his or her tendency toward sleep-related breathing disorders.

Caffeine

Stimulants such as coffee, tea or soft drinks that contain caffeine will be detrimental to sleep and should be avoided late at night. Many people think that they can drink a strong cup of coffee immediately before going to bed and have little difficulty in sleeping. However, most research has shown that caffeine intake before sleep does cause an increase in sleep fragmentation compared with avoiding caffeine. A typical cup of coffee contains about 100 milligrams of caffeine, and a bottle of cola drink has about 50 milligrams of caffeine.

Caffeine was probably one of the first medications used for the treatment of excessive sleepiness. However, it is not recommended for this purpose since it can produce cardiac stimulation with palpitations and hypertension as well as heightened irritability or nervousness. For patients who have disorders of excessive sleepiness, more effective stimulant medications, such as modafinil (Provigil), methylphenidate (Ritalin) or amphetamines, are available by prescription.

Nicotine

Like caffeine, nicotine is a stimulant that can be detrimental to sleep habits. Nicotine is contained in cigarette tobacco; it is also present in chewing tobacco. If taken immediately prior to sleep, nicotine may cause a condition known as sleep onset insomnia. It is certainly not recommended when people awaken during the night that they smoke as it may contribute to difficulty in falling back to sleep again.

Nicotine produces an alerting pattern in the electroencephalogram. It may also cause hand tremor, decreased skeletal muscle tone, and reduction in deep tendon reflexes.

People who are very sleepy or who have sleep disorders such as obstructive sleep apnea syndrome could fall asleep while smoking in bed, possibly causing a fire. This can be a major cause of accidental death during sleep.

Alcoholic Beverages

Alcohol has been used as a sleep aid, and there is evidence that small amounts of alcohol do help. Unfortunately, once alcohol is metabolized it tends to become stimulating and will disrupt sleep with an increased number of awakenings, particularly in the second half of the sleep episode. The routine use of alcohol as a sedative produces an improved onset time, often with a deeper sleep in the first third of the night, but then sleep becomes lighter and more fragmented.

After the ingestion of alcohol, people often will awaken the next morning feeling less rested. They may also awaken with headaches, particularly following excessive alcohol use.

Alcohol can also exacerbate particular sleep disorders, such as sleep apnea, by reducing arousals related to episodes of cessation of breathing during sleep at night and therefore may be dangerous. It will also increase the amount and loudness of snoring.

Alcoholism is associated with an increased number of sleep-related disturbances including sleepwalking, night terrors and bed-wetting (sleep enuresis).

People who chronically use alcohol for getting to sleep may develop alcohol-dependent sleep disorder. This disorder is not associated with heavy alcohol ingestion during the daytime, and it is not a symptom of alcoholism. As tolerance develops, the amount of alcohol ingested increases, but those with alcohol-dependent sleep disorder usually do not go on to become alcoholics.

Sleep Medications

Much has been written about the use of sleep medications. There are strong opinions on whether sleep medications should be avoided or whether they can be helpful. Fortunately, the sleep medications that are now available, such as zaleplon (Sonata) and zolpidem (Ambien), are much safer than those of only a few years ago. They are not as likely to be addicting and have fewer detrimental effects upon health. Older sleeping pills, such as the barbiturates, can be dangerous and even cause death if taken in excess, whereas the newer medications are not life-threatening, even in high doses.

The careful use of sleeping pills can be very helpful in relieving sleep disturbances for many individuals. Prior concerns about the development of tolerance, that is, a need to keep increasing the amount of medication in order to get an effect, is not a factor with the new medications, which do not need any dose escalation to be effective. Also, the newer medications are much easier to withdraw from, when it is time to stop them. In the right setting, and under the right conditions, sleeping pills can be an extremely valuable aid in promoting and enhancing good sleep patterns. Self-medication, however, is definitely to be avoided. A person should be under the care of a qualified medical professional if it is determined that a sleep medication is recommended for treatment of his or her sleep disorder.

Naps

In general, if you are very sleepy during the day, a nap is the most effective way of relieving that sleepiness. A nap is strongly encouraged if you are sleepy and you need to perform any type of activity that requires concentration and alertness, such as driving or operating dangerous machinery. Of course, in some cultures, the taking of an afternoon nap or siesta, is a routine habit. This makes sense in climates where a hot midday sun prevents working effectively.

But in most modern societies, a single episode of nocturnal sleep and two-thirds of the day spent in full wakefulness is the preferred pattern. Furthermore, if you have a sleep disturbance at night, you may find that a nap during the daytime is detrimental to developing good sleep habits.

With the increased widespread problem of sleep deprivation in the United States and in other countries, however, taking a 15-to-20-minute nap at work is a concept and practice that is gaining favor. A brief nap can improve concentration, mood, alertness, memory, productivity and energy, as well as lower stress.

10 Tips for Getting a Good Night's Sleep

1. Maintain a regular bedtime and a regular time for awakening, even on weekends.
2. Stay in bed just the right number of hours for *you*—too much time in bed may cause frequent awakenings at night or an inability to go to sleep, and too little time asleep can lead to daytime sleepiness and exhaustion.
3. Avoid excessive mental stimulation for the hour before going to bed. But you can read a book, have a hot bath, do some light relaxing exercise such as yoga or rest.
4. Exercise may improve sleep, particularly if it is done in the late afternoon or early evening, rather than immediately before bedtime or upon awakening in the morning, except for sexual activity before bed, if this typically helps you and your partner to sleep.
5. Although you can become conditioned to your typical sleep environment so noise or light does not affect your sleep, in an unfamiliar environment such as a hotel room, noise or light should be minimal or eliminated or it may keep you awake.
6. Avoid going to sleep when you are hungry or after a large meal. A light snack before bed may help promote sleep.
7. Stay away from alcohol, caffeine or nicotine right before bed since all may increase sleep fragmentation, the number of awakenings during the night, or cause you to wake up the next morning feeling less rested.
8. In the right setting and under the right conditions, including being under a doctor's care, sleeping pills may be useful in promoting good sleep and enhancing desirable sleep patterns.
9. Unless there are cultural reasons for a nap, or you are so exhausted that a nap is required for alertness, especially if driving a car or operating dangerous machinery, eliminating nap time may actually improve your nighttime sleep.
10. Deal with and, ideally, eliminate the worries, stress, anxiety or rage that may be interrupting your sleep. If necessary, write down your concerns before you get into bed so you can deal with them the next day rather than ruminating throughout the night.

Psychologist and napping advocates Bill Anthony and his wife, Camille, have written two books on napping, *The Art of Napping* and *The Art of Napping at Work*. They have conducted original research on napping through surveys that are posted at their informative website, http://www.napping.com.

If you do nap after lunch, the time of the day when most day workers may feel an energy dip, keep the nap to 20 minutes or you will go into the slow wave sleep stage of sleep, which makes you feel more lethargic when you are awoken out of it.

A nationwide study conducted in 2000 by the National Sleep Foundation of 1,154 adults found that 46% of those who are allowed to nap at work do so. (One out of six adults in the survey noted that their employers allow them to take a nap.) One-third of the adults (33%) noted that they would nap at work if it were allowed.

SLEEP DISORDER TREATMENT OPTIONS

Treatments for sleep disorders vary widely, depending upon the type of disorder under management. For patients with insomnia, consideration is given to either behavioral treatments of insomnia, which involve lifestyle changes, or pharmacological treatment. Pharmacological treatment may involve the use of sleeping pills, also known as hypnotics, or the use of other medications, such as sedating antidepressant medications. Treatments for disorders such as sleep apnea might involve behavioral treatments (particularly weight loss), mechanical treatment such as the use of a CPAP device or various oral appliances that are inserted into the mouth or may involve upper airway surgery. Either behavioral treatments or pharmacological medications can treat narcolepsy.

When to Seek Help

The chart that follows, developed by Dr. Michael J. Thorpy, may help you to decide whether, according to the experts, you should seek help. Look over the list of 10 symptoms in the column on the left side of the chart and rate your symptom, from very mild to severe, with gradations in between as noted across the top of the chart. Then, depending upon the shading (light, medium or dark) you may assess whether treatment is definitely needed (dark), recommended (medium) or not necessarily needed (light).

CATEGORIES OF SLEEP DISORDERS

There are five main categories of sleep disorders:

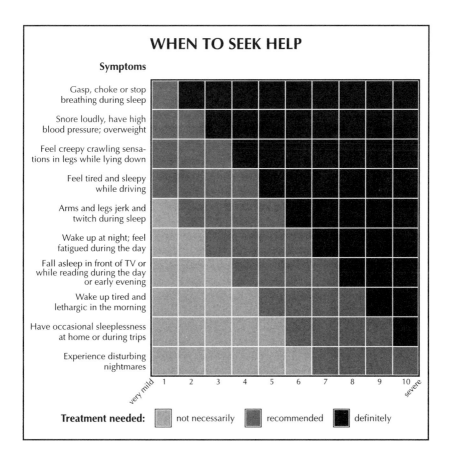

WHEN TO SEEK HELP

Symptoms

Symptom	1 very mild	2	3	4	5	6	7	8	9	10 severe

Gasp, choke or stop breathing during sleep

Snore loudly, have high blood pressure; overweight

Feel creepy crawling sensations in legs while lying down

Feel tired and sleepy while driving

Arms and legs jerk and twitch during sleep

Wake up at night; feel fatigued during the day

Fall asleep in front of TV or while reading during the day or early evening

Wake up tired and lethargic in the morning

Have occasional sleeplessness at home or during trips

Experience disturbing nightmares

Treatment needed: ▨ not necessarily ▨ recommended ■ definitely

---

• disorders that cause insomnia
• disorders that cause excessive daytime sleepiness
• movement disorders, including restless legs syndrome and periodic limb movement disorder
• disorders that cause abnormal events during sleep at night, also known as parasomnias, including sleep terrors and sleepwalking.
• disorders associated with alteration in the timing of sleep in relation to underlying biological (circadian) rhythms, including jet lag and shift-work sleep disorder.

All of the approximately 80 sleep disorders will fit into one or more of these five categories. In the next six chapters, you will find a discussion of some of the most common sleep disorders. Each chapter includes a description of the problem, a typical case history and a range of possible treatment options.

SLEEP DISORDERS MEDICINE

. . . We have created a new clinical specialty, sleep disorders medicine, whose task is to watch over all of us while we are asleep.

—William Dement (1985)

Several books on sleep had a major influence on the development of sleep disorders medicine. Pieron's *Le Problème Physiologique du Sommeil* in 1913 summarized the scientific sleep literature at that time. A similar approach was taken by Kleitman, who produced his monumental treatise *Sleep and Wakefulness* in 1939 (updated in 1963 to contain 4,337 references).*

Organized sleep disorders medicine in the United States began with the founding of the Association for the Psychophysiological Study of Sleep (APSS) in 1961, an association composed of sleep researchers, many with clinical interests. Sleep research led to the investigation of sleep disorders, which resulted in the establishment in the early 1970s of clinical sleep disorder centers for the diagnosis and treatment of patients. In 1976, the Association of Sleep Disorder Centers (ASDC) was founded. The first sleep disorder center to be engaged in active patient evaluations and treatment was that established at Stanford University in California by Dement.

The Association of Sleep Disorder Centers classification committee chaired by Howard Roffwarg produced the *Diagnostic Classification of Sleep and Arousal Disorders* in 1979; it ushered in the modern era of sleep diagnoses and became the first classification to be widely used. The *Principles and Practices of Sleep Disorders Medicine,* published in 1989 and edited by Meir Kryger, William C. Dement and Thomas Roth, was the first comprehensive textbook on basic sleep research and clinical sleep medicine.

An accreditation process for sleep disorders centers was established by the ASDC, and the first to be accredited in 1977 was the Sleep-Wake Disorders Unit, headed by Weitzman, at Montefiore Medical Center in New York. In 1978, the medical journal *Sleep* was created to present research and clinical articles on sleep, and in 1979 a complete issue was devoted to the *Diagnostic Classification of Sleep and Arousal Disorders.*

In 1978, the Association of Polysomnographic Technologists, founded by Peter McGregor, set standards of practice for polysomnographic technologists. In 1983 the Association for the Psychophysiologic Study of Sleep was renamed the Sleep Research Society (SRS), and in 1984 the Clinical Sleep Society (CSS) was founded as the membership branch of the Association of Sleep Disorder Centers. In 1986, the Association of Sleep Disorder Centers, the Clinical Sleep Society, the Sleep Research Society and the

*For a detailed account of the history of sleep and man from prehistoric and ancient times till the present by Michael J. Thorpy, M.D., see "History of Sleep and Man," pages xi–xxxii, in *The Encyclopedia of Sleep and Sleep Disorders, Second Edition, Updated and Revised* by Michael J. Thorpy, M.D., and Jan Yager, Ph.D. (New York: Facts On File, 2001).

Association of Polysomnographic Technologists formed a federation called the Association of Professional Sleep Societies (APSS). The Association of Sleep Disorder Centers changed its name to the American Sleep Disorders Association in 1987. Then, in 1999, it was renamed the American Academy of Sleep Medicine (AASM).

The term *sleep specialist* usually applies to a physician involved in the treatment of sleep disorders. Although this term is also applied to psychologists with expertise in sleep, by far the majority of sleep specialists are physicians, usually pulmonary physicians, neurologists or psychiatrists. In the United States, the American Board of Sleep Medicine credentials physicians in the practice of sleep medicine. These physicians must undergo intense training in sleep medicine for at least one year, and certification requires passing both a written and practical examination. The main professional sleep organization in the United States is called the American Academy of Sleep Medicine (AASM). Several of the professional medical organizations also have sections devoted to sleep medicine, among them the American Thoracic Society and the American Academy of Neurology.

The American Academy of Sleep Medicine (AASM) credentials sleep disorders centers to ensure that they meet the highest-quality conditions for the diagnosis and treatment of sleep disorders. There are more than 1,000 sleep disorders centers accredited by the AASM in the United States. (For a state-by-state listing, consult their website, http://www.aasmnet. org.)

Sleep disorders centers usually evaluate patients for sleep problems by taking a medical history and performing a physical examination. Sometimes treatment is initiated at that point, especially for patients suffering from insomnia. Patients with other disorders, such as obstructive sleep apnea syndrome or narcolepsy, may need to return to the sleep disorders center for an overnight sleep study. The study, which is usually performed in a bedroom that is not unlike a hotel room, measures the physiological variables discussed above, during a whole night of sleep. Patients with narcolepsy may require testing during the daytime to determine their level of alertness. The Multiple Sleep Latency Test (MSLT), a test that measures how quickly an individual falls asleep on four or five nap opportunities, is performed at two-hour intervals throughout the day. How quickly the person falls asleep and whether REM sleep occurs are important in determining a diagnosis of narcolepsy.

CHAPTER 3

INSOMNIA

WHAT IS INSOMNIA?

The term *insomnia* is derived from the Latin words *in,* meaning "not," and *somnus,* meaning "sleep." *Insomnia* strictly means *the inability to sleep.* Everybody at some time suffers from sleep disturbance, but when it becomes a problem, night after night, we call it insomnia. Although insomnia has been used to refer to a disorder in which sleep disturbance can be objectively documented, it is more generally used for any disorder associated with a complaint of disturbed or unrefreshing sleep.

In the A-to-Z entries section of this book, you will find a discussion of specific insomnias as well as sleep disorders characterized by insomnia such as altitude insomnia, pregnancy-related sleep disorder, psychophysiological insomnia, adjustment sleep disorder, idiopathic (or childhood) insomnia and menstrual-associated sleep disorder. However, in this chapter we will discuss the condition of insomnia, or the inability to fall asleep, or stay asleep, in a more general way.

In terms of insomnia, key questions you should consider are: When should you seek help for insomnia? When is insomnia regarded as a problem?

For example, occasional difficulty in being able to sleep well at night was something that Jane was used to. However, after she turned 30, it became a problem that persisted every night for several weeks, and she knew she had to get help. Her marriage was not going well, and she was under a lot of pressure at work. She became withdrawn and would cry over even the littlest thing that went wrong. Her physician diagnosed her as being depressed. She started a course of Elavil (amitriptyline), a tricyclic antidepressant with sedating effects that is commonly used in the treatment of insomnia due to depression, at night. Just a small dose of 50 milligrams was sufficient to improve her sleep at night and gradually the depression resolved.*

In trying to understand insomnia we have to first understand the factors involved in producing it. Typically, insomnia is a difficulty in falling asleep or frequent awakenings during sleep that leads to feeling tired or exhausted the next morning. Common causes of insomnia in most healthy individuals include anxiety, stress, worries, pain or discomfort. At

---

*Cautionary note: As stated in the disclaimer at the beginning of this book, you need to seek medical help for treatment, especially medication; in terms of type of medication or dosage, do not self-medicate.

some stage, everybody experiences these potential causes of insomnia. Fortunately, for most people, a night of sleep disturbance is usually followed by a night of better sleep; the sleep disruption does not become an ingrained habit, and does not turn into chronic insomnia. The prevalence of insomnia increases with age, from young adulthood to old age.

Medically, chronic insomnia is defined as insomnia that lasts for three weeks or longer. The tendency these days is to prevent more acute forms of insomnia from becoming chronic. Therefore, treatment for insomnia should be started well before the sleep disturbance has lasted three weeks.

Treatment Options

Why should we treat insomnia? There are two main reasons. One is to prevent the insomnia from becoming chronic. Think of insomnia as a conditioned response; that is, it becomes an ingrained habit. The more sleep disturbance you have, the more likely you are to have sleep disturbance. It is like a snowball rolling down a hill that tends to get bigger and bigger as it goes. If we can prevent the sleep disturbance from becoming a habit, then chronic insomnia is less likely to ensue.

The other reason for treating insomnia is to prevent the symptoms that are directly related to it, such as tiredness and fatigue during the daytime. Typically, people do not like being awake during the night when they would rather be sleeping. Therefore, they become restless, start to worry about their inability to sleep and fear that they may be more tired and less able to concentrate or be effective the following day.

All of these symptoms are amplified in the person who has chronic insomnia. Typically, people with chronic insomnia become preoccupied with sleep, and so from the moment they wake up in the morning, they worry about the next night of sleep. There is also evidence that insomnia can contribute to impaired social relationships and contribute to many types of accidents, including motor vehicle accidents. For all of these reasons, experts feel that insomnia should be prevented, and certainly if there is a means of preventing the onset of chronic insomnia, it is preferable to living with it.

A night or two of sleep disturbances in relation to some underlying stress is extremely common, and in this situation most people do not seek specific treatment. However, there are some situations when even the expectation of a night of sleep disturbance might cause an individual to consider some anticipatory treatment. For example, if one hears of a death in the family and knows they are unlikely to sleep the next night, he or she might request a sleeping pill. Or, if somebody is traveling in an airplane across time zones, he or she may request a sleeping pill to make it easier to sleep in the airplane or at the new environment. So the question arises: When is treatment necessary for insomnia and under what circumstances?

It is important to recognize that insomnia differs according to the age of the individual. Insomnia in children may be very different from insomnia in middle age. Insomnia in the elderly may more likely be associated with underlying medical or psychiatric disorders, or may be the result of medications taken to treat those medical or psychiatric disorders. The treatment strategies mentioned above are primarily for people who are otherwise in good health and who suffer from primary forms of insomnia.

Although we all recognize that anxiety, stress or discomfort can contribute to insomnia, most chronic forms of insomnia are not related to these transient problems. The most common causes of chronic insomnia are depression and anxiety disorders, but there are some forms of chronic insomnia that are not secondary to psychiatric or medical disorders. These types of sleep disturbance are often termed primary insomnia. One of the major forms is known as psychophysiological insomnia, a conditioned form of insomnia that usually develops from an acute episode of sleep disturbance. The acute episode causes anxiety and disruption of the sleep-wake process that then becomes an ingrained behavior, and so the sleep disturbance becomes chronic. Reconditioning the patient to good-quality sleep usually treats this type of insomnia.

We often hear about individuals who have not slept for many years. These stories are typically reported in the tabloid press and often consist of dramatic stories about someone not having slept for 10 or 13 years. However, the inability to sleep for prolonged periods of time is extremely rare and usually associated with specific and obvious neurological disorders. Most people who feel that they do not sleep, in fact, do sleep for some period of time. It is important to recognize the process that occurs. Sleep itself is usually perceived as being relatively instantaneous. It is very difficult for us to judge how long we have been asleep at night, and typically we do this by assessing changes in our environment. For example, if you fall asleep in front of the television and later awaken to find a different program playing, you know that you have been asleep for a period of time. Or, if you fall asleep when it is light outside and wake up when it is dark, again you know you have been asleep. However, if you have no cues as to how much time has passed, it is extremely difficult to judge exactly how long you have been asleep.

Contrast this with being awake in bed at night. If you are trying to fall asleep, every second counts. You are aware of every moment that you are awake. A few minutes can seem like hours. If you fall asleep and then awaken, typically you do not recognize the fact that you have been asleep but only remember being awake. As a result, most people with insomnia are totally unaware of the exact amount of time they slept. In a sleep laboratory, this is very evident as most patients with insomnia will report having slept a much shorter time than is shown objectively by the sleep testing. This is an important aspect of insomnia to understand. Most people with sleep disturbance underestimate the amount of time that they have spent asleep and should be reassured that they have probably slept longer than they believed. However, this knowledge does not help the individual who would like to fall asleep rapidly and sleep soundly until his or her time of awakening the next morning. Sleeping longer than one believes one is sleeping is not going to solve the problem.

Insomnia due to psychiatric or medical disorders usually will respond to the treatment of the underlying disorder. For example, if depression is the cause of the insomnia, then the depression should be treated first. However, the sleep disturbance associated with the depression can be helped by specific treatments directed to the sleep disruption in addition to treating the depression. As mentioned earlier, psychophysiological, or conditioned insomnia, is the form of chronic insomnia that occurs in most healthy people who otherwise do not have an underlying medical disorder. Treatment for conditioned insomnia can be specific and very effective.

All patients who have sleep disruption benefit from sleep hygiene. It is important to emphasize that the most important thing for someone with insomnia to understand is that the time of going to bed, the time of getting up in the morning and the amount of time spent in bed are absolutely crucial when dealing with the problem.

However, when sleep disruption, or insomnia, occurs, the typical reaction is to try to stay in bed longer the next morning in order to make up for lost sleep the night before. Also, if you have had very little sleep, the tendency is to go to bed earlier the next night because you are tired, in the hope that you will make up for some of the sleep that you lost the previous night. It is therefore not unusual for someone to spend an excessive amount of time in bed, anywhere from perhaps 8 P.M. to 8 A.M. A primary treatment strategy is to reduce the amount of time spent in bed. A set bedtime, independent of whether the person slept the night before, and a set time of waking in the morning, is absolutely crucial. The amount of time in bed for most people with chronic insomnia should not exceed $7^1/_2$ hours.

Sleep Restriction Therapy

Sleep restriction therapy is a very specific behavioral treatment that has been used for treating sleep disturbance. This treatment is based on the fact that spending an excessive amount of time awake in bed at night can be counterproductive to developing good sleep habits. In its strictest form, patients estimate the amount of time that they spend in bed each night and then average it out over a two-week period. During the two weeks they also estimate the amount of time spent asleep each night. If the amount of time spent asleep averages only six hours, for example, then the person would be placed on a bedtime and wake time schedule that corresponds to six hours; for example, 12 midnight to 6 A.M. After keeping to these bedtime limits for five days, if the person fills the designated time with sleep, the amount of time available for sleep is extended by 15 minutes. Then, every five days, an additional extension by 15 minutes is made if the person fills the new limits with sleep. By this means, the person fills the time with good sleep, with few awakenings, and usually the total amount of sleep increases.

Sleep restriction therapy has the advantage of conditioning someone back to good sleep and maintaining stable wake times and bedtimes. To a lesser extent, this process can be applied to the average person who has chronic sleep disturbance. If someone has insomnia and spends eight hours in bed, he or she should reduce the amount of time in bed by approximately one hour so the sleep becomes consolidated. The time of awakening should be fixed, but bedtime should be delayed to the appropriate time. For example, if the person is put on a schedule of seven hours in bed, it may mean getting up at 7 A.M., but not going to bed until midnight. This bedtime can be gradually extended by 15 minutes every five days when the person starts to fill that time with sleep.

Although sleep restriction therapy can be carried out rigorously under the supervision of a sleep specialist, it can also be carried out in a limited way, as described above, by the average person suffering from insomnia. Generally, this will produce some sleep improvement. However, in many situations the sleep process needs to be enhanced by medication. The primary aim is that the individual will learn to sleep well and therefore reduce a lot of his or her anxiety around sleep. Sleep medications can facilitate this process. Commonly used sleeping pills are zolpidem (Ambien) and zaleplon (Sonata). These medications, when taken within 30 minutes of going to bed at night, can greatly enhance the ability to sleep and usually are free of side effects. They help the person become reconditioned back to good sleep; once the sleep pattern has improved, the medications can be gradually withdrawn. This treatment strategy requires monitoring by a physician.

Although numerous sleep medications are available, the two main ones that are prescribed in the United States are zolpidem and zaleplon. These medications are very similar, although zaleplon has a much shorter half-life than zolpidem, which means that the effect of the medication wears off more quickly. Zaleplon only acts for two or three hours and, therefore, can be taken in a second dose, if necessary, in the middle of the night. Ambien has a longer duration of effect and generally acts over the seven or eight hours of the normal nocturnal sleep episode. In certain individuals, either of these medications can result in feelings of tiredness or fatigue the next day. This is more common in the elderly, who tend to metabolize medication less rapidly.

Antidepressant Treatment

In patients who have depression as a primary cause of their insomnia, treatment with an antidepressant medication is usually indicated. Unfortunately, many of the newer antidepressant medications, such as Prozac, tend to have sleep disturbance as part of their effect. Although they are effective in treating the underlying depression, they may initially worsen the sleep disturbance. Several antidepressant medications, including Remeron or trazodone, are more effective in improving sleep without causing disruption of the sleep process. Some of the older antidepressant medications, such as amitriptyline (Elavil), can be very effective in improving the sleep quality of people who are depressed. These older medications, the tricyclic antidepressant medications, tend to have significant side effects. These side effects, called anticholinergic effects, consist of dry mouth, tiredness upon awakening, constipation, blurring of vision and sexual dysfunction. These side effects are most typically seen in the high doses used to treat depression, but are less commonly associated with the lower dosages used in the treatment of insomnia. In some patients, amitriptyline may be a very effective agent, although it is contraindicated in elderly patients who have heart disease.

Unfortunately, some physicians who are not knowledgeable about the treatment of sleep disturbance are unaware of the most effective way of giving Elavil to patients with insomnia. This medication should be given well before the sleep episode, typically at least one hour, if not two hours, before the planned bedtime. The advantage of this is that it helps to relax the patient before it is time to go to bed. Also, the dose must start very low, typically with the lowest strength of the medication, which is 10 milligrams. This dose can be increased every third night by 10 milligrams until the patient gets a beneficial response, or until he or she takes a maximum dose of 50 milligrams, at which time the dosage should be discussed with a physician. Most patients respond to only 10 or 20 milligrams of amitriptiline. Dry mouth and initial tiredness may occur, but usually these symptoms will go away within two to three days of starting the medication.

Melatonin

Sleeping pills and antidepressants are the most effective medications used in the treatment of insomnia. However, other compounds, such as melatonin, have also been recommended. Melatonin, a hormone, initially received much attention because it was demonstrated to be helpful for the treatment of insomnia in elderly patients.

Melatonin is very effective in altering the timing of the sleep process and is receiving much attention now for the treatment of shift-work disorder or jet lag disorder. However, low doses of melatonin may be helpful for some people with insomnia since there is evidence that melatonin has a slight sleep-inducing effect. Since the effect is not strong, however, it is not effective for most people with chronic forms of insomnia. Because there is limited research on the potential for adverse reactions to melatonin, it should not be used regularly unless recommended by a physician.

Stimulus Control Therapy

In addition to medications and sleep restriction therapy, stimulus control therapy is another form of behavioral treatment that can be very helpful. This is a technique that typically involves leaving the bedroom when awake at night in order to go to another room to get the mind off the need for sleep. The usual recommendation is that when you are awake at night, you should leave the bedroom and go read a book or watch television until you feel tired, and then go back to bed.

This is an effective treatment for many people and should be incorporated into any treatment regime, even if sleep medications are also used. One important element is to reduce the amount of time spent awake in bed at night, so that you only go to bed when sleepy. However, you should arise at exactly the same time every morning, and should avoid daytime naps. This can be used as a sole treatment for primary insomnia, or can be used as an adjunct to medication treatment for insomnia.

CHAPTER 4

SNORING AND SLEEP APNEA

The leading sleep disorder today, obstructive sleep apnea syndrome, was described in 1836, not by a clinician but by the novelist Charles Dickens (1812–70). Dickens published a series of stories entitled *The Posthumous Papers of the Pickwick Club* in which he described Joe, the fat boy, who was always excessively sleepy. Joe, a loud snorer who was obese and somnolent, may have had right-sided heart failure that lead to his being called "young dropsy."

More than 100 years followed Dickens's description before obstructive sleep apnea syndrome became a well-recognized clinical entity. However, a number of writers in the 19th century did allude to some of the features of sleep apnea in their publications. William Wadd, surgeon to the king of England, in 1816 wrote about the relationship between obesity and sleepiness. George Catlin, a painter and lawyer, in 1861 described the breathing habits of the American Indian in his book entitled *The Breath of Life*, in which he graphically portrayed the effects of obstructed breathing during sleep. William Henry Broadbent (1835–1907) in 1877 was the first physician to report the clinical features of the obstructive sleep apnea syndrome, and William Hill in 1889 observed that upper airway obstruction contributed to "stupidity" in children. The most notable description was by William Hughes Wells (1854–1919) in 1878; he cured several patients of sleepiness by treatment of upper airway obstruction.

Following the reports of snoring, sleepiness and obesity in the 19th century, Sir William Osler (1849–1919) in 1907 referred to Dickens's description of Joe: "An extraordinary phenomenon in excessively fat young persons is an uncontrollable tendency to sleep, like the fat boy in Pickwick."

Charles Sidney Burwell in 1956 brought general recognition to obstructive sleep apnea syndrome, which he called the "Pickwickian Syndrome"; and Henri Gastaut reported the first objective documentation of polysomnographic features in 1965. Though the tracheotomy had been performed since the time of Asclepiades (first century B.C.), Wolfgang Kuhlo and Erich Doll in 1972 reported that it provided an effective treatment of the obstructive sleep apnea syndrome. Tanenosuke Ikematsu in 1964 popularized uvulopalatopharyngoplasty (UPP) surgery for the treatment of snoring, which was subsequently applied to the obstructive sleep apnea syndrome by Shiro Fujita in 1981. That same year, nasal continuous positive airway pressure (CPAP) treatment was described by Colin Sullivan and subsequently became the treatment of choice.

SNORING

His loud snoring was something that Paula could not bear, and so, after his 40th birthday, she decided that her husband, John, would have to sleep in the guest room. Being separated from his wife at night led John to realize that he needed professional help in dealing with his snoring, so he saw his physician.

Sleep studies showed that not only did John snore loudly at night but also he would stop breathing up to 100 times during the night. His blood oxygen level also fell below normal. He was diagnosed as having sleep apnea. Treatment involved sleeping with a mask over his nose attached to a continuous positive airway pressure device (CPAP). Although the device was cumbersome, Paula was pleased that John's snoring was eliminated, that the CPAP machine had improved his physical health and that they could resume sleeping together.

Most middle-aged men snore. Snoring is a sign of upper airway obstruction occurring during sleep at night. Usually, snoring is of no consequence. However, when it is loud, it can be very disturbing for a bed partner or other household members. It can also be associated with impaired sleep quality at night with resulting daytime tiredness, fatigue and sleepiness. It can even have more severe consequences when associated with cessation of breathing during sleep. At worst, snoring can cause sudden death during sleep at night.

Snoring can occur at any age. However, it is most commonly seen in the middle-aged male. In this age group the upper airway is partially narrowed because of loose soft tissues in the upper airway, or narrowness of the upper airway, that has occurred over a period of years. Many people with loud snoring have had a long history of nasal congestion or nasal obstruction. This, in part, can lead to thickening of the tissues of the upper airway, thereby contributing to obstruction. In children, a common cause of upper airway obstruction is enlarged tonsils, which narrow the upper airway, thereby contributing to obstruction during sleep. Removal of the tonsils in children is usually associated with improved breathing and a reduction of snoring.

Snoring is produced by vibration of the tissues of the upper airway. Typically, as a person starts to breathe in, the upper airway will collapse and the airflow will become obstructed. This causes turbulence of the airflow and the soft tissues of the soft palate and uvula tend to vibrate, thereby causing the sound of snoring. We know that people who are loud snorers have times when their breathing is not just partially obstructed but completely blocked off. When the episodes of obstruction last 10 seconds or longer, we call it sleep apnea. It is now recognized that the syndrome of repetitive cessation of breathing during sleep at night, associated with snoring and daytime sleepiness, is called obstructive sleep apnea syndrome.

For most people snoring is not a significant problem and not one that requires any medical intervention. Patients usually seek help when loud snoring bothers a family member, or because episodes of cessation of breathing have been noticed during sleep at night, or because the snorer is aware of increasing daytime tiredness, fatigue and sleepiness. Loud snoring and reports of episodes of cessation of breathing, or symptoms of tiredness and sleepiness, suggest the possibility of obstructive sleep apnea syndrome, and the individual needs appropriate diagnostic medical testing.

TYPES OF SLEEP APNEA

Apnea is derived from the Greek word meaning "want of breath." An apnea has occurred if breathing stops for at least 10 seconds as detected by the airflow at the nostrils and mouth. Sleep apnea is when apnea, or the cessation of breathing, occurs during sleep.

Central Sleep Apnea Syndrome

There are several types of sleep apneas or breathing disturbances during sleep at night, which sometimes causes confusion. One type is called central sleep apnea syndrome. In its pure form, it is produced by episodes of complete cessation of breathing during sleep at night that are not associated with upper airway obstruction. These episodes occur because the brain does not send the correct message to breathe in sleep. This is typically associated with brain disorders such as stroke. Central sleep apnea syndrome may also be produced by cardiac disorders associated with impaired circulation time that leads to an oscillation of the breathing pattern, thereby producing central apneas. In addition to these pure forms of central sleep apnea syndrome, many patients with obstructive sleep apnea have episodes of central apnea where the breathing is stopped for 10 to 40 seconds without upper airway obstruction. These episodes usually occur less commonly than the episodes of obstructive sleep apnea syndrome and they usually end once the obstructive sleep apnea syndrome is treated.

Upper Airway Resistance Syndrome

In addition to central sleep apnea syndrome, there is a recently described disorder called upper airway resistance syndrome. This disorder can be considered a minor manifestation of upper obstructive sleep apnea syndrome because there may not be episodes of upper airway obstruction or drop in the oxygen saturation during sleep. However, an increased effort to breathe during sleep leads to brief arousals that are usually not perceived by the snorer. These brief arousals contribute to feelings of daytime tiredness and fatigue, and treatment is usually the same as for obstructive sleep apnea syndrome.

Obstructive Sleep Apnea Syndrome

Obstructive sleep apnea syndrome is the most common sleep apnea. Obstructive sleep apnea syndrome is present in 24% of middle-aged males and 9% of middle-aged females. It becomes more common in females after the menopause. Although obstructive sleep apnea syndrome can occur in infants, it is less common in this age group, and most cases of sudden infant death syndrome are not associated with obstructive sleep apnea syndrome.

The diagnosis of obstructive sleep apnea syndrome is made by sleep studies. An all-night polysomnogram will demonstrate the number of apneas during sleep at night, their duration, and whether they occur in relation to body position or a particular sleep stage. Typically, these apneic episodes occur more severely when the person is supine or in the REM sleep stage. Associated cardiac arrhythmias are looked for, and the oxygen level in the blood is monitored to determine the severity of the drop in oxygen saturation. The quality of sleep is determined, and the number of arousals that occur in relationship to the altered breathing episodes is counted.

Several measures of breathing are monitored during sleep at night. Typically, the movements of the chest and abdomen demonstrate whether there is any obstruction to airflow and whether the chest can be inflated. In addition, a measure of airflow at the nostrils or mouth will show whether apneic episodes occur. Further to episodes of complete cessation of breathing, there are also shallow episodes called hypopneas. Hypopneas can also be associated with arousals during sleep at night or a drop in the blood oxygen level. Sometimes a test is performed the next day following the overnight sleep test to determine the level of tiredness and sleepiness. The Multiple Sleep Latency Test (MSLT) can demonstrate whether pathological daytime sleepiness exists. Usually these tests are performed in the sleep laboratory of an accredited sleep disorders center. However, occasionally these tests may be performed in the patient's own home. The information obtained in the home, however, is usually less reliable than that obtained in the laboratory.

Since those suffering from obstructive sleep apnea syndrome rarely get a good night's sleep, the next day they tend to feel tired and fatigued. Sleepiness can come on at any time and is of most concern when the person is driving a motor vehicle. Studies have shown that there is a greater risk of motor vehicle accidents in people who have obstructive sleep apnea syndrome. Sleepiness can also interfere with daily activities and impair concentration and memory.

Typically people with obstructive sleep apnea syndrome are not aware of having frequent awakenings at night, though some may recall waking up gasping and choking. When the upper airway closes off, usually during inspiration, there is an inability to bring oxygen into the lungs and therefore the oxygen level in the blood falls. At some point, after the cessation of breathing, the person will awaken, usually 20 to 40 seconds later. However, some episodes of sleep apnea can last several minutes. Usually the episodes of cessation of breathing terminate spontaneously, and the chance of the individual dying because of not breathing again is extremely remote. When the person resumes breathing, gasping and choking sounds can be audible to somebody nearby, but may not be perceived by the snorer. An observing bed partner, who sees a frightening display of repetitive episodes of cessation of breathing and gasping, may encourage the snorer to seek medical help.

Cessation of breathing creates an inability to move air in or out of the lungs. Therefore, the oxygen in the blood will get used up because it is not refreshed. This fall in the oxygen level can have severe consequences. Recent evidence has demonstrated that people with sleep apnea are more likely to develop high blood pressure, in part related to the stressful response to the episodes of cessation of breathing. A drop in the oxygen saturation can also cause the heart to produce an abnormal rhythm. Typically, a slowing and speeding up of the heart is seen during sleep, but some individuals may develop major heart irregularities and potentially fatal abnormal heart rhythms.

Body weight plays a major part in the development of obstructive sleep apnea syndrome. Most males tend to put on weight during middle age. This weight gain is associated with the increasing severity of snoring and the development of obstructive sleep apnea syndrome. Body weight plays a part by narrowing the upper airway and causing the tissues of the tongue and neck to collapse, thereby contributing to the obstruction. In addition, abdominal weight prevents movement of the respiratory muscles during sleep at night. This contributes to a pattern of shallow breathing that can predispose the person to developing apneas. Losing weight can reverse the process, although usually not completely.

In addition to enlarged tonsils, anything that narrows the upper airway can contribute to the development of obstructive sleep apnea. Some people have a small jaw, or a jaw that is placed slightly posteriorly, and this contributes to obstruction at the base of the tongue. The clinical features involved in the development of sleep apnea can usually be determined during a medical evaluation.

Treatment of Obstructive Sleep Apnea Syndrome

Treatment of obstructive sleep apnea syndrome depends upon the severity of the underlying disorder. For some people, treatment may be required just for snoring. In these cases, behavioral changes are usually the first line of treatment, and the most important of these is to try to attain an ideal body weight. Because weight is so closely associated with snoring, everyone who snores and who is overweight should be encouraged to try to attain an ideal body weight.

Episodes of cessation of breathing are more common when sleeping on the back, and therefore attempting to train oneself to sleep on the side can be helpful. Sometimes a body pillow can be used to help promote sleeping on the side.

Other means, such as sewing a tennis ball into a pocket on the back of a pajama jacket, have also been reported to be helpful.

Alcohol ingested before sleep will usually make obstructive apnea episodes more severe, and therefore should be avoided, as should any sedative medication. Before adjusting any prescribed medications, snorers should discuss it with their physician.

Elevating the head of the bed, by putting something under its legs so that the whole bed is on a slight incline, may be helpful for some people. Although sleeping in a semireclining position may be useful in reducing snoring, it may also contribute to impaired sleep quality and add to daytime sleepiness.

Colds and nasal congestion should be treated promptly to prevent their making the sleep apnea worse.

Other behavioral measures may include avoiding large meals before bedtime, and stopping smoking. Smoking irritates the upper airway, thereby contributing to narrowing of the upper airway and promoting obstructive sleep apnea.

There are no medications that can help obstructive sleep apnea. The main form of treatment is usually nasal continuous positive air pressure (CPAP). CPAP consists of a pump that can be likened to a vacuum cleaner in reverse. A pump blows air through a tube to a small mask that goes over the nose. The mouth is free and can be open. The airflow through the nose prevents the episodes of upper airway obstruction. The principle is very simple. As one breathes in, the upper airway tends to suck together. If a positive air pressure is applied through the nose, then there is no suction effect on the upper airway tissues, and one can breathe in and out against a slow flow of air pressure without the upper airway being obstructed.

The snorer has to use the CPAP every night in order to remain free of apneic episodes. Usually the treatment becomes routine, just like brushing one's teeth before going to bed, and the individual is not bothered by the treatment. The CPAP is put on as the person turns out the light. After falling asleep, usually the snorer is only aware of the CPAP when it is time to take it off upon awakening in the morning.

Although many patients use CPAP effectively and without any concern, there are some patients who find it very disturbing and have great difficulty sleeping with a mask over their nose. Some patients who have difficulty in tolerating nasal CPAP can use a device called bilevel CPAP. This larger and heavier device allows the airflow to be reduced when breathing out. The airflow is therefore not continuous but cycles with each breath. Some patients find that breathing out against a lower incoming airflow easier. It also may be particularly helpful for some patients who have heart problems that cause impaired blood return to the heart.

Another variation on CPAP is called automatic CPAP. This device automatically senses the pressure required during sleep, and the airflow pressure applied through the nose varies depending upon whether apneas are present. Although these newer devices have received a lot of attention, at this time they appear to be less effective than standard CPAP. Hopefully, with future advancements these may become a more effective means of treating sleep apnea.

For patients who cannot sleep with the CPAP, other treatment options must be considered, including the use of an oral appliance or surgery. An oral appliance is like a bite plate that is placed in the mouth that usually moves the upper jaw forward, thereby preventing obstruction at the base of the tongue. Oral appliances are less effective than CPAP and may also be less tolerated during sleep. However, oral appliances are a useful alternative for people who, for one reason or another, are unable to use nasal CPAP.

For some patients, surgical management is the primary means of treatment. If severe obstruction occurs in the nose to the extent that the person has great difficulty in breathing in or out through the nostrils, then reduction of the size of the turbinates or correction of a deviated nasal septum may be recommended. Surgery for milder degrees of nasal impairment is usually not associated with any improvement in the underlying sleep apnea.

In children, the primary treatment is removal of the large tonsils and adenoids. In most adults, the tonsils and adenoids are not present and therefore this treatment is less commonly performed.

In the early 1980s, a treatment called uvulopalatopharygoplasty (UPP) was the most commonly performed surgical procedure. An uvulopalatopharygoplasty was a means of shortening the soft palate at the back of the mouth. This procedure is very effective in mild sleep apnea, where the primary concern is snoring, because it removes the soft tissues that vibrate. However, most patients with obstructive sleep apnea have obstruction, not only at the level of the soft palate, but also at the base of the tongue, and UPP surgery does not relieve this obstruction. More recently, the UPP operation has been performed via laser. Laser-assisted uvulopalatoplasty (LAUP) is a simpler procedure than UPP and can be performed in the doctor's office on an outpatient basis. The procedure takes only about 20 minutes, but may need to be repeated several times in order to get a good response.

The major disadvantage of LAUP is discomfort, as it can leave the throat sore for several weeks. A variation of the laser-assisted procedure is performed by radio frequency. This procedure involves putting a needle into the soft palate. The radio frequency waves cause the tissue to die around the needle, and over a period of several weeks the soft palate may shrink in size. Therefore, snoring is reduced.

None of these surgical procedures are primarily indicated in obstructive sleep apnea syndrome, as they are more effective for snoring, rather than relieving the upper airway obstruction. However, sometimes these procedures are recommended in conjunction with using CPAP, and may be considered in patients who are unable to use CPAP to help reduce the severity of the sleep apnea.

More extensive surgical procedures might involve trying to relieve the obstruction at the base of the tongue. Various surgical procedures alter the position of the lower jaw in relationship to the upper jaw. These are more experimental procedures. However, if the sleep apnea is due to a small lower jaw, or a lower jaw that is obviously placed back further than the upper jaw, then these procedures may be indicated. Sometimes radio frequency procedures are performed at the base of the tongue to help shrink the tongue tissues.

Other procedures that are rarely performed now are tracheostomy and gastroplasty. Tracheostomy—placing a hole in the wind pipe—was performed when there was no other way to avoid the obstruction to airflow in the upper airway. This procedure was the sole means of treatment for severe apnea syndrome 20 years ago, but now has largely been replaced by the procedures mentioned above. Occasionally, in rare situations, a tracheostomy may still be indicated.

Reducing severe body weight contributing to sleep apnea can be achieved by stomach surgery or gastroplasty. This is usually reserved for people with morbid obesity, that is, people weighing more than 300 pounds, when other (behavioral) attempts to lose weight have been unsuccessful. Usually, such patients also require some other treatment for their sleep apnea syndrome, such as a CPAP device.

Treatment of sleep apnea syndrome is very rewarding not only for the patient but also for the clinician. Patients often have a dramatic response. They are more energetic and awake during the daytime, they sleep better at night, their blood pressure may improve and treatment of sleep apnea syndrome may prevent sudden death during sleep for some patients.

Ways to Help Snoring or Sleep Apnea

1. Attain an ideal body weight, if you are overweight or obese.
2. Retrain yourself to sleep on your side since episodes of cessation of breathing are more common when sleeping on the back.
3. Use a body pillow to help promote sleeping on the side.
4. Avoid drinking alcohol before sleep.
5. Avoid sedative medications before sleep since they may worsen the obstructive sleep apnea episodes.
6. Elevating the head of the bed may be helpful for some people.
7. Treat colds or nasal congestion promptly to prevent their worsening the sleep apnea.
8. Avoid large meals before bedtime.
9. Stop smoking.
10. If necessary, your doctor may require that you use a continuous positive air pressure (CPAP) device. (Other treatment options include surgery.)

CHAPTER 5

EXCESSIVE DAYTIME SLEEPINESS AND NARCOLEPSY

Excessive sleepiness (also referred to as excessive daytime sleepiness or somnolence) is the inability to remain awake during the awake portion of an individual's sleep-wake cycle. Excessive daytime sleepiness is a symptom of numerous sleep disorders including narcolepsy, described below. It also occurs with sleep disorders associated with psychiatric disorders including mood disorders as well as other sleep disorders such as post-traumatic hypersomnia or insufficient sleep syndrome, both discussed in the A-to-Z entries section. Furthermore, poor sleep hygiene and erratic sleep habits, as well as disorders of the sleep cycle such as shift-work sleep disorder, can lead to excessive daytime sleepiness.

EXCESSIVE DAYTIME SLEEPINESS (EDS)

Tiredness, fatigue and sleepiness are common symptoms that everybody can relate to. The most common cause of daytime tiredness and sleepiness is an insufficient amount of sleep at night. It is possible to cut yourself short of sleep at night without realizing that the reduction in total sleep time is the cause of daytime tiredness. This can happen if you slip into a pattern of being active late at night and arising early, and do not realize that your short sleep episode is the reason that you are tired or sleepy during the daytime. Extending the duration of nocturnal sleep, for at least two weeks, results in improved daytime alertness.

Poor sleep quality may also be the reason for tiredness during the daytime. Sleep disruption as a result of underlying sleep disorders such as sleep apnea or insomnia may produce daytime tiredness and sleepiness. However, it is important to recognize that significant daytime sleepiness that causes the patient to fall asleep at inappropriate times of the day does not usually occur in patients with insomnia. Insomnia can be likened to a 24-hour-a-day disorder of inability to sleep insomuch as the sufferer is unable to sleep at night as well as during the daytime. If significant sleepiness occurs during the daytime, then one has to look for explanations other than insomnia. In addition to disorders that affect the quantity or quality of sleep at night, other primary sleep disorders may be the cause of daytime sleepiness.

NARCOLEPSY

Perhaps the greatest clinical contribution in the field of sleep disorders medicine was the first description in 1880 of narcolepsy by Jean Baptiste Edouard Gelineau (1828–1906), who derived the term *narcolepsy* from the Greek words *narkosis* ("benumbing") and *lepsis* ("to overtake"). The term *cataplexy,* for emotionally-induced muscle weakness (a prominent symptom of narcolepsy), was coined in 1916 by Richard Henneberg. Although Gelineau was the first to clearly describe the clinical manifestations of narcolepsy, several apparently narcoleptic patients had previously been described by Caffe in 1862, Carl Friedrich Otto Westphal (1833–90) in 1877 and Franz Fischer in 1878.

Narcolepsy is a major cause of daytime tiredness. An uncommon condition that occurs in approximately 250,000 people in the United States, narcolepsy is a neurological disorder that can produce severe daytime sleepiness. The cause of narcolepsy has recently been discovered to be a loss of a certain nerve cells in the base of the brain. These cells, called hypocretin cells, are located in the part of the brain called the hypothalamus. Recent research has demonstrated that in people with narcolepsy, these cells are reduced or absent. This reduces the level of hypocretin in their cerebrospinal fluid.

The primary symptom of narcolepsy is sleepiness during the daytime. Sufferers are unable to remain fully alert for extended periods of time and must take brief naps, which may last only seconds to minutes, intermittently throughout the day. Narcolepsy generally occurs in the second decade of life at a median age of onset of 16 years. The initial symptoms can occur prior to puberty. Some patients with narcolepsy have had symptoms since infancy; rarely the disorder may occur as late as in the 70s. There are some families in which many family members are affected, although this is uncommon. Most cases of narcolepsy appear to be isolated cases.

For example, Mary, a 19-year-old college student, was unable to stay awake in classes. Although many of her college friends were sleepy because of being up late at night, Mary knew that her problem was different. Even when she got plenty of sleep, she would still have to take several brief naps. Several years later she developed weakness in her legs when she laughed and on one occasion fell to the ground. She underwent sleep studies that showed that she had narcolepsy. Treatment with Provigil made a dramatic difference to her ability to stay awake.

As in Mary's case, the initial symptom of narcolepsy is tiredness or sleepiness. Sometimes, when the disorder begins in childhood, children may become hyperactive during the daytime and occasionally have been misdiagnosed as having attention deficit disorder. The sleepiness is present every day and is not relieved by extending nighttime sleep. Motor vehicle accidents are more common in undiagnosed narcolepsy patients. Narcolepsy interferes with concentration, memory and daytime activities. It can impair social relationships, and patients with narcolepsy have great difficulty in remaining awake during concerts, meetings and movies.

Narcolepsy has a peculiar symptom called cataplexy that is quite specific to the disorder. Cataplexy is an emotionally induced muscle weakness. It is most evident when people are laughing, hearing or telling a joke or becoming angry. At these times, the person may experience a weakness that is usually felt in the legs. At worst, patients may fall to the ground suddenly in response to an emotional stimulus. For many people with narcolepsy, the weakness is just perceived as an abnormal sensation in the legs or in the back. Sometimes, the cataplexy is very subtle, and the patient does not recognize that there is anything wrong.

Cataplexy, which can occur with any emotion, not only when laughing or angry, but also sudden surprise or during sporting events, is a manifestation of disrupted REM sleep. Typically in REM sleep, our muscles become relaxed; in cataplexy, this relaxation is induced by the emotional stimulus.

Other manifestations of narcolepsy include sleep paralysis and hypnagogic hallucinations. Sleep paralysis is characterized by a feeling of immobility that typically occurs upon awakening in the morning. Episodes may occur before falling asleep or when awakening during the night. Typically the sufferer will feel immobility and is unable to move the arms or legs. Because of an inability to attract anyone's attention, sleep paralysis becomes a very frightening sensation. Fortunately, it only lasts for a few seconds or minutes at most. Episodes of sleep paralysis may occur very infrequently or may occur on an almost daily basis in narcolepsy. These symptoms can also be present in individuals who do not have narcolepsy, although much less frequently.

Hypnagogic hallucinations are vivid hallucinations that occur before sleep onset. Typically, the person will be lying in bed and may see an object or people in the bedroom. Sometimes, these hallucinations may be auditory in that voices can be heard. The hallucinations are a manifestation of dreaming that occurs while the patient is still awake. Both sleep paralysis and the hypnagogic hallucinations are manifestations of disrupted REM sleep—a component of REM sleep that occurs without the complete features of REM sleep.

Narcolepsy is diagnosed by recognition of the typical symptoms as mentioned above. In addition, patients need to undergo an all-night polysomnogram followed in the daytime by a Multiple Sleep Latency Test. During the overnight sleep study, the patient will fall asleep quickly and may go into REM sleep more quickly than a patient without narcolepsy.

Also, there may be an increase in the lightest stage of sleep (stage one sleep) and more frequent awakenings and arousals than is seen in normal sleepers. The amount of REM sleep at night is usually normal.

One reason for performing the overnight sleep test is to ensure that other sleep disorders, such as obstructive sleep apnea syndrome, are not present and do not account for the daytime symptoms. Following the overnight sleep study is a daytime Multiple Sleep Latency Test. This test can be diagnostic for narcolepsy. Typically, patients with narcolepsy will fall asleep rapidly on each of the four or five nap opportunities, usually in less than 5 minutes. Normal individuals will take more than 15 minutes to fall asleep. Patients with narcolepsy will also go into REM sleep during two or more of the nap opportunities, whereas this is not likely to happen in normal sleepers.

Because narcolepsy is a lifelong disorder without any cure, patients often require a lot of emotional support to deal with the illness throughout their life. Advice regarding education and occupation is needed. For this reason, it is important that this disorder is diagnosed early enough so that appropriate intervention can be established.

Narcolepsy places a big burden on other family members who may require advice and assistance on how to best help the family member who has narcolepsy. (For suggested resources, see the listings in Part III, Resources, in the back of the book, especially for the Narcolepsy Institute at the Sleep-Wake Disorders Center of Montefiore Medical Center, the Narcolepsy Network and the Stanford University Center for Narcolepsy.)

Treatment

Narcolepsy is treated by medications. Typically, two medications are required, one for the treatment of the sleepiness and one for the treatment of the cataplexy. Sometimes, other medications may be required for treating the symptoms of hypnagogic hallucinations and sleep paralysis.

Usually, the medications used for the treatment of narcolepsy are stimulants such as Ritalin, Dexedrine and Cylert. Cylert is currently not recommended because of concern regarding possible liver damage.

A new nonstimulant medication called Provigil is now available for the treatment of narcolepsy. This medication is a wake-promoting agent that appears to improve alertness without any of the general body stimulant effects that are seen with medications such as Ritalin or Dexedrine. Provigil has now become the primary medication for the treatment of narcolepsy in the United States. This medication is relatively free of side effects although it may cause headaches or nausea in some individuals. The usual dose ranges between 200 to 600 milligrams a day, usually given once in the morning. For younger patients or elderly patients, 50 milligrams may be the starting dose. For some patients, Provigil is not strong enough, in which case they may need to use the stimulants Ritalin or

Dexedrine. These medications can produce general body stimulation and tend to have a higher rate of side effects than Provigil. However, they can be very effective in improving alertness. Usually they must be taken several times a day. People with cardiovascular disorders may not be able to use Ritalin or Dexedrine.

Usually a different medication is required for the treatment of cataplexy. In the past, the medications used have been of the tricyclic antidepressant class, such as Vivactil or Anafranil. These medications can be very effective at preventing the cataplexy episodes. However, they have a high rate of side effects. These side effects are called anticholinergic symptoms and typically consist of daytime tiredness, drowsiness, sexual dysfunction, constipation or blurring of vision. Newer medications such as the selective serotonin reuptake inhibitors (SSRIs), which include medications such as Prozac or Zoloft, have been used for the treatment for cataplexy. The SSRIs may take up to two weeks to affect the cataplexy. Most patients with cataplexy can be effectively treated with either the tricyclic antidepressants or SSRIs.

Sometimes patients with narcolepsy have disturbed nocturnal sleep. A medication may be required to improve sleep quality at night. This may be either a sleeping medication such as Ambien or a sedating antidepressant medication such as Tofranil taken at night to suppress the paralysis or hypnagogic hallucinations. Sometimes patients with narcolepsy can have an excessive amount of activity during sleep as a result of disrupted REM sleep at night. This has been called REM sleep behavior disorder and usually responds to the medication Klonopin.

CHAPTER 6

MOVEMENT DISORDERS DURING SLEEP

Movement disorders during sleep can be produced either by discomfort in the limbs or unrecognized abnormal movements. Leg jerking during sleep at night is relatively common and may not be associated with any untoward symptoms. A bed partner may notice the jerking movements.

Most people are aware of a whole body jerk that occurs at the beginning of sleep and is usually associated with a sensation of falling. These episodes are called sleep starts or hypnic jerks and usually occur in the transition between wakefulness and sleep. Very rarely, sleep starts are associated with an inability to sleep at night and cause insomnia. However, for most people they occur very infrequently and, although unpleasant, are not usually disabling.

PERIODIC LEG MOVEMENTS AND PERIODIC LIMB MOVEMENT (PLM) DISORDER

If the individual suffers from insomnia or excessive daytime sleepiness, the leg-jerking activity during sleep may need to be treated. This type of activity is called periodic leg movements. When the disorder is associated with insomnia or excessive sleepiness it is called periodic limb movement disorder. The jerking movements of the legs occur every 20 to 40 seconds during sleep at night and typically occur in the non-REM sleep stages. It is unusual for leg jerking to occur during REM sleep.

The exact cause of leg jerks is unknown, although they are more common in people who have body chemistry abnormalities, such as that seen in association with kidney disease. Sometimes hundreds or even thousands of leg jerks may occur during sleep at night. When sleep is disrupted or sleepiness occurs during the daytime, treatment may be required. Typical treatment used to involve reducing the arousals or awakenings associated with the leg movements. Several of the benzodiazepine medications similar to Valium, such as Klonopin, have been used. However, these medications do not stop the leg movements, but only stop the awakenings associated with the leg movements.

More recently, it has been recognized that a class of medications called dopamine agonists, among them L-Dopa or Sinemet, can be useful in suppressing the leg activity during sleep. Now newer dopamine agonists such as pramipexole or ropinirole are more effective. However, it is important to stress that most people with periodic leg movements in sleep do not require any specific treatment.

RESTLESS LEGS SYNDROME

The most common and most disabling form of movement disorder associated with discomfort is called restless legs syndrome (RLS). Swedish neurologist Karl A. Ekbom described and named this disorder in the mid-1940s. Today, researchers estimate that this movement disorder may affect more than 12 million Americans or anywhere from 10% to 15% of the population.

Restless legs syndrome is always associated with the following symptoms. (Discomfort can occur in the arms, although most typically it is in the legs.) The feeling in the legs is often described as a creepy, crawly sensation in the skin, or it may be described as an itching, tingling, searing, aching or even painful sensation. Usually these symptoms occur when the person is sitting or lying down. For this reason it is most evident when patients are in bed at night. The sensations are usually felt in the calves of the legs but can occur in the feet or the thighs. Jerking movements of the legs and periodic leg movements can also occur during sleep at night in people with restless legs syndrome.

When the symptoms occur, patients feel that they need to get up and move around and will typically get out of bed and start to walk about. Because of the disruption to sleep onset, often patients will complain of insomnia. Since the symptoms may occur intermittently through the night, preventing the person from being able to fall back to sleep, he or she may complain of tiredness or sleepiness the next day.

Restless legs syndrome can occur at any age but most commonly begins within the first two decades of life. The symptoms then gradually increase and are usually at their severest in middle or late age. It is known that restless legs syndrome can occur in families, and there are families where most members are affected to some extent.

RLS more commonly occurs in certain disorders, as in patients who have kidney disease, and can occur in women during pregnancy. It has also been associated with iron deficiency, in which case replacement of iron can sometimes be helpful. However, for most patients, the cause of restless legs syndrome is unknown. The diagnosis of restless legs syndrome is usually dependent upon the clinical symptoms. Sometimes sleep studies may be required to show the excessive movement during sleep at night, although usually this is not necessary.

CHAPTER 7

PARASOMNIAS

There are a number of behavioral disorders during sleep that usually do not cause symptoms of insomnia or excessive sleepiness. Known as the parasomnias, these are potentially some of the most dramatic of the sleep disorders, including sleepwalking, sleep terrors, headbanging and sleep-related eating disorder.

Parasomnias produce mental disorientation and sufferers are not usually responsive to being awoken during the episodes. They often have complete amnesia afterwards about the episodes, unable to recall any of their behavior during sleep.

The term *disorder of arousal* has been used to describe several of these behavioral disorders, including the confusional arousals, sleep terrors and sleepwalking. Typically, these disorders occur from the deepest stages of sleep and the person has no memory for the events the next morning.

CONFUSIONAL AROUSALS

Confusional arousals, also called sleep drunkenness or excessive sleep inertia, cause a person to become briefly aroused during sleep at night with a little confusion. Episodes in children may be associated with talking or sitting up in bed, and even crying. The child goes back to sleep and has no memory of the episode. Episodes may last from several minutes to several hours. Usually, confusional arousals do not require any specific treatment. However, these episodes may progress to more severe sleep terrors or sleepwalking behavior that may require treatment to prevent injuries.

First mentioned by Roger J. Broughton in 1968, confusional arousals are most typical in childhood, often before puberty, less common in older children or adolescents and even rarer in adults.

SLEEP TERRORS

Sleep terrors are sudden arousals from sleep with a piercing scream or cry and intense fear. Sleep terrors occur out of the deepest sleep stages, stage three or stage four, and when they occur in children, the child is inconsolable. There may be violent activity, such as jumping out of bed and rushing for the door. Injuries are common.

The difficulty in arousing is because the brain is still in a deep sleep state. For this reason, after the episode ends and the child goes back to sleep, there is usually no memory of the episode the next morning. The cause of sleep terrors is unknown. Usually no treatment is required unless the child has frequent episodes and is in danger of injuries. Dangerous objects should be removed to prevent injury. Sometimes a bedroom door or window may need to be secured. If treatment is required, Paxil or Klonopin have been shown to be effective in some patients.

SLEEPWALKING

Sleepwalking consists of a series of complex behaviors that are initiated during the deepest stages of sleep and result in walking during sleep. Because the deepest sleep usually occurs in the first third of the night, these episodes are more likely to happen at that time.

It may be very difficult to awaken the sleepwalker because of the deepness of the slow wave sleep. The sleepwalker may return to bed, like the patient with sleep terrors, go to sleep and have no memory for the episode the next morning. Sleepwalking episodes may need to be distinguished from nocturnal seizures. However, nocturnal seizures are more likely to occur in people who have daytime seizure episodes, and in most cases nocturnal seizures do not pose any diagnostic difficulty.

Similar to sleep terrors, sleepwalking episodes usually do not require any specific treatment. For example, 14-year-old Evan was just about to walk out the front door in his pajamas when his mother heard the door open and jumped out of bed just in time to stop him. Evan had been sleepwalking since he was 10 and it was becoming an almost nightly behavior. He was referred by his pediatrician for a sleep study where it was discovered that he had many abrupt awakenings out of stage four sleep. This was a sure sign of the tendency for sleepwalking.

Evan's parents were advised to secure the bedroom so Evan would not injure himself. They installed an electric eye sensor across his bedroom door, connected to a buzzer, to alert them when he walked out of his bedroom. By the time Evan was 16, he had spontaneously stopped his sleepwalking behavior, although he still occasionally sat up abruptly in bed during the night.

For sleepwalkers like Evan, the environment should be secured and potentially harmful objects removed. Windows and doors should be locked so that the sleepwalker does not accidentally go outside. Treatment with medication, if necessary, may require benzodiazepines such as Valium, or the use of Paxil, although medication is usually not very effective.

HEADBANGING

Another type of parasomnia is rhythmic movement disorder or head-banging. Usually this disorder occurs in children and involves a rhythmical, repetitive movement of the head or neck. Typically, these episodes happen prior to sleep onset and may help the child to fall asleep. Sometimes the movements may be very violent. The whole bed or crib may rock and the child may suffer injuries from banging the head against the wall or the side of the crib. The exact cause of rhythmic disorder is unknown.

The majority of children with rhythmic movement disorder do not require any specific treatment. Padding the crib or environment may be necessary to prevent injury. Psychosocial support may be helpful, particularly as these children often worry about sleeping away from home. (You may recall the example of 31-year-old Michelle, a physician, described in the Author's Note, who had been headbanging since infancy and the life-long negative impact it had had on her social relationships until treatment helped reduce the frequency of the movements.)

A variety of treatments have been used to help rhythmic movement disorder. Many of them have been successful in some individuals, but not in most. Medications, such as the benzodiazapines, may be helpful for some children. However, no effective pharmacological treatment has been discovered. Fortunately, most children will outgrow this disorder although, rarely, it may persist into adulthood.

REM SLEEP BEHAVIOR DISORDER

It was three o'clock in the morning when Cheryl felt her 65-year-old husband, Charles, start to move in bed. Charles began to talk, softly at first, but then more rapidly and loudly. His movements became more violent, as if he was trying to get away from someone. Cheryl soon realized that Charles was dreaming. She unsuccessfully tried to awaken her husband, then got out of bed, afraid he might accidentally hit her.

As these episodes became more frequent over several months, she accompanied him to a sleep specialist who advised a sleep study. The test showed that Charles would start to move about whenever he went into the REM sleep stage, a time when his body should have been motionless. He was diagnosed as having REM sleep behavior disorder and started on Klonopin, 0.05 milligram before bedtime. The episodes immediately reduced in intensity and ceased completely once the dosage was raised to 0.1 milligram.

Charles had REM sleep behavior disorder, a disorder of acting out dreams during REM sleep. The activity may be very violent and may include fighting or running movements that occur while the person is still asleep. Often, a bed partner may be influenced by these movements and may accidentally be hit during the night. REM sleep behavior disorder is more common in patients with narcolepsy, but also can occur in people without any particular cause. For some patients, REM sleep behavior disorder may be the initial symptom of Parkinson's disease. Sleep studies show that the normal reduction of muscle activity during REM sleep does not occur in patients who have REM sleep behavior disorder. Most commonly, the disorder occurs in males, usually those over the age of 60 years. The bedroom may need to be secured to prevent injuries.

REM sleep behavior disorder can also be induced by various medications. It can occur in association with withdrawal of alcohol or sedative medications, such as barbiturates or benzodiazepines. Some of the newer antidepressant medications, including SSRIs, particularly venlafaxine (Effexor), may be a cause of REM-sleep behavior disorder.

Other than securing the environment, the most effective treatment is the one used for Charles: prescribing Klonopin 0.5 milligram to 1.5 milligram for most patients. This medication is very effective. However, other medications, including Neurontin, an anticonvulsive, may be necessary if Klonopin does not help. Recent evidence has suggested that melatonin may be helpful.

SLEEP-RELATED EATING DISORDER

One final form of behavioral disturbance during sleep is called sleep-related eating disorder (also known as nocturnal eating [drinking] syndrome). This disorder has features in common with sleepwalking and can occur in patients who have sleepwalking or sleep apnea. It can also occur in patients with eating disorders. Typically, sleep-related eating disorder is associated with almost nightly eating and an absence of daytime binge eating. It is more likely to occur in females and usually occurs between 20 and 30 years of age.

For example, Alison was 27 and concerned about her increasing weight. But what distressed her most was the fact that she was getting up at night to eat. Because of the weight gain, Alison cut back on her food intake in the daytime, but found that she continued to awaken at night. She would then go to the kitchen and eat large amounts of food. Sometimes she did not realize that she was eating during the night and could only tell by the signs of crumbs found in the kitchen the next morning.

Her physician diagnosed her as having sleep-related eating disorder and recommended that she eat small, frequent meals during the day to prevent hunger and take 0.5 milligrams of Klonopin before bedtime. Despite increasing the dose over the next few weeks to 1.5 milligrams, her nightly eating behavior persisted, but to a slightly lesser degree. She sought counseling to help deal with the problem.

Most patients with this sleep disorder, like Alison, will awaken at night, go to the kitchen, get something to eat and have no memory of doing so the next day. They may only see the evidence the following morning. Usually these patients worry over weight gain and typically do not overeat during the daytime. The behavior is most often described as an automatic form of behavior out of the patient's control, driven by an obsessive urge to eat. Usually alcohol is not taken at these times, and there is a preference for milk products and heavy foods. Smoking rarely occurs during these episodes. The compulsion to get food at night exists in any environment. In some cases, other family members have gone to great lengths to lock up the refrigerator and cupboards. However, usually the patient finds a way of obtaining food, despite attempts to secure access to it. Patients have even been known to leave their hotel bedroom in the middle of the night, get into a car and search for food.

As with Alison, psychological counseling is indicated for treating many of these patients. However, some can respond to medication such as Klonopin or dopamine agonist medications.

CHAPTER 8

CIRCADIAN RHYTHM SLEEP DISORDERS

Circadian rhythm sleep disorders were recognized in the late 1970s, partly due to recognition of the chronobiological features of jet lag and shift work. In 1978, Elliot David Weitzman and Charles Czeisler demonstrated the internal organization of temperature, neuroendocrine rhythms and the sleep-wake cycle in subjects who were monitored in an environment free of time cues for periods of up to six months. However, it was not until the 1980s that Czeisler and colleagues demonstrated the importance of the light-dark cycle in the entrainment of human circadian rhythms.

The atypical, sleep-onset insomnia called delayed sleep phase syndrome, discovered by Weitzman and colleagues in 1981, led to a radically different form of treatment called *chronotherapy* which was based on chronobiological principles.

JET LAG

Jet lag and shift-work sleep disorder are transient sleep disorders, also known as circadian rhythm sleep disorders, that are associated with an alteration in the timing of sleep in relation to underlying biological rhythms. Typically, the timing of sleep and wakefulness is altered in relation to body temperature, cortisol and other biochemical and hormonal factors. The consequences of these disorders are difficulty in sleeping when the person would like to sleep, and fatigue and sleepiness when they want to be awake. (Other circadian rhythm sleep disorders include delayed sleep phase syndrome, advanced sleep phase syndrome and non-24 hour sleep-wake pattern.)

The number of time zones crossed and the direction of travel determine the intensity of jet lag. Traveling to the east will shorten the day to less than 24 hours, whereas traveling to the west will lengthen it. As it is easier for us to delay the time that we go to bed rather than be able to fall asleep earlier than usual, travel to the west is associated with a quicker adaptation and readjustment than travel to the east.

The duration of our sleep is determined by the timing of sleep in relationship to the underlying circadian rhythms, rather than how long it is since we last slept. Typically, we tend to awaken as our body temperature starts to rise. If we go to bed when our body temperature is very low, we will only sleep a short period of time before we are awakened as the body temperature rises. Consequently, people traveling to the west generally will go to bed later but will awaken earlier. The underlying biological rhythms of body temperature and cortisol may take up to two weeks to readjust to the change in sleep pattern. It is during this time that we feel the effects of jet lag.

Treatment

A number of factors are involved in trying to ease the adjustment to crossing time zones. If we travel to the west across three time zones, say from New York City to Los Angeles, some adjustment can take place before departing on the journey. If the stay in Los Angeles is only a few days, it is usually better not to adjust, but to try to keep on New York time. There will be less disruption to sleep upon returning to New York. If the stay in Los Angeles were to be several weeks or longer, then promoting a rapid readjustment to the new time zone would be beneficial.

As 12 midnight in New York is 9 P.M. in California, there is little point in someone who usually goes to bed at 12 midnight in New York trying to go to bed at 12 midnight in California. It would be the same as if they went to bed at 3 A.M., a time when they would already be extremely sleepy. However, if they go to bed at their usual New York body clock time, it would mean going to bed at 9 P.M. in California. That would not be a problem, unless the person has evening commitments that prevent them from going to bed at 9 P.M.

A better situation would be to reach a midway point so that the person goes to bed at about 10:30 P.M. in California, which would be equivalent to going to bed about 1:30 A.M. in New York. In the morning, because 6 A.M. in California is the same as 9 A.M. in New York, the individual is likely to awaken prior to 6 A.M. in California. Therefore, the sleep episode may be a little shorter than that which they are accustomed to in New York.

In order to promote the ability to sleep later in the morning in California, the person could take a sleeping medication, such as Ambien, to prolong the sleep episode, thereby preventing some sleep loss. A sleep medication for the first few days in California may be helpful to ensure an adequate duration of sleep.

Traveling to the east poses greater difficulties. The time difference from Los Angeles to New York means that 9 P.M. in California is the same as 12 midnight in New York. Someone traveling east would probably have difficulty in being able to fall asleep at that time, although falling asleep may be helped by using a short-acting hypnotic medication, such as Sonata, or using 3 milligrams of melatonin taken one hour before bedtime. Melatonin has been shown to be helpful in altering the timing of sleep episodes, although the long-term safety of this medication is unknown. There appears to be little evidence of any untoward effects of melatonin when taken in the short term.

Some adjustment to the sleep pattern can be made prior to departing on the trip. If traveling to California from New York, the person could start going to bed a little later in New York for a few days before departure, in order to delay the sleep episode by one or two hours. Conversely, the person traveling from California to New York can go to bed a little earlier for the few days before departure, so as to have little difficulty falling asleep at an appropriate time in New York.

If traveling across five or six times zones, such as traveling from New York to London, a number of factors must be taken into consideration. First, the timing of travel is very important. If it is a night flight, sleeping during the flight can be very beneficial. Using a short-acting hypnotic medication during a flight may be beneficial for some people and help promote three or four hours of good-quality sleep during the trip. Making the trip as comfortable as possible, by either traveling business or first class or using eyeshades or earplugs, can help promote better quality sleep during a flight.

For example, if arriving in London at 6:30 A.M. London time, it is best to keep active in order to readjust to the new time zone. However, a midafternoon nap may help relieve some effects of the prior night's sleep loss. A hypnotic taken in the new time zone will help promote sleep, although it should be realized that sleeping at midnight in London would be the equivalent of going to bed at 6 P.M. in New York. It would be difficult to fall asleep at this time unless there was some effect of the prior night's sleep loss. A sedative medication taken one hour before bedtime can help.

Despite all of the above measures, the treatment of jet lag is not always effective. Up to two weeks may be required for the body to readjust to the new time zone. For most people it is a matter of having to put up with some symptoms of tiredness and fatigue and poor-quality sleep until the body readjusts to the new time zone.

SHIFT-WORK SLEEP DISORDER

Shift work poses similar difficulties to jet lag, although full adjustment to shift work may never occur. Typically, individuals who work from 11 P.M. to 7 A.M. five days a week never fully adjust to this pattern. Usually, they go to sleep at approximately 8 A.M., sleep for about four hours, then may take a two- to three-hour nap in the late evening prior to going back to work at 11 P.M. Sleep is therefore broken up into two episodes during the work week. Adjusting to a schedule of 11 P.M. to 7 A.M. is possible if one keeps to a regular sleep pattern seven days a week. However, most shift workers revert to a more socially acceptable sleep pattern on the weekends—that is, they go to bed at 11 P.M. and awaken at 7 A.M. Usually, they try to be awake during the daytime part of the weekend, a time during which they would normally be sleeping. Consequently, full adjustment to the shift work never occurs.

The problems of shift work can be compounded if workers are on a changing shift pattern. That is, if they move from a night shift to an evening shift, and then to a day shift, the sleep patterns may become even more disrupted, making it even more difficult to adapt.

Accidents are not uncommon. There is concern about night shift workers having to drive home after their night shift, a time when they are significantly tired. Caffeine has been shown to be helpful in improving alertness for workers on the night shift, as has exposure to bright lights. An exhausted shift worker should not attempt driving, however, just because he or she had a cup of coffee. A nap at work or even a longer sleep period may be required before a shift worker can safely drive home.

Dealing with Shift Work

If you are an "owl"—a night person or evening person—you may find it easier to adapt to evening or night shift work than someone who is a "lark," or morning person.

Unfortunately, there is no ideal solution for the sleep-related challenges facing those who work the evening or night shift. All shift workers suffer from some daytime tiredness and sleepiness, especially when changing from a day shift to a night shift for the first time. For example, after spending three months on his new job at a construction site, James was asked to work a night shift from 11 P.M. to 7 A.M. Since leaving school six months ago, James had only worked days, from 8 A.M. to 4:30 P.M., so working nights was going to be a big change. He liked the idea of having his days free but was concerned about not being able to have late nights with his friends.

Following the first two weeks on the new shift, he was starting to settle down to the routine. He would get home at 8 A.M., sleep for about four hours until noon, and then take a brief nap at 7 P.M. for three hours returning to work at 11 P.M. On his days off, he would go out with his friends and usually slept from 1 A.M. until 10 A.M. the next morning.

It took some initial adapting to the new routine, but all was working fairly well until he had been on the night shift for about six months. He started to have difficulty sleeping when he came home from work at 8 A.M. and often would stay up until he took a three-hour nap at 7 P.M. He started to get sleepy on the job, and had difficulty remaining energetic. He would sneak an occasional brief nap while at work. He became more irritable and felt depressed. Everything started to bother him, and he spent less time with his friends on his days off. Furthermore, he could not sleep

How to Get a Good Major Sleep Episode Despite Your Night Shift Work Schedule

1. For your daytime sleep episode, create an environment that is conducive to good sleep. Eliminate noise and light by wearing earplugs and closing the blinds.
2. Make sure the temperature in the room is not too hot or warm, but slightly on the cool side. This will promote sleep.
3. If an adequate sleep period cannot be obtained following a night of shift work, it may be preferable to break the sleep period into two portions with an initial four-hour sleep episode after the shift, in the morning, and another two-to-four hour period, at night, prior to going to the shift.
4. Make sure the work performed on the night shift is stimulating and not monotonous or boring, to help in maintaining full alertness.
5. If possible, maintain the same sleep pattern seven days a week. Try to avoid switching back to the more traditional pattern of sleeping at night and being awake throughout the day on weekends.
6. Rotations in a clockwise direction are preferable to counterclockwise rotations. Therefore, try to rotate from day to evening to night shift rather than the reverse.
7. Keep the evening or night shift as short as possible; there is an increased tendency for greater sleepiness in the final hours of night shifts that are 12 hours long compared to night shifts that are only six- or eight-hour shifts.
8. A short course of a short-acting hypnotic or sleep medication may enhance a shift worker's daytime sleep episode and lead to improved alertness during the waking portion of the sleep-wake cycle.
9. New treatments are being explored include melatonin to alter sleep onset and modafinil to improve alertness.
10. Caffeine and exposure to bright lights may help improve alertness.
11. If you are tired at the end of your shift, make sure you take a nap or go to sleep at work before attempting to drive home.

as well on his days off and often would spend long periods in bed, but not sleeping.

It was clear to his family that his mood was greatly changed, and they recommended that he see a physician. Physically he was well but emotionally it was clear that he needed psychological help. It was recommended that he take an antidepressant medication when he awoke and that he keep to regular sleep times with a brief nap on awakening in the morning and another before going to work, as he had done when starting the night shift.

But now he could not sleep well at any time of the day. In between times he was tired, irritable and depressed. After several attempts at adjusting the medication and the sleep times, it was clear that James was not improving. The recommendation was made to his company that he be placed back on a regular daytime shift.

The company was supportive and allowed James to return to the day shift, 8 A.M. to 4:30 P.M. After two weeks, there was a noticeable difference in James: his mood and demeanor greatly improved. One month later, James returned to his former good health; it was recognized that he was one of those individuals who is not able to cope with shift work without it strongly affecting his psychological health.

However, switching back to daytime work may not be an option for you. First of all, working the night shift may be a requirement of the job you have which might not exist during the day, such as a radio or television announcer for an all-night or early morning talk show. Some couples with young children, either out of choice or necessity to avoid hiring part-time or full-time child care, will work two different shifts enabling one parent to be available for child care at all times. Your company may only have openings for the night shift, leaving night work or unemployment as your only options.

If working the night shift is a short- or long-term job requirement, there are some ways you can increase the likelihood you can make it work without debilitating exhaustion or sleepiness.

DELAYED SLEEP PHASE SYNDROME

Delayed sleep phase syndrome and advanced sleep phase syndrome are more persistent alterations in the timing of sleep. People with delayed sleep phase syndrome have a tendency to sleep at a later hour and across the first part of the morning. For example, an adolescent with delayed sleep phase syndrome may have difficulty in falling asleep before 2 or 3 A.M. and therefore have great difficulty in awakening at an appropriate time the next morning. Consequently, he or she may miss morning classes and only awaken at 11 A.M. or 12 noon. Attempts to get to bed early are associated with difficulty in being able to fall asleep until a much later hour. This pattern may persist for months or years and pose great hardships because of the disruption in daytime activities, particularly morning activities.

ADVANCED SLEEP PHASE SYNDROME

The elderly are more likely to suffer from advanced sleep phase syndrome, that is, the inability to remain awake until the desired time. People with this disorder will tend to get sleepy and have difficulty staying awake after 9 P.M., and consequently will awaken earlier in the morning than they would desire. The whole sleep pattern is advanced to an earlier time, although the total amount of sleep attained may be normal, as in the delayed sleep phase syndrome patients.

NON-24-HOUR SLEEP-WAKE PATTERN

Very rarely, some individuals may have a non-24-hour sleep-wake pattern in which their tendency is to go to bed later every day so that their sleep pattern rotates around the clock. Although this is a rare disorder, documented patients have been shown to sleep later each day by approximately one hour for a period of months and even years. Obviously, this is extremely disruptive, as several times per month the individual would be sleeping across the middle of the day.

Treatment for Delayed, Advanced and Non-24-hour Sleep Phase Syndromes

Treatment of the delayed and advanced sleep phase syndromes usually involves behavioral manipulations of the timing of sleep, medications or light therapy. The person with delayed sleep phase syndrome who falls asleep at 3:15 A.M. can try making 15-minute advances on a nightly basis, so that the first night they might go to bed at 3 A.M., the next night 2:45 A.M., the next night 2:30 A.M., etc. These gradual advances may allow the person to adjust to the changing sleep-wake pattern. Sometimes this can be enhanced by taking hypnotic medications half an hour before sleep at night to advance the sleep onset. Short-acting hypnotics are useful in this situation. Other alternatives might include 3 milligrams of melatonin taken three to six hours before the sleep time. Bright light exposure in the morning can help prevent persons with delayed sleep phase syndrome from delaying their sleep further, and may help sleep occur at an earlier time at night.

Elderly patients with advanced sleep phase syndrome may benefit from bright light exposure in the late evening and a gradual 15-minute per day delay in their sleep pattern. Gradual attempts to shift the sleep pattern to a later time can be successful and allow the person to sleep later and awaken at a more appropriate time the next day.

Treatment for non-24-hour sleep-wake pattern is difficult and no specific treatments have been determined. The above measures, coupled with slight changes to the sleep pattern in combination with the use of medications and bright light therapy may be helpful.

CHAPTER 9
SLEEP ACROSS THE LIFE CYCLE

INFANCY

We often hear the phrase "sleeping like a baby." In general, we think that this indicates really good quality deep sleep but as all parents know, it is not always like that. At birth, most full-term babies will sleep between 16 and 18 hours a day. That may sound good, but unfortunately there is as much wakefulness at night as there is sleep during the daytime. It is the parents who suffer as a result of this alternating pattern of sleep and wakefulness because they have to attend to the child when he or she awakens. Of course, the infant needs to be fed, but large feedings at night can contribute to more frequent awakenings. Frequent feedings mean extra fluid intake, which means wet diapers and increased discomfort that unsettles the infant. Unfortunately, in the otherwise healthy infant, two conditions can increase the frequency of awakenings and disturbance. Colic produces crying and the infant can be inconsolable. That can be very distressing, particularly to a new parent. Fortunately, colic tends to go away by the time the infant is three to four months old. However, the disruption to the sleep process may continue after that time and there may be more frequent awakenings. The other disorder is a food allergy insomnia that may be caused by an allergy to cow's milk. When treated by milk protein formulas, the sleep disturbance tends to settle.

Fortunately, by six months of age, most infants have started to sleep through the night and the longer sleep episode is now increased to 6 hours. The night is usually made up of two long sleep episodes interrupted by a brief awakening for a nighttime feed. Unfortunately, sleep disruptions tend to become more prominent after the first six months of life. It is at this time that good sleep habits are very important in ensuring that a child will continue to sleep well. When the child is put down at night, it should be in a quiet environment that is conducive to good sleep. Of course, during the daytime there should be adequate stimulation so that the infant is alert and active at appropriate times. The periods of wakefulness during the daytime gradually lengthen and consolidate and they are only briefly interrupted by a short sleep episode.

By 12 months of age, the infant will have one or two daily naps, but most of the day will be spent awake. Brief awakenings still occur at night and it is important that the parents realize that these are normal awakenings and that the infant will naturally return to sleep. If the parent intervenes because of excessive concern, an increase in awakenings may occur and the child may come to expect some intervention during the night. In most cases, less is better. That is, the infant should be left alone when he or she briefly awakens, even if there are brief episodes of crying or disturbance during sleep at night. Generally, the infant will fall asleep again, and this will help promote a healthy pattern of sleeping.

If the parents interact excessively, the child will start to develop what is known as a sleep onset association disorder that may continue through the next few years. That is, the child now becomes dependent upon a certain association with the episodes of wakefulness. Associations with rocking the child, giving the child a pacifier or other interventions may become a necessary part of the child's life. The most important thing is to have the child learn that sleep can occur without these particular associations.

For example, Simon had just turned six months of age and his sleep had been getting lighter at night over the last couple of weeks. He was waking more during the night and had more frequent crying episodes. He slept about 6 hours at a stretch and required one feeding during the night.

As Simon was June's first child, she began to worry about his sleep and discussed it with her pediatrician. She was reassured that infants often have more disturbed sleep at night around six months of age. As Simon was a healthy baby, she was told that she should keep things stable until he outgrew the problem. June ensured that Simon had a regular schedule of rest and activity. By the time he was nine months of age, his sleep had improved and he started to sleep through the whole night with rare awakenings.

Sudden Infant Death Syndrome

The main concern of most parents regarding the newborn infant is the possibility of sudden infant death syndrome (SIDS). This condition tends to peak between two and four months of age. Fortunately there have been major advances in our understanding of sudden infant death syndrome, and the incidence is decreasing. It is now known that the infant may smother when placed face down, particularly if there is soft, loose bedding. The recommendation now is that infants should be placed on their backs to sleep. The possibility of sudden infant death syndrome is greatly reduced by this simple manipulation. Also, there is evidence that some infants can have a cardiac abnormality that can be detected by an electrocardiograph.

Other than the electrocardiographic changes, there are no features that readily identify the child who is at risk of sudden infant death syndrome. Fortunately, the risk is very low and it is not something that most parents need to be concerned about, especially if they place the infant on the back when sleeping. Previously it was thought that some infants with sudden infant death syndrome had obstructive sleep apnea syndrome, but this is most unlikely and is only a very rare cause of sudden infant death. In most cases, infants with sleep apnea can be easily recognized because of difficulty in breathing, with gasping and choking that is evident soon after birth. Cosleeping, which is sharing the parents' bed, has been reported to be a cause of sudden infant death syndrome because of accidental smothering of the infant. However, this rarely happens, and in some cultures cosleeping is normal behavior.

CHILDREN

In addition to sleep onset association disorder, described above, the young two- and three-year-old child may develop a limit-setting sleep disorder. This is due to efforts of the young child to delay going to bed at night. The child may refuse to either remain in bed or try to fall asleep. The child may stand up in the crib, or an older child may come out of the bedroom and call out to the parents. The parents must be firm and not give in to this behavior, because every time they give in to it, the bad behavior is reinforced. Limits must be set, even if this means allowing a child to cry for a few minutes. Setting the rules and limits of the sleep time are very important in these first two or three years of life.

The older child may also develop fears and nightmares that can be associated with sleep disturbance. These may take the form of monsters or intruders in the bedroom. Again, limit setting is very important in this situation. However, the child also needs support. Rewards may be given for staying in bed during this time. If the anxieties and concerns become intense, then professional counseling may be required.

The young child may have a disorder characterized by repetitive body activity during sleep called headbanging (discussed previously in the section on movement disorders during sleep). Fortunately, this type of rhythmical behavior reduces around the age of four years though, some cases may persist until adulthood. Most of the time, it does not require any intervention until it persists into the preteen years. Some forms of rhythmical rocking or movements during sleep are commonly seen in healthy children.

Sleep disorders that occur in the prepubertal child include confusional arousals, sleepwalking and sleep terrors. Confusional arousals usually occur when the child awakens during the night. Fortunately, in most cases the child can be consoled and will return back to sleep without difficulty. Episodes of sleepwalking may occur when the child is in the deepest stage of sleep and unaware of what is happening. There may be no memory of the episode the next morning. Treatment usually consists of ensuring that the environment is free of any factor that may harm the child, i.e. securing the bedroom. Usually the episodes will subside spontaneously as the child gets older. Sleep terror episodes can be very disturbing to parents as the child may suddenly scream in the middle of the night. Again, these episodes occur out of the deepest slow wave sleep and fortunately tend to resolve as the child gets older. In children, these are not associated with any underlying psychiatric disorder, so the parent can be reassured that these are normal behavioral phenomena that generally will stop as the child gets older.

Of course, children may also develop uncommon sleep disorders. An example of this was 12-year-old Sam, whose parents worried about what the night would bring since his sleep had become more and more bizarre over the last two years. Sam had become increasingly restless during sleep at night. He did not have insomnia, but during sleep his limbs would twist and writhe. Extensive neurological testing did not reveal the cause of his problem, so he was sent to a sleep center for help.

At the sleep center, sleep studies showed that the activity would occur out of non-REM sleep, and the movements were termed *choreic* and *athetotic.* These were signs of the rare disorder called paroxysmal nocturnal dystonia. Although there is no known cure, the medication clonazepam helped to reduce the activity during sleep, but at times Sam would continue to have minor episodes.

Bed-wetting

The sleep disturbance that is of most concern to parents in the toddler stage is bed-wetting. Bed-wetting is defined as episodes that occur in a child at least five years of age. In most cases, it is not associated with any physical disorder. Usually, the child will grow out of the behavior, as the disorder is a maturational disorder (one that spontaneously resolves as the child gets older). About 15% of children will improve with each year of age.

John, however, was still bed-wetting at age six. His parents were concerned, not just because of the bed-wetting, but because they tried to awaken him in the middle of the night to take him to the bathroom but found this almost impossible. His pediatrician reassured them that the difficulty in awakening John was normal and not reflective of any abnormal sleep problems. John would have been in the deep slow wave sleep, a stage during which it is very difficult to awaken anyone.

To treat John's bed-wetting, his parents were advised to get him a urine sensor with an alarm to attach to his underwear during the night. The alarm woke John when he first started to urinate, and he would go to the bathroom to finish urinating. Over a nine-month period, John's bed-wetting was reduced, and it rarely occurred by the time that he turned seven.

There are some medical causes of enuresis and this should be suspected in the child who has previously not been bed-wetting but then starts bed-wetting for no apparent reason. Urinary tract infections, epilepsy, diabetes and sleep apnea are possible causes. Treatment of bed-wetting is either by pharmacological agents or behavioral treatments. Behavioral treatments usually are safer and more effective for most children. Using a urinary alarm that awakens the child is the most common means of treating bed-wetting. Other behaviors, such as stream interruption, which requires stopping the urine flow at least once during the daytime, helps strengthen the appropriate muscles. Medications have included the tricyclic antidepressants, such as Tofranil, that reduce the contraction of the bladder muscle. Adverse effects can occur with medications, and they should be used strictly under the guidance of a physician. Alternatives to the antidepressant medications are the antidiuretics such as DDAVP. However, the effectiveness of DDAVP is not clear, and the treatment is also very expensive. This compound replaces a normal agent called vasopression that prevents urination during sleep at night.

ADOLESCENCE

Michael was a typical 15-year-old who enjoyed Rollerblading in the summer and snowboarding in the winter. He was an excellent student who liked to stay out late with his friends on the weekend and often would listen to music or watch videos after doing his homework during the week. He found that he was having increasing difficulty falling asleep before 11 P.M. and by the time he was 16, he was unable to get to sleep before 2 A.M. Consequently, he had difficulty awakening in the morning, and he was often late for school.

His grades began to suffer. His parents took him to a sleep center where he was diagnosed as having delayed sleep phase syndrome. He was placed on a regular schedule and advised to get plenty of bright light exposure first thing in the morning. He was also told to take melatonin at 6 P.M.

Gradually his sleep pattern improved to the point where he could fall asleep more easily at 11 P.M. He recognized the importance of keeping regular hours, with little late night TV watching or listening to music. His grades improved and he awoke more refreshed in the morning.

Fortunately, most adolescents sleep well although their bedtime tends to get later. It is important for parents to recognize that as children go through puberty they often require more sleep, and can need as much as nine or 10 hours of sleep on a nightly basis. If they do not achieve this amount of sleep, they can be excessively sleepy during the daytime. Again, setting limits by the parents is very important to ensure that the child gets an adequate amount of sleep at night and does not stay up late at night watching television or playing music. Control of the sleep habits before the time of puberty will often help parents as their children go through adolescence. Sometimes, the delay in the sleep time can be of such an extent that the child suffers from delayed sleep phase syndrome. This disorder occurs in a child who can't fall asleep before midnight, even though bedtime is early. In some cases, the child cannot fall asleep until 3 A.M., 4 A.M. or even 5 A.M. Consequently, there is great difficulty in getting up for school the next day. This delay in the sleep pattern can be corrected by various manipulations that might involve delaying the sleep pattern around the clock, the use of bright light therapy or even melatonin. If the sleep pattern cannot be reestablished by setting regular limits to the time of going to bed and the time of waking in the morning, then professional help should be sought.

Although the most common cause of sleepiness in adolescents is insufficient sleep at night, there can be other possibilities, such as narcolepsy. Narcolepsy often will appear before puberty but most commonly appears around the age of 16 years. The child may erroneously be diagnosed as having attention deficit disorder because the sleepiness makes the child act out at school. There may be difficulty concentrating, studying and remembering things. If the parent recognizes that the child sleeps well at night and yet is sleepy during the daytime, then professional help should be sought. Another symptom that may be seen by parents is an abnormal weakness in the child when the child becomes emotional, a symptom called cataplexy. The presence of this symptom in a sleepy child should immediately cause concern, and the parent should bring it to the attention of a physician.

Insomnia is rare in adolescents. However, if insomnia does occur and the child not only reports difficulty falling asleep, but also frequent awakenings at night and early morning awakening, then this raises the possibility of an underlying stressful situation or psychiatric disorder. Professional help should be sought. Fortunately, there are very effective medications available for depression. Counseling is also likely to be required and so a visit with a child psychologist or psychiatrist may be indicated.

Around the time of puberty, snoring and gasping episodes may occur during sleep. This may occur in association with large tonsils and raises the possibility of obstructive sleep apnea syndrome. If a parent is concerned about the possibility of this condition, he or she should mention it to the pediatrician. It may be necessary for the child to have an all-night sleep study to determine his or her breathing pattern during sleep at night. Treatment in the child usually involves removing the tonsils, although in some situations when the tonsils are not the cause of the breathing disturbance, an artificial ventilation device such as a CPAP (continuous positive airway pressure) machine may be necessary.

ADULTHOOD

In college, Jason had no difficulty sleeping; in fact he usually slept soundly and would need an alarm clock to awaken. After leaving college and getting his first job, Jason developed difficulty in falling asleep and would have frequent awakenings at night. His physician recognized that the stress of Jason's new job and the stress of moving to a new city were important factors in the development of the sleep disturbance. He prescribed a sleeping medication for Jason to use until he settled down to the new environmental changes and gave Jason some relaxation exercises to do before bedtime. After several months Jason adapted to his new environment and was able to sleep without the need for the sleep medication.

Jason's case is typical in that the primary sleep complaints of adulthood consist of insomnia or excessive daytime sleepiness. Insomnia is more common in women than in men and is most commonly seen in the young adult female. Typically the insomnia is associated with stress, anxiety or depression. Lifestyle changes that are produced because of leaving home and entering the workplace are contributing factors to insomnia. Maintaining regular, and good, sleep hygiene is very important in preventing stress-related insomnia from becoming chronic. If there are elements of depression, they may need to be treated with specific antidepressant therapy.

In males, excessive daytime sleepiness is most often associated with either sleep deprivation due to social or work commitments, or obstructive sleep apnea syndrome. Young adults tend to reduce the amount of time available for sleep by staying up later at night and getting up early for work in the morning. Sleep is usually made up on the weekends when the individual will stay in bed longer.

Obstructive sleep apnea syndrome becomes evident as an adult starts to put on weight. The peak incidence of obstructive sleep apnea syndrome is between the ages of 40 and 60 and is often associated with a longstanding history of chronic nasal breathing difficulties and increasing body weight. Treatment may involve mechanical means, such as CPAP, or surgical means, such as upper airway surgery. Weight reduction is always important.

In women, sleep may be disturbed because of pregnancy and childbirth. Initially in pregnancy a woman may feel increased tiredness and sleepiness during the daytime. Then, towards the last trimester of pregnancy, this gives way to sleep disruption, in part related to pain and discomfort because of the pregnancy. After delivery, sleep disturbance is common, as a result of frequent nocturnal awakenings to nurse the infant, and in some patients, postpartum depression may play a part. Not only mothers, but also fathers, are affected by the arrival of a new member in the family. Throughout early adulthood sleep is often disrupted because of child-related factors such as night fears or children coming into the parents' bedroom.

In middle age, menopause is a factor associated with sleep disruption in women. Loss of ovarian hormones is associated with frequent awakenings, in part related to hot flashes. Sleep disturbance may be improved by hormonal replacement therapy, although for most women the sleep disturbance is only temporary and generally subsides. With menopause can also come an increased tendency for snoring and obstructive sleep apnea syndrome. This time of life may also be associated with increasing weight gain. Features of loud snoring and excessive daytime sleepiness, around the time of menopause, should raise the suspicion of sleep apnea syndrome. For example, Angela had always been a little overweight, but after menopause she was unable to control her weight gain. She began to snore loudly and her husband noticed that she had irregular breathing during sleep. Her physician sent her to a sleep center where she underwent an overnight apnea syndrome test. The test showed that she stopped breathing 105 times for as long as 40 seconds and her blood oxygen level dropped to 85%. She was diagnosed as having obstructive sleep apnea and advised to lose weight and commence treatment with a CPAP machine. Although Angela was unable to lose weight, the CPAP machine allowed her to sleep more restfully.

For women like Angela who have sleep disorders in menopause, treatment may produce some improvement in feelings of well-being and reduction of daytime tiredness.

ELDERLY

Mildred, who is in her mid-70s, has sleep problems that are typical of the elderly who are more likely to have sleep disturbances characterized by difficulty falling asleep and frequent awakenings at night. Her high blood pressure was under control with medication but severe arthritis limited her ability to get out of the house in the daytime. She would take frequent daytime naps. To help Mildred with her sleep-related problems, her physician put her on a regular sleep schedule and advised her to reduce the amount of time spent in daytime napping. She was also advised to get more exposure to bright light during the daytime and told to keep herself as active as possible during daytime hours. Her blood pressure medication was changed to one that did not adversely affect her sleep, and a small dose of a sleeping medication helped to get her back into a regular nighttime sleep pattern.

As men and women age, the potential for sleep-related difficulties gets much greater. There is also an increase in obstructive sleep apnea syndrome or periodic leg movements in sleep, contributing to sleep disruption. The elderly also have a decreased ability to remain in deep sleep during the night; therefore, sleep becomes lighter and more disrupted with frequent awakenings. In addition, daytime sleepiness gradually increases and the tendency to nap during the day becomes more common than in middle age. If the elderly individual is not careful, sleep may occur intermittently throughout the 24-hour period with long awakenings at night and frequent daytime naps. This tendency must be corrected by ensuring that regular sleep onset and wake times are maintained, and that most of the sleep occurs during the nocturnal hours.

With advancing age, it is important that elderly individuals are exposed to plenty of bright light, an important factor in maintaining regular sleep patterns. In addition, exercise during the waking portion of the day is important. Frequent social interaction is also important, particularly for the wheelchair-bound or bedridden elderly patient.

Although sleep apnea may be a significant factor in the elderly, generally, because of increasing weight loss as one becomes elderly, the tendency for sleep apnea lessens.

Prescription medications taken for a variety of medical disorders can disrupt sleep, and many medications can lead to daytime tiredness and sleepiness. Medical disorders, particularly Parkinson's disease, can be associated with a disrupted sleep-wake pattern.

In addition to degenerative neurological disorders, cardiac and respiratory disorders are also major factors in causing sleep disruption. Assisted breathing devices such as CPAP machines may be necessary in those elderly who have impairment of ventilation during sleep at night. Cardiac disorders can also be associated with variation in breathing tendency throughout sleep, and optimum management of the cardiac disorder may be necessary to improve sleep quality at night.

Finally, dementia is usually associated with disruption of the sleep-wake process. Sleep becomes fragmented and difficult to attain at night, and there may be an increased tendency for tiredness and sleepiness during the daytime. Sleep medications become less useful in this age group, and around-the-clock nursing care is often necessary. The disruption of the sleep-wake pattern is a major reason for institutionalization of the demented elderly.

CHAPTER 10

THE INTERPLAY BETWEEN PSYCHOLOGY AND SLEEP

by Arthur J. Spielman, Ph.D. and Paul B. Glovinsky, Ph.D.*

Both the psychology and physiology of sleep have profound influences on waking life. Daytime experience has a direct effect on what transpires during sleep. By the same token, nocturnal activity is connected to waking thought and action. In this chapter, we will review our understanding of the interplay between sleep and our psychological lives.

The one-third of our lives that we spend asleep is clearly not "time-out" from a psychological point of view. That sleep is a psychologically active state is perhaps most clearly manifested by our dreams. While the function of dreaming for daytime activities is still hotly debated, it does appear that many of the same neural circuits or mental capacities that serve us during the day, such as our recall of specific memory traces or our tendency to organize perceptions into narrative, have been recruited in the service of the dream. During sleep, other mental processes, including memory, mood and, most fundamentally, alertness, are also being primed for the new day.

The significance of sleep for our general psychological well-being is most apparent when sleep loss occurs. When sleep loss occurs, sleepiness, fatigue, lack of mental clarity and general malaise wash over us as we struggle through the day.

The interdependence of psychology and sleep is also appreciated from another direction; it is easy to see how our state of mind during the day affects subsequent sleep. Poets and playwrights of the human condition, as exemplified by Shakespeare's fitful Lady Macbeth, have long known that the guilty, the scheming, the overwrought, the sad and even the ecstatic struggle with sleep rather than find repose.

In addition to these well-known aspects of the relationship between psychology and sleep, we will discuss less obvious areas, such as the interaction of self-image and sleep and the contributions of an inherent rhythm of sleepiness and alertness.

*Dr. Arthur Spielman is in the Department of Psychology, The City College of New York, and Sleep Disorders Center, New York Methodist Hospital, Brooklyn, New York. Dr. Paul Glovinsky is at the Capital Region Sleep/Wake Disorders Center, Albany, New York. Drs. Spielman and Glovinsky are both in private practice, 420 East 51st Street, New York, New York 10021.

EXTERNAL STRESSORS

Sleep resonates with the plucks of the day. We expect to be sleepless during states of emergency—during times of war, natural disaster, life-threatening illness or other catastrophes. Yet the turmoil churned up in the course of more pedestrian experiences is not easily put to rest. The history of patients with chronic insomnia often begins with stresses inherent to modern life. The trigger could be a performance error or merely the anticipation of a flub. Relocation to a new town, a harried commute, shift work, struggling to meet sales quotas, unrelenting rent or mortgage payments, the strains of raising a family, maintaining a harmonious marital relationship or coping with catastrophic illness, are just some of the typical challenges of contemporary living that can lead to sleep problems.

The trigger to sleep problems was no mystery when one of our patients presented for evaluation of an acute insomnia. His sleep problems had begun when he lost a large portion of his savings in the stock market. Looking for immediate relief for his situation, this middle-aged man knew too well that his mind was overactive. He was furious at his advisers and belittled himself for his poor decisions. This traumatic loss had real and wide-ranging consequences for his life and on his psyche. His plans for an early and comfortable retirement were dashed. Each night, rather than allowing himself to drift off to sleep, he set up an inquisition on his pillow, second-guessing his every turn and judgment, extracting imagined confessions of ignorance from his former advisers. Even when he did manage to fall asleep, he would awaken in the middle of the night with a start, as he replayed the same negative transcripts running through his head.

This patient's trouble falling asleep, and his intermittent awakenings, began to ease when he came to grips with his active role in his financial calamities and his sense of victimization was relinquished. Although the acknowledgement of personal responsibility was not without an accompanying intense psychic pain of shame, he gradually gained mastery over his financial setback. As he started to see his way to another path, he began expending more energy on ways in which he could meet the challenges of his new situation. With incremental progress in this direction, his insomnia at last subsided.

Insomnia becomes more prevalent as we get older in part because of the increased stresses and declining coping capacities associated with advancing age. Direct losses that are typically suffered, in addition to the deaths of peers, include the loss of physical capabilities and the loss of normal routines that accompanies aging or illness. There are also significant psychological blows to be dealt with, including worries about infirmity, increased dependence and the loss of self-esteem. Even with recovery from illness and relief from physical pain, the residual awareness of vulnerability and anticipation of future declines are hard to shake and are likely to impact sleep quality.

Sleep is also stressed by our modern version of the good life. We are desirous of leisure time and use our late-night hours to gratify those desires, whether that includes listening to jazz, working out at the gym or losing ourselves in the labyrinth of the Internet.

Our sleep schedules are in part determined by the work and leisure choices that we make. Technology has multiplied these options way beyond the light bulb that pierces the night. "24/7" has become the battle cry of armies of jet-lagged consultants, caffeinated techies, retailers, both traditional and online, plugged-in managers and, perhaps under increasing protest, their e-mail tethered employees. Acknowledgement of the need for sleep is, unfortunately, too often taken as an admission of weakness.

This brief survey of the interplay between psychology and sleep should make it clear that we are unlikely to successfully shield our sleep from these disrupting stressors. They can appear from all directions, arising from the customary as well as the extraordinary. But whatever their origin, these stressors are potent suppressors of sleep, with readily apparent consequences for daytime mental cognitive functioning, mood and overall zest.

EMOTIONAL TROUBLES

That the troubled mind has difficulty sleeping is a truism recognized in myths and history across cultures. This ancient theme has been taken up by many authors; it also underlies the practice of the current diagnostic manual of the American Psychiatric Association, which utilizes insomnia as a symptom for many psychiatric disorders.

Images of the depressed, unable to sleep and awake in the early morning hours, and of the anxious, ruminating late into the night, have been sufficiently reinforced to become popular stereotypes. Professional consensus is forming that these sleep-related manifestations of psychiatric disorders arise from a combination of vulnerability, psychological mechanisms and altered brain chemistry. However, the specific details of how or why this occurs have not been worked out.

SLEEP STAGES, SLEEP DEPRIVATION AND DEPRESSION

Interestingly, numerous sleep phenomena have guided investigators in the search for underlying mechanisms of the depressive disorders. The early appearance of REM sleep in the nocturnal sleep of depressed individuals has been dubbed one of the "biological markers" of depression. Instead of taking 80 minutes to go into REM sleep, as is typical of young to middle-aged adults, in the seriously depressed, REM sleep may appear in less than 50 minutes.

Another key component of sleep, slow wave sleep, makes up a smaller proportion of sleep in the depressed.

The pattern of secretion of the stress hormone cortisol is also different in the depressed compared to normal individuals.

A striking difference between depressed and nondepressed individuals is in their response to sleep deprivation. Following one night of total sleep deprivation, the average person will seem depressed, sad, irritable and lacking in motivation. In stark contrast, the seriously depressed will enjoy a respite from dysphoria (depression) following a sleepless night. Ironically, their depression lifts and their good spirits return. One curious aspect of this conversion from sad to glad is that the switch usually occurs in the early morning hours, before each individual's typical wake-up time. However, the reprieve is all too brief. After their next episode of sleep, the plague of depression returns.

EVERYDAY ACTIVITIES THAT AFFECT SLEEP

Pick up a popular magazine, turn to the health section, and you will often see a list of "Tips for Good Sleep." The popularity of these lists is due to the prevalence of insomnia and other sleep-related problems, and the search for getting a good night's sleep.

What are some of the everyday activities that affect sleep? The spread of specialty coffeehouses with their potent elixirs may be a boon to daytime output and performance, yet a cost is incurred at night when the heart still races and wakefulness will not yield to sleep. Similarly, it may seem a good idea to freshen up for the theater or a late party with a nap, especially if one has been short of sleep lately. Yet the ability to initiate sleep again later that night, and the quality of the sleep obtained, may be seriously compromised by this innocent adjustment.

Physical workouts, especially in the early evening, can increase the deep type of sleep called slow wave sleep. Unfortunately, this benefit may be limited to those who are already physically fit. The change in the composition of sleep has been attributed to the increase in body temperature that is produced by increased physical activity. While there are undoubtedly many differences in the benefits afforded by exercise, as opposed to lolling about in a Jacuzzi, passively heating the body in a hot tub has been shown to accomplish the same increase in deep slow wave sleep. However, the details of optimum timing, temperature and duration of exposure to the bath have yet to be completely specified. One cautionary note: Both strenuous exercise and passive body heating occurring too close to bedtime may make it more difficult to fall asleep.

For many people, the ability to sleep late into the morning (or even afternoon!) is one of the prime attractions of the weekend. The luxury of "sleeping in" may in fact redress sleep loss accumulated during the harried workweek. This may be of considerable value beyond the pleasurable, considering the dangers of sleepiness. However, altering the timing of sleep and wakefulness over the weekend may make it more difficult to get back one's regular weekday schedule. As discussed in the previous chapters as well as below, an endogenous pacemaker or "biological clock" in part governs the timing of our propensity for sleep. Oversleeping by several hours or more, two mornings in a row, begins to reset this clock towards a later sleep pattern—a trend that is difficult to abruptly reverse as the new workweek begins.

SLEEP AND PSYCHOLOGICAL WELL-BEING

Poor-quality sleep, as well as insufficient sleep, produces a host of specific deficits with far-reaching consequences. The amount of sleep loss does not have to be large to be keenly felt. Shortfalls in sleep accumulate if suffered nightly. Sleep loss disrupts a host of distinct cognitive and affective functions including memory consolidation, attention, concentration and mood regulation. A more general sense of ineffectiveness and incompetence gradually builds as these various functions are affected, with far-ranging consequences.

Not as well appreciated is the effect of reduced sleep on creativity. The sleep-deprived cannot fully exploit all that was learned while in a better frame of mind. Retrieval blocks, difficulty formulating new viewpoints or considering alternate angles, and problems maintaining a critical eye, are the kinds of deficiencies that make it very difficult for the sleep-deprived to synthesize something both new and worthwhile.

Many of us are familiar with the experience of pushing on valiantly through the night in order to finish writing an important assignment, exultantly collapsing into bed upon its completion, only to realize after a few hours of sleep that what looked brilliant at 4 A.M. has lost much of its sheen. This loss of accurate self-appraisal can become a chronic deficit in the personalities of the sleep-deprived. Individuals with troubled sleep, as well as those who voluntarily restrict their sleep, may be figuratively in the dark with regard to the impact of sleep loss of their functioning.

Many years ago we studied a man who described himself as a normal "short sleeper." He reported that he slept only three hours a night regularly and claimed to suffer no ill effects. He held down two jobs and on cursory inspection he indeed appeared to be without major problems. We studied this man in a special facility designed to eliminate time cues, which had been constructed to help investigate biological rhythms. No windows or clocks were present, the television shows were all taped with references to time of day eliminated, and male technicians were even instructed to shave on a random schedule so as not to appear clean-shaven only in the morning.

With all indications of time of day absent, this self-described "short sleeper" now slept for about seven and one-half hours per night! Interestingly, he was not aware that he was sleeping more than usual. After a few days, he asked us if we were putting drugs in his food. In this case, our subject was not just being paranoid—he was just feeling so good that he did not know how else to account for his newfound zest. He guessed that "it must be drugs that were doing it." It was, in fact, the additional sleep that was doing it.

The lesson of this vignette can be extended. We all have a tendency to assume our habitual practices to constitute a baseline, to be beyond reproach when it comes to ferreting out the causes of our complaints. If we are heavy coffee drinkers and are motivated to come to a sleep-disorders center because of poor sleep, invariably we have tried to cut back on coffee in the past, found that it made no difference, and thus are loathe to consider that drinking coffee might still be contributing to our problem. Similarly, if we select a lifestyle that affords little sleep (or in the case of our laboratory subject, if economic circumstances, necessitating two jobs, appear to dictate such a choice) it is not lack of sleep that we believe makes us irritable or unable to concentrate. We attribute our complaints to other features of our lives, or perhaps feel that they have arrived "out of the blue."

If a contrast to our normal methods of operation can be engineered, even on a trial basis, it may enable us to realize that things do not have to be the way they are. In the case of our "short sleeper," a time-isolation facility enabled us to circumvent the man's preconceptions and thereby provide him with more sleep. The contrast was dramatic. He realized that with more sleep he could feel so much better, and ultimately is more productive. This led to a wholesale reappraisal of his life. Fortunately, for the rest of us, transformational experiences do not usually require such an esoteric or scientifically monitored setting.

THE CHICKEN AND THE EGG: THE CONUNDRUM OF CHRONIC INSOMNIA

We have seen that poor days follow poor nights, which are followed in turn by poor days again. Individuals with poor sleep, regardless of its origin, begin to worry about the upcoming night because of the negative impact sleeplessness will have on their daytime mood and functioning. The irony, of course, is that worrying about insomnia becomes a self-fulfilling prophecy. It does little good and potentially much harm to anticipate a bad night's sleep. Thus dread of insomnia produces sufficient hyperarousal to perpetuate the sleep disturbance. Asked by the well-meaning clinician, "What worries do you have?" the frustrated insomniac replies, "Sleep is my only worry."

It is one of the critical, and sometimes elusive, tasks of the clinician to help the insomniac reduce his or her apprehension about sleeplessness. The worries of the insomniac with regard to reduced daytime efficacy and productiveness are certainly not groundless, but they often are exaggerated. It is often helpful to stress the point that all those days following sleep loss are somehow muddled through and that the chronic insomniac is in fact an expert at coping with sleep loss. Lowering the stakes becomes a tactic hopefully leading to a calmer outlook and a greater likelihood of achieving sleep.

The Self-Image of the Insomniac

Constantly contending with the compromised effectiveness that comes from sleep loss eventually affects an individual's self-image. He or she begins to identify as "an insomniac," rearranging schedules and limiting obligations so as not to place too much of a burden on sleep. Demeaning thoughts about the self proliferate, for example, deciding that "I'm not up to hosting a dinner party" or "I'd better not take on any high-visibility assignments at work, because I'm not very effective these days."

Over time, these self-imposed put-downs lead to a sense of helplessness and hopelessness and to the general dysphoria (depression) that regularly accompanies insomnia.

Psychological Treatments of Insomnia

Some of the most common recommendations for better sleep are based on learning theory. These include such advice as "Don't get into bed before going to sleep" and "Get out of bed if you are not asleep quickly." Establishing sleep habits that regularly combine sleep cues, such as getting into bed or turning off the light, with actually falling asleep quickly helps an individual relearn the sleep response. However, an individual with insomnia is not permitted to stay in bed tossing and turning because this inappropriately pairs sleep cues with being awake and restless in bed.

A short list of instructions to help individuals relearn the sleep response by reestablishing the connection between bedtime cues and sleep was developed by Richard Bootzin of the University of Arizona. Here, excerpted, are Bootzin's rules:

1. Use the bed only for sleep. (Having sexual relations is exempt from this rule.)
2. Go to bed only when sleepy.
3. If you do not fall asleep within about 15 minutes of getting into bed, then get out of bed. Do not return to bed until you are sleepy or feel you can fall asleep.
4. When you return to bed, abide by rule #3.

The following additional rules keep sleep in line with principles of good sleep hygiene, previously discussed in Chapter 1:

5. Get up at the same time every morning.
6. Do not nap.

A different view sees trouble in sleeping as reflecting increased physiological arousal. One way to increase sleep drive in order to overcome or dissipate this hyperarousal is with more strenuous exercise, as discussed above. Another way to increase sleep drive and thereby counter hyperarousal is to mildly deprive the individual of sleep for a short period of time. This treatment, known as sleep restriction therapy and developed by Arthur Spielman and colleagues, begins by curtailing the time in bed. If an individual reports sleeping six hours on average, for example, then he or she would be allowed to stay in bed for only six hours at the start of treatment.

Mild sleep loss will result from this bedtime restriction and over time this will enhance the depth and continuity of sleep. As sleep onset becomes more rapid and sleep less interrupted, the patient's worried anticipation regarding the upcoming night's sleep tends to diminish. As sleep improves, the patient is permitted to spend progressively more time in bed.

A direct way to dampen hyperarousal is through relaxation exercises. The goal of progressive muscle relaxation is to increase the awareness of muscle tension. The patient practices contracting specific muscle groups, holding the tension in order to heighten awareness. The patient then relaxes the muscles and concentrates on the perception of decreasing tension. These two steps, tensing and relaxing, are repeated for the major muscle groups. Relaxation training helps patients counteract the chronic muscular tension that typically accompanies hyperarousal.

In addition to physiological hyperarousal, many insomniacs must also contend with an overactive mind. They will often say, "My mind is racing," or complain of an inability to "shut off" worrisome thoughts. Cognitive therapies, championed most recently by Charles Morin of the University of Laval (Canada), have been devised that train patients to exert more mastery over their thought processes. Specific time can be set aside for worry, well before bedtime and away from the bedroom, so as to reduce the potential of these worries to disrupt sleep later that night. Similarly, thoughts can be restructured so as to minimize the salience of distressing experiences. These and other cognitively based therapies aim at establishing the reasonably calm mental state that is required for a smooth transition to sleep, and to ensure that sleep is refreshing.

THE RHYTHM OF SLEEP AND WAKEFULNESS

One of the most promising new areas in sleep research is the investigation of the role of biological rhythms in the regulation of sleep at night and daytime alertness. In humans and all other mammals studied, a neural pacemaker or biological clock that fluctuates with a periodicity near 24 hours, called *circadian,* has been located. The clock controls daily fluctuations of sleep as well as a vast array of other functions. In part, the function of this clock is to coordinate biological processes.

A major theory of the control of sleep and alertness suggests that there are two separate systems involved. This understanding derives from many investigators, most notably Alexander Borbely of the University of Zurich. The first system, of which we all have firsthand experience, promotes sleep as we stay awake and promotes wakefulness by discharging during sleep. In this model, a sleep need builds up gradually during wakefulness and is satisfied by sleep. The longer one stays awake, the greater the need for sleep.

The second system is regulated by circadian rhythms and promotes sleep at night and alertness during the day just as a pendulum swings back and forth. This second circadian system explains how alertness actually improves during the day after we have stayed awake all night. During such an "all-nighter," we get sleepier until a little before our habitual wake-up time. Then, without any accumulated sleep, we begin to get a second wind and sleepiness is lessened. If only the first system were operating, then the degree of sleepiness we experience would be directly related to how long we have been awake. This two-system theory also explains how we can maintain alertness throughout the day. As sleep need is building up through extended waking hours, the circadian system is countering the drive for sleep with a well-timed boost of alertness.

DREAMING

In the almost 50 years since Nathaniel Kleitman and colleagues discovered the relationship between rapid eye movement (REM) sleep and dreaming at the University of Chicago, we have learned much about these unique phenomena. The physiological components of REM sleep have been closely observed, and the typical 90-minute cycle of REM sleep and vivid dreaming throughout the night has been well described. Freud's view that that dreams originate from and reflect unconscious conflict has found many challengers among those who are based in sleep laboratories. However, most of the fundamental questions regarding both REM sleep and dreams are still unanswered, still matters for conjecture and experimentation. How are dreams constructed during the REM sleep state? What is the function of dreaming? What does REM sleep do?

In *The Promise of Sleep,* William C. Dement provides these answers: "Years of experimentation strongly suggest that in REM, the brain is acting very much as it does in waking life, sending out signals to move muscles in response to the scenario that is being played out in the dreams . . .

To certain parts of the brain, there is no difference between waking life and dreaming life. When we are dreaming of eating or fighting or thinking, the brain is sending out the same signals it would if we were awake and eating or fighting or thinking. . . . in dreams what we experience is limited only by the brain itself and not organized and driven by sensory input from the outside world."

Most of us can attest to the interplay between psychology and sleep that is demonstrated by dreams. Daily experience, whether monumental or trivial, is often recapitulated in some form or another during REM sleep. While dreams typically appear to have less effect on our daily outlook—oftentimes seeming to vanish from memory within seconds of awakening—now and then we may experience a dream that profoundly alters our waking life. In *The Promise of Sleep,* William C. Dement recounts a vivid dream he had in the early 1960s, when he was still a two-pack-a-day chain-smoker. It was a terrifying dream about getting diagnosed with lung cancer, and Dement recalls that when he awoke from the dream, it changed his life. "I stopped smoking right then and have never lit another cigarette," Dement writes.

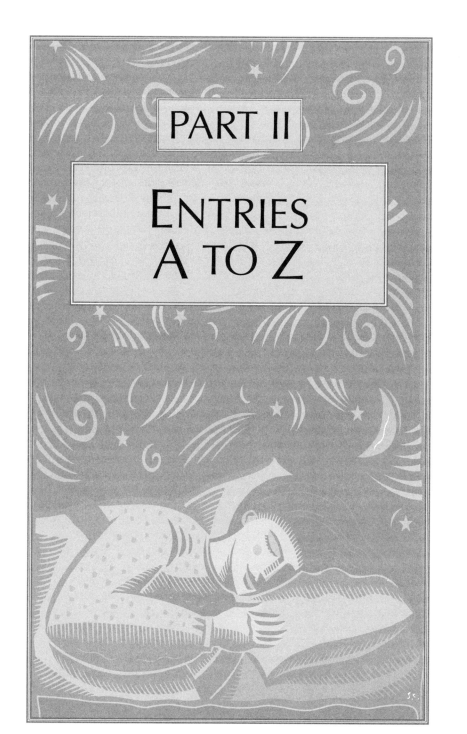

PART II

ENTRIES
A TO Z

A

abnormal movements Some sleep disorders are characterized by atypical limb movements. For example, movement occurs in response to the creepy, crawly feeling in the legs due to the disorder known as *RESTLESS LEGS SYNDROME (RLS). The relief that these movements bring, however, is only temporary.

Repetitive, abnormal movements of the legs or arms during sleep, occurring as frequently as every 10 seconds, are typical of PERIODIC LIMB MOVEMENT DISORDER (PLMD). These leg or arm movements are often powerful enough to cause an awakening as well as to disturb a bed partner because of the shaking of the bed or accidentally being kicked. Those suffering from REM SLEEP BEHAVIOR DISORDER, in which dream content is acted out during the REM (dreaming) stage of sleep, display movements such as punching, kicking or running, sometimes inadvertently causing injury.

The presence of abnormal movements during sleep that cause INSOMNIA or lead to EXCESSIVE SLEEPINESS during the day should be discussed with a physician to see if tests need to be performed, such as POLYSOMNOGRAPHY (sleep test).

accidents Common in persons with sleep disorders, especially those who suffer from EXCESSIVE SLEEPINESS. Sleepiness produces impaired ALERTNESS and awareness, and this can be a problem for those who operate dangerous machinery or drive cars. See CAFFEINE, DROWSY DRIVING, NAPS, SEIZURES, SLEEP TERRORS, SLEEPWALKING, and SNORING.

accreditation standards for sleep disorder centers In 1975, the Association of Sleep Disorder Centers (ASDC) began to develop guidelines and standards for the practice of SLEEP DISORDERS MEDICINE. These standards resulted in the accreditation of the first sleep disorder center in 1977. Since that time, the Association of Sleep Disorder Centers has merged with the CLINICAL SLEEP SOCIETY to form the American Sleep Disorders Association (now called the American Academy of Sleep Medicine), which is responsible for producing guidelines for sleep disorder centers. An accreditation committee visits sites and ensures that sleep disorder centers throughout the United States meet appropriate standards for the practice of sleep disorders medicine. The standards involve a review of the following areas: the relationship of the center to the host medical institution, to ensure that there is a stable relationship among the medical structure of

---

*Capitalized words or terms within an entry indicate that there is a separate entry for that term, concept, or disorder in the A to Z section of *Sleeping Well*. For further information, you are directed to that separate entry, arranged alphabetically.

the sleep disorder center, the physical environment and the personnel; the way in which patient referrals and evaluation procedures are handled; the polysomnographic and other monitoring procedures; the interpretation and documentation of the polysomnographic data; and the physical equipment of the recording laboratory.

By 2000, more than 500 sleep disorder centers had been accredited by the American Academy of Sleep Medicine. In this way, the development of sleep disorder centers in the United States has proceeded in an orderly and appropriate manner, with the highest standards of patient care being maintained. (See also SLEEP DISORDER CENTERS.)

actigraphy   A biomedical instrument capable of monitoring motor activity in order to identify the presence or absence of body motion during sleep or wakefulness. Activity monitoring by means of an actigraph is useful in detecting sleep episodes and differentiating periods of sleep and rest from periods of wakefulness.

Actigraphy is commonly employed for long-term CIRCADIAN RHYTHM studies to document the pattern of sleep and wakefulness with little inconvenience to the patient. A typical actigraph has a simple-to-wear, easily programmable microprocessor device, which is usually attached to the non-dominant wrist, but can also be attached to one or both legs. The device works on the principle that movement of the non-dominant wrist is correlated with wakefulness, whereas long, quiescent periods are associated with rest or sleep. Studies have demonstrated an 88.9% correlation of accuracy with polysomnographically measured sleep. Special computer programs interpret the information recorded, and it can be displayed in many different formats.

New forms of actigraphs include light-detecting monitors for measuring light exposure and actigraphs that include radio frequency transmitters for relaying information cordlessly to a distant computer.

Wrist activity monitors have also been used to measure abnormal movements that can occur in patients suffering neurological disease, such as Parkinson's disease or other types of movement disorders. (See also SHIFT-WORK SLEEP DISORDER.)

active sleep   The low voltage, mixed frequency EEG and rapid eye movement (REM) activity. This term, a phylogenetic and ontogenetic term for REM SLEEP, is synonymous with the term "activated sleep."

activity monitors   Devices used to detect motion as a way of differentiating periods of wakefulness or rest. (See also ACTIGRAPHY.)

activity-rest cycle   Term used to describe the cyclical pattern of activity that alternates with rest in animals and humans; it is commonly considered to be the same as wakefulness and sleep. The activity-rest cycle is usually determined in animal research studies of CHRONOBIOLOGY and CIR-CADIAN RHYTHMS; it is more easily measured than sleep and wakefulness. The activity-rest patterns of rodents alternate wheel running activity with rest periods.

In addition to the 24-hour pattern of activity and rest there is a BASIC REST ACTIVITY CYCLE (BRAC) that has a shorter period length, of approximately three hours, than the activity-rest cycle. BRAC is believed to be indicative of an underlying ultradian cycle that is manifest during sleep by the NREM-REM SLEEP CYCLE.

acute mountain sickness   See ALTITUDE INSOMNIA.

adjustment sleep disorder   INSOMNIA resulting from an acute emotional stress that can be related to conflict, loss or a perceived threat, for example, a death in the family, an upcoming examination, marital, financial or work stress. Typically, adjustment sleep disorder lasts for a few days, and always less than three weeks, after which the sleep pattern returns to normal.

Features of adjustment sleep disorder are prolonged SLEEP LATENCY, frequent awakenings, or EARLY MORNING AROUSAL. There may also be a tendency for excessive SLEEPINESS during the day. In acute circumstances, there can be loss of the ability to maintain normal social activities or employment until the acute reaction is over. Intense anxiety or depression may be associated with the stress response and the sleep disturbance. The sleep pattern returns to normal with the resolution of these acute psychological symptoms.

Polysomnography or a multiple sleep latency test may help diagnose a condition either of hyperarousal or of excessive daytime sleepiness. Treatment is essential soon after the sleep disturbance begins to prevent its development into chronic PSYCHOPHYSIOLOGICAL INSOMNIA. Hypnotic medication therapy, lasting only several days, is recommended. Attention to good SLEEP HYGIENE is essential, not only during the time of the stress reaction, but also in the days immediately following.

Adjustment sleep disorder, synonymous with transient psychophysiological insomnia and situational insomnia, is the preferred term.

advanced sleep phase syndrome   A CIRCADIAN RHYTHM SLEEP DISORDER characterized by difficulty in remaining awake until the desired bedtime, and getting up too early, or early morning INSOMNIA. This disorder, which is seen typically in elderly persons, often causes embarrassment due to an inability to remain awake in social situations in the mid-evening hours. The patient may also be at risk of ACCIDENTS, for instance, by falling asleep at the wheel of a car. After a late night out, the inability to delay the time of the final awakening often produces a tendency to daytime sleepiness. Inappropriate daytime napping may result.

Polysomnographic studies have demonstrated an early onset in the tim-ing of the low point of the circadian body temperature rhythm. Sleep onset time occurs at a time earlier than desired, and a normal duration and quantity of sleep follows. The spontaneous awakening is typically earlier than desired.

The origin of advanced sleep phase syndrome is unknown, but, as it seems more common in the elderly, it has been suggested that it is due to degeneration of the nerve cells of the circadian pacemaker, so that the cir-cadian pacemaker is unable to induce a delay of the sleep pattern. As with the delayed sleep phase syndrome, the advanced sleep phase syndrome may be due to an abnormality of the phase response curve. The disorder is apparently rare.

Advanced sleep phase syndrome differs from other causes of early morning awakening. Mood disorders, particularly depression, are associ-ated with early morning awakening but are also associated with sleep onset and sleep maintenance difficulties. The advanced sleep phase syn-drome needs to be differentiated from INSUFFICIENT SLEEP SYNDROME, which typically can also produce evening sleepiness but is caused by a forced early morning awakening. Individuals who are classified as short sleep-ers may have an early morning awakening but do not have evening sleepiness.

The diagnosis of advanced sleep phase syndrome is usually made by the typical complaint of an inability to stay awake till the desired bedtime, and an inability to remain asleep till the desired time of the morning. The dis-order must be present for at least a three-month period. When the person is not required to remain awake till the desired bedtime (that is, goes to bed early), then the sleep episode is of normal quality and duration. The final awakening is always earlier than desired.

Mild disturbances can be treated by close attention to maintaining a regular sleep onset and waketime. Incremental delays of sleep onset on a daily basis, by 15 to 30 minutes, may assist in delaying the sleep pattern. One patient has been reported to have been treated by CHRONOTHERAPY, which involved advancing the sleep pattern by three hours per day. The sleep pattern was rotated around the clock so that a more appropriate sleep onset time was reached. Exposure to bright light prior to sleep onset may assist in producing a more normal sleep onset time. (See also AGE, LIGHT THERAPY.)

affective disorders Term describing mental disorders characterized by mood disturbances, typically DEPRESSION or mania. More recently, the terms MOOD DISORDERS and ANXIETY DISORDERS have been applied to this group of psychiatric disorders.

age See Chapter 9: Sleep Across the Life Cycle. (See also SLEEP EFFICIENCY, SLEEP NEED, TOTAL SLEEP TIME.)

airway obstruction   The predominant cause of OBSTRUCTIVE SLEEP APNEA SYNDROME. This disorder is associated with obstruction at any site from the nose to the larynx. Upper airway obstruction is assessed by means of cephalometric radiographs and FIBEROPTIC-ENDOSCOPY; treatment may be by surgical or mechanical means. (See also CONTINUOUS POSITIVE AIRWAY PRESSURE, MANDIBULAR ADVANCEMENT SURGERY, SURGERY AND SLEEP DISORDERS, TONSILLECTOMY AND ADENOIDECTOMY, TRACHEOSTOMY; UPPER AIRWAY OBSTRUCTION, UVULOPALATOPHARYNGOPLASTY.

alcohol   Commonly used to help insomnia sufferers get to sleep at night—with very deleterious effects on sleep. Drinking alcohol in the evening may help sleep onset, but headaches upon awakening the next morning are typical, particularly with excessive alcohol use. The routine use of alcohol as a sedative produces an improved sleep onset time, often with a deeper sleep in the first third of the night, but then sleep becomes lighter and more fragmented.

ALCOHOL-DEPENDENT SLEEP DISORDER occurs in people who chronically use alcohol for its sleep-inducing effects. This disorder is *not* associated with heavy alcohol ingestion during the daytime and is not a symptom of alcoholism; as tolerance develops, the amount of alcohol ingested increases, but persons with alcohol-dependent sleep disorder usually do not go on to become alcoholics. Alcohol will shorten the SLEEP LATENCY and increase the amount of stage three and four SLEEP (see SLEEP STAGES), but REM SLEEP is reduced and becomes fragmented. Awakenings frequently intrude into the second half of the nocturnal sleep episode.

It is commonly recognized that alcohol will increase the amount and loudness of SNORING, but it can also exacerbate OBSTRUCTIVE SLEEP APNEA SYNDROME. ALCOHOLISM is associated with an increased number of sleep-related disturbances, such as NOCTURNAL ENURESIS, NIGHT TERRORS, SLEEP-WALKING.

Alcohol has detrimental effects on daytime alertness. The sleep fragmentation and disruption at night can lead to excessive sleepiness and diminished alertness during the daytime. The effects of alcohol upon performance, particularly driving, may be greatly influenced by the amount of the prior night's sleep so that ACCIDENTS due to alcohol abuse are often, in part, related to the soporific effects of alcohol.

The effects of alcohol are exacerbated by the ingestion of other drugs, particularly sedatives. This combination may be dangerous and lead to stupor and even coma or death.

Alcohol will impair the arousal and ventilatory response to the apneic episodes in obstructive sleep apnea syndrome, causing the apneas to be longer and the oxygen desaturation to be more severe. The association of alcohol with exacerbation of obstructive sleep apnea may lead to serious cardiovascular consequences that could prove fatal.

Treatment of obstructive sleep apnea syndrome often involves use of a CONTINUOUS POSITIVE AIRWAY PRESSURE device (CPAP), and alcohol ingestion can be a common cause of failure of an adequate CPAP response. A patient who consumes alcohol on a nightly basis may fail to do so in a sleep laboratory and therefore the adjustment phase of CPAP may lead to an inadequate pressure setting. Following alcohol ingestion, a higher than usual pressure may be required in order to overcome the apneic events. There is also evidence that alcohol can produce obstructive sleep apnea syndrome in persons who otherwise would not have apneic events.

Alcohol can exacerbate other sleep disorders, such as JET LAG and SLEEP-RELATED EPILEPSY. Epilepsy may also be exacerbated by the disruptive sleep pattern caused by alcohol, which leads to sleep deprivation and possibly the precipitation of epileptic seizures.

alcohol-dependent sleep disorder   Disorder characterized by the chronic drinking of alcohol for its soporific effect. The self-prescribed use of ethanol (ALCOHOL) as a sedative is the cause of this disorder that often results from an underlying insomnia, such as an ADJUSTMENT SLEEP DISORDER or INADEQUATE SLEEP HYGIENE. Typically, alcohol is drunk late in the evening, a few hours before bedtime, usually in quantities of up to eight drinks. However, in this disorder, the alcohol ingestion is rarely associated with excessive alcohol intake during the daytime, or the development of chronic ALCOHOLISM.

The sedative properties of the alcohol are greatest at the onset of the pattern of alcohol ingestion. However, with chronic usage, tolerance develops and there is a loss of the sleep-inducing effect. In addition, withdrawal effects occur in the second half of the nocturnal sleep episode, so that a pattern of frequent awakenings and difficulty in maintaining sleep often results. Other symptoms of alcohol withdrawal, such as headaches, dry mouth, fatigue and tiredness upon awakening, may also occur.

In addition to the ingestion of alcohol, other sedative agents may be taken, although more typically the alcohol is the sole sedative ingested. The use of alcohol is generally longstanding and most often occurs in individuals after the age of 40 years.

Polysomnographic monitoring shows an increase in stage three and four sleep (see SLEEP STAGES) and a short SLEEP ONSET latency; however, REM SLEEP fragmentation is present with frequent awakenings, sometimes with early morning awakening.

Treatment of the alcohol dependency is the same as for any other drug dependency. A gradual drug withdrawal, with the institution of SLEEP HYGIENE measures, is essential to prevent further sleep disruption. In some situations, it may be necessary to supplant the alcohol with a more effective hypnotic agent during the alcohol withdrawal phase, and then the prescribed hypnotic can be gradually withdrawn.

alcoholism   Chronic alcohol intake with alcohol abuse and dependency. Sleep disturbances are a common feature of alcoholism, particularly INSOMNIA as well as EXCESSIVE SLEEPINESS during the day.

Alcohol produces an increased tendency for sleepiness that lasts for approximately four hours after drinking (depending upon the amount actually consumed). When taken before bedtime, it will reduce the SLEEP LATENCY and reduce wakefulness in the first third of the night, but as the alcohol is metabolized, there can be withdrawal effects, with increased sleep fragmentation. Individuals who drink chronically and excessively find that sleep disruption occurs with abstinence from alcohol, and very often alcohol is used to improve sleep. The chronic alcohol abuser may also suffer from NIGHTMARES and other REM phenomena as a result of REM SLEEP fragmentation during chronic ingestion of alcohol as well as abstinence. Alcoholics are susceptible to other sleep disrupting factors, such as environmental stimuli. Alcohol in alcoholics will often induce increased amounts of slow wave sleep in the first half of the night, and REM fragmentation and decrease is typically seen in the second half of the night. Sleep becomes so fragmented that stage two SLEEP SPINDLES and increased muscle tone can occur during REM sleep.

Associated features of alcoholism include an increased incidence of BED-WETTING, SLEEP TERRORS, SLEEPWALKING, nightmares and exacerbation of SNORING and OBSTRUCTIVE SLEEP APNEA SYNDROME. Alcoholic liver disease and encephalopathy with the development of a Korsakoff psychosis are common results of chronic alcohol ingestion. The direct effect of these disorders can also contribute to sleep disturbances. (See also ALCOHOL for other effects of chronic drinking.)

The alcoholic, when withdrawing from alcohol, can develop delirium tremors within a week of stopping the alcohol intake. This state is marked by severe autonomic hyperactivity, with tachycardia, sweating and tremulousness. Withdrawal seizures, called "rum fits," can occur within the first few days of alcohol withdrawal and always precede the development of delirium. During the time of delirium and hallucinosis, sleep is severely disrupted.

There may be an excessive amount of REM sleep that occurs in the first few days after alcohol withdrawal, although it may be fragmented. Slow wave sleep can be reduced and may recover very gradually following abstinence from alcohol, often never returning to pre-alcohol levels. Disturbed sleep may continue to be present for up to two years following complete abstinence.

Treatment of the alcohol-induced sleep disturbance is usually restricted to managing alcohol abstinence and may involve the use of short-term HYPNOTICS to reduce the severe sleep disruption. Attention to good SLEEP HYGIENE is essential. (See also ALCOHOL-DEPENDENT SLEEP DISORDER.)

alertness   Opposite of SLEEPINESS. Ideally, alertness should be full for the approximately two-thirds of the day when we are awake. Persons who have sleep disorders often notice an increased tendency for sleepiness in the midafternoon, an exaggerated form of a natural dip in alertness that occurs at that time. This midafternoon dip is part of the biphasic CIRCADIAN RHYTHM of sleep, which is reflected in the major sleep episode at night and the increased tendency for sleepiness that occurs 12 hours later, in the midafternoon. Some cultures take advantage of this decreased alertness by scheduling a SIESTA for several hours. The decrease in alertness also can be exacerbated by a large lunch or the ingestion of ALCOHOL.

Subjective measures of alertness include the STANFORD SLEEPINESS SCALE (SSS), which rates the degree of alertness and sleepiness on a scale from one to seven, and the EPWORTH SLEEPINESS SCALE. Objective alertness measures include PUPILLOMETRY, a measure of fluctuations in pupil diameter size that reflects changes in alertness. Decreased pupil size and oscillations of the pupil indicate decreased alertness. The most widely used objective measure of alertness, however, is the MULTIPLE SLEEP LATENCY TEST, which measures at two-hour intervals the tendency to fall asleep throughout the day. Five nap tests are scheduled from 10 A.M. to 6 P.M. and the electro-physiological measures of sleep are monitored for SLEEP STAGES. A short SLEEP LATENCY to the first epoch of sleep indicates decreased alertness and the presence of sleepiness, particularly if the mean sleep latency over the five naps is 10 minutes or less.

Daytime alertness can be influenced by a number of factors, including the quality and quantity of the prior night's sleep as well as medications or drugs taken during the daytime. Caffeine found in coffee and many sodas is a commonly-used central nervous system stimulant that will increase daytime alertness. STIMULANT MEDICATIONS, often used to improve alertness in persons with excessive sleepiness due to disorders such as NARCOLEPSY, include amphetamines, methylphenidate hydrochloride and pemoline. These agents improve alertness but have less of an effect on multiple sleep latency measures of sleepiness. Methylphenidate and amphetamines have been objectively shown to produce a reduction in sleepiness.

The cycle of daily alertness appears to be independent of the cycle of daytime sleepiness. This is most evident in a person's ability to maintain alertness unless placed in an environment conductive to sleep, where severe sleepiness may readily become apparent. The findings on the multiple sleep latency test for the effects of stimulant medications tend to support this notion of two independent processes.

For this reason, the MAINTENANCE OF WAKEFULNESS TEST was developed. This test measures the ability to remain awake and is performed in a manner similar to the multiple sleep latency test.

Measurement of alertness following treatment of some sleep disorders can be valuable in establishing whether or not an individual is sufficiently alert to drive a motor vehicle or operate dangerous machinery, for instance. (See also EXCESSIVE SLEEPINESS, VIGILANCE TESTING.)

alpha-delta activity   Term describing the presence of the alpha EEG rhythm, which occurs simultaneously with the slower delta EEG pattern of sleep. Alpha-delta activity is typically seen in disorders that disrupt nocturnal sleep, such as INSOMNIA, and is also a characteristic feature of the FIBROSITIS SYNDROME. (See also ALPHA RHYTHM.)

alpha rhythm   ELECTROENCEPHALOGRAM (EEG) wave activity that occurs with a frequency of 8 to 13 hertz (cycles per second) in adults. This activity occurs in the central to posterior portions of the head and is indicative of the awake state in humans. ALPHA ACTIVITY is usually present during relaxed wakefulness when visaual input is reduced (for instance, when the eyes are closed). The activity tends to be slower in children and the elderly compared to young and middle-aged adults. It may occur during sleep stages if sleep is disrupted, as is seen in the many disorders of insomnia. Alpha activity during slow wave sleep is a particular characteristic of the FIBROSITIS SYNDROME.

altitude insomnia   An acute INSOMNIA that occurs with the ascent to high altitudes; also known as acute mountain sickness. Altitude insomnia typically occurs in individuals, such as mountain climbers, who ascend to levels higher than 4,000 meters (13,200 feet) above sea level. Some symptoms may be evident at levels above 2,500 meters (8,250 feet), although the most predominant symptoms occur within 72 hours of exposure to higher altitudes. The disorder is characterized by difficulty in initiating and maintaining sleep, as well as other symptoms, such as headaches and fatigue.

This disturbance appears to be related to the low level of atmospheric oxygen that produces HYPOXEMIA and associated APNEA. The apnea is due to a post-hypoxemic period of hyperventilation that lowers the carbon dioxide to produce the central apneic episode.

People with lung disorders, anemia or impaired cardiac function are more likely to develop altitude insomnia.

The disorder may be treated by means of RESPIRATORY STIMULANTS, such as acetazolamide, and may be improved by breathing a high level of inspired oxygen. After a few days at altitude, changes in body chemistry occur that lead initially to alkalosis, but the condition gradually corrects itself. Severe hypoxemia at altitude may lead to the development of cardiac complications, with acute pulmonary edema, and lead to compensatory changes such as a stimulation of red blood cell production.

Altitude insomnia can be differentiated from other sleep or respiratory disorders by means of polysomnographic investigations. The usual pattern consists of 10 to 20 seconds of apnea followed by three to five breaths of hyperventilation, with associated arousals or awakenings. Arterial blood gases will demonstrate hypoxemia and reduced carbon dioxide levels.

The syndrome rapidly resolves itself upon return to lower altitudes. (See also CAHS [CENTRAL ALVEOLAR HYPOVENTILATION SYNDROME], CENTRAL SLEEP APNEA SYNDROME, OBSTRUCTIVE SLEEP APNEA SYNDROME.)

alveolar hypoventilation   Inadequate VENTILATION of the terminal units of the lungs, the alveoli. Patients who suffer from alveolar hypoventilation have inadequate gas transfer across the lungs to and from the blood and therefore have elevated carbon dioxide and lowered oxygen levels in their blood.

Alveolar hypoventilation can be produced by disorders that affect the lung directly or harm ventilation because of impaired respiratory drive. Typically, patients with alveolar hypoventilation have deterioration of ventilation during sleep. Daytime alveolar hypoventilation may be due entirely to SLEEP-RELATED BREATHING DISORDERS, such as OBSTRUCTIVE SLEEP APNEA SYNDROME, CENTRAL SLEEP APNEA SYNDROME, or CAHS (CENTRAL ALVEOLAR HYPOVENTILATION SYNDROME).

ambulatory monitoring   The continuous measurement of physiological variables in a patient who is not confined to bed or a specific room. Typically, ambulatory monitoring employs a portable recording device that records data while attached to the patient.

Ambulatory monitoring techniques have been used for many years for the continuous measurement of heart rhythm by Holter monitoring. More recently, ambulatory techniques have been developed for the continuous recording of ELECTROENCEPHALOGRAM activity to detect seizures. Ambulatory monitoring devices have also been developed for the measurement of a variety of other physiological variables and the assessment of sleep disorders.

Twenty-four-hour ambulatory sleep-wake monitoring can determine the presence of the sleep pattern in patients who have INSOMNIA or patients who complain of EXCESSIVE SLEEPINESS. Continuous monitoring may also be helpful for the daytime assessment of unintended sleep episodes in patients with NARCOLEPSY or IDIOPATHIC HYPERSOMNIA. Continuous monitoring throughout the 24-hour period has some advantages over the usual intermittent nap testing by means of a MULTIPLE SLEEP LATENCY TEST, as it detects sleepiness that might be missed between naps. However, it is less standardized and therefore less useful for comparison purposes among patients or for comparing a patient's status at different times. Ambulatory monitoring is particularly useful for the documentation of abnormal events and can be used for screening of such disturbances as episodes of APNEA or PERIODIC LEG MOVEMENTS during sleep. This form of monitoring can be helpful in detecting events that occur infrequently, as patients can wear the monitoring device for several days or even weeks. Activities such as SLEEPWALKING, SLEEP TERRORS or abnormal SEIZURE episodes may be detected on ambulatory recorders.

Ambulatory monitoring is also useful for determining disturbed patterns of sleep and wakefulness, such as are seen in the CIRCADIAN RHYTHM SLEEP DISORDERS. It is particularly useful for the detection of the rest-activity cycle of shift workers and individuals who undergo frequent time zone changes (see JET LAG).

Several ambulatory monitoring systems are currently available in the United States. Typically they consist of a microcomputer digital system that monitors respiration, oxygen saturation, electrocardiography, and body temperature, position and movement. Some monitors are capable of detecting electroencephalographic activity for the measurement of sleep.

Ambulatory monitoring has the potential to become the ideal means of recording physiological information from a patient in his usual environment. However, present systems are unable to measure a number of physiological variables accurately, especially given the risk of sensors malfunctioning when the patient is not under constant supervision.

Because of the major disadvantages of current ambulatory monitoring, it cannot be applied to the routine clinical evaluation of patients with most sleep disorders. Its usage currently is primarily for screening purposes, follow-up evaluations after treatment has been initiated, research experimentation or for determining patterns of rest and activity. (See also ACTIVITY MONITORS, POLYSOMNOGRAPHY.)

American Board of Sleep Medicine   In 1978 the Association of Sleep Disorder Centers formed a committee to produce an examination for the purpose of establishing and maintaining standards of individual proficiency in clinical POLYSOMNOGRAPHY. This committee, which became the Examination Committee of the American Sleep Disorders Association, directed by Helmut S. Schmidt, M.D., had certified 432 physicians and Ph.D.s as accredited clinical polysomnographers (ACPs) by the middle of 1991. By the end of 2000, some 1,500 sleep specialists had been board certified in sleep medicine.

Culminating many years of planning, the American Board of Sleep Medicine was incorporated by WILLIAM C. DEMENT, M.D., Ph.D., as an independent, nonprofit, self-designated board on January 28, 1991.

For up-to-date and more specific details on examination requirements or to apply for board certification in sleep medicine, contact: American Board of Sleep Medicine, 6301 Bandel Road, Suite 101, Rochester, Minnesota 55901. E-mail: absm@absm.org; Web: www.absm.org.

amitriptyline   See ANTIDEPRESSANTS.

amphetamines   See STIMULANT MEDICATIONS.

Anafranil   See ANTIDEPRESSANTS.

anorectics   See STIMULANT MEDICATIONS.

antidepressants   Medications used for the treatment of the psychiatric disorders associated with DEPRESSION. These disorders, previously called affective disorders and currently called mood disorders, can have pronounced effects upon sleep. INSOMNIA is a typical feature of mood disorders, as are altered sleep-wake patterns. The antidepressant medications can be useful for treating not only the predominant mood disorders but also the underlying sleep disturbance. The group of antidepressant medications most commonly used are the SEROTONIN reuptake inhibitors; however, other medications, including the tricyclic antidepressants and the monoamine oxidase (MAO) inhibitors, are frequently recommended. In addition to their role in treating sleep disturbance related to depression, the antidepressant medications are commonly used for the treatment of CATAPLEXY in patients who have NARCOLEPSY.

antipsychotic medication   See NEUROLEPTICS.

anxiety   A feeling of dread and apprehension regarding one or more life circumstances. A common cause of sleep disturbance, anxiety may be a short-lived, acute stress, such as that related to an examination or a marital, financial or work problem. Acute anxiety in these situations can lead to an ADJUSTMENT SLEEP DISORDER, which typically resolves itself within a few days of the acute anxiety, but it may persist for several weeks. Chronic anxiety often indicates an ANXIETY DISORDER and may lead to an enduring and pervasive sleep disorder.

Individuals with chronic sleep disorders, such as PSYCHOPHYSIOLOGICAL INSOMNIA, may become anxious as a secondary feature of the sleep disorder. Treatment of the underlying sleep disorder in these situations usually leads to resolution of the anxiety. (See also PANIC DISORDER.)

anxiety disorders   Psychiatric disorders characterized by symptoms of anxiety and dread, and avoidance behavior. Sleep disturbance commonly occurs in association with anxiety disorders. Anxiety disorders include PANIC DISORDER, with or without agoraphobia, phobias, obsessive-compulsive disorder, post-traumatic stress disorder and general anxiety disorder.

Patients with general anxiety disorder typically have a sleep onset or maintenance INSOMNIA, with frequent awakenings that may be associated with anxiety dreams. Typically there is ruminative thinking that occurs at sleep onset or during the awakenings. Individuals often complain of being unable to "turn off their minds" because of the flood of thoughts and concerns, many of which are trivial in nature. Following the disturbed night of sleep, there may be feelings of unrest, tiredness, fatigue and sleepiness. Often during the daytime there is intense anxiety over the thought of another impending night of inadequate sleep. Associated with the daytime anxiety is evidence of increased muscle tension, restlessness, shortness of breath, palpitations, dry mouth, dizziness, trembling and difficulty in concentration. Most patients with anxiety disorders have little ability to take daytime naps, as the difficulty in being able to fall asleep persists around the clock.

The anxiety disorders characteristic of early adulthood are more common in females than in males. There appears to be a familial tendency for general anxiety disorder. Polysomnographic studies demonstrate a prolonged sleep latency, with frequent awakenings during the night, reduced sleep efficiency and increased amount of lighter stages one and two sleep, with reduced slow wave sleep. REM SLEEP latencies are normal although REM sleep may be reduced in percentage (see SLEEP STAGES).

The chronic nature of anxiety differentiates patients with anxiety disorders from those who are experiencing an ADJUSTMENT SLEEP DISORDER, which is typically seen in association with acute stress. Sleep disturbance associated with anxiety disorders should be distinguished from that seen in patients who have PSYCHOPHYSIOLOGICAL INSOMNIA; the anxiety in psychophysiological insomnia is less generalized and is more focused on the sleep disturbance, which, when effectively treated, leads to resolution of the anxiety. Patients with generalized anxiety disorders have more pervasive anxiety that may persist even though the sleep disturbance is otherwise resolved.

Anxiety disorders are treated either by pharmacological means or through counseling and psychotherapy. Pharmacological agents used to treat anxiety disorders include HYPNOTICS and BENZODIAZEPINES; the use of ANTIDEPRESSANTS may be required if elements of depression coexist. Good SLEEP HYGIENE and treatment of the sleep disturbance by behavioral means, such as STIMULUS CONTROL THERAPY or SLEEP RESTRICTION THERAPY, are usually necessary in patients with sleep disturbance because of anxiety disorders.

Case History

A 39-year-old male high school teacher had a long history of sleep disturbance, a condition that had deteriorated in the prior three years. In addition to teaching, he also had a part-time job as a landlord, which contributed a number of anxieties and rather complicated his life. His sleep pattern was disrupted by a constant feeling that he couldn't turn off his mind. He became very annoyed and angry at his inability to fall asleep. Occasionally, he would perform RELAXATION EXERCISES before getting into bed at night and would avoid any activities that might be stimulating or disruptive to his sleep. He usually was unable to sleep for more than an hour at a time before awakening, and then he would be in and out of sleep for the rest of the night. Occasionally he tried drinking a small amount of ALCOHOL to improve his sleep but stopped this when he found it did not produce any benefit. Upon awakening in the morning, he would be tired and had difficulty in maintaining concentration, which affected his conversations. He found that he would often have to repeat himself. He became slightly depressed and irritable because of the sleep disturbance.

His problem with initiating and maintaining sleep was finally diagnosed as secondary to chronic anxiety and depression. There was no evidence of major depression; the anxiety features were more prominent. Treatment was initiated by scheduling his time for sleep within the limits of 10:45 at night with an awakening at 6:45 in the morning. With 0.5 milligrams of alprazolam (Xanax; see BENZODIAPENES) the sleep disturbances abated but were not resolved. After several weeks of treatment, combined with close attention to his hours, a small dose of sedating antidepressant medication was added to his treatment. He commenced 50 milligrams of amitryptiline (see ANTIDEPRESSANTS) taken one hour before sleep.

On the new treatment regime, he dramatically improved and the quality of sleep was the best he had had in years. In addition, the intermittent feelings of daytime depression were eliminated and he did not suffer from fatigue and tiredness. He was maintained on the medications with strict adherence to a regular sleeping-waking schedule.

apnea   Derived from the Greek word that means "want of breath," apnea has occurred if breathing stops for at least 10 seconds, as detected by airflow at the nostrils and mouth. Respiratory movement may or may not be present during an apneic episode. Typically there are three forms of apnea, depending upon the degree of respiratory movement activity: obstructive, central and mixed.

Obstructive apnea is associated with upper airway obstruction and is characterized by loss of airflow while respiratory movements remain normal. Airflow is usually measured by means of a nasal thermistor (a temperature-sensitive metal strip) that records changes in air temperature with inspiration and expiration, whereas respiratory muscle movement activity can be measured by means of the electromyogram, strain gauges or by a bellows pneumograph. Obstructive apnea is usually accompanied by sounds of snoring.

Central apnea is cessation of airflow associated with complete cessation of all respiratory movements. The diaphragm and chest muscles are immobile. This type of apnea can occur among those who have diseases such as poliomyelitis or spinal-cord injuries.

Mixed apnea typically has an initial central apnea component for about 10 seconds followed by an obstructive component.

Apnea during sleep can produce a lowering of the blood oxygen level, increased blood carbon dioxide levels, cardiac arrhythmias, and sleep disruption with resulting excessive sleepiness. If the number of apneas becomes frequent enough to produce clinical symptoms and signs, then the patient may have either an OBSTRUCTIVE SLEEP APNEA SYNDROME or CENTRAL SLEEP APNEA SYNDROME.

apnea-hypopnea index   The number of obstructive, central and mixed APNEA episodes, plus the number of episodes of shallow breathing (HYPOPNEA), expressed per hour of total sleep time, as determined by all-night polysomnographic recording. Most clinicians believe that the apnea-hypopnea index is a more reliable measure of apnea severity than the APNEA INDEX because it monitors all three types of respiratory irregularity during sleep. The apnea-hypopnea index is sometimes referred to as the RESPIRATORY DISTURBANCE INDEX (RDI).

apnea index   A measure of APNEA frequency most commonly used in determining the severity of respiratory impairment during sleep. The number of obstructive, central and mixed apneic episodes is expressed per hour of total sleep time as measured by all-night polysomnographic recording. Occasionally an obstructive apnea index, which is a measure of the obstructive apneas per hour of total sleep time, or a central apnea index, is stated. Typically an apnea index of 20 or less is regarded as mild apnea, an index of 20 to 50 as moderate and above 50 as a severe degree of apnea. The term "apnea index" is only one index of apnea severity because the duration of apneic episodes and severity of associated features, such as oxygen saturation and the presence of electrocardiographic abnormalities, are also important in determining apnea severity.

If the number of episodes of shallow breathing during sleep (HYPOPNEA) are added to the apneas in calculating the index, then an APNEA-HYPOPNEA INDEX is produced, an index preferred by many clinicians.

apnea monitor   A biomedical device developed primarily for detection of episodes of cessation of breathing that occur in infants and young children. An apnea monitor detects respiratory movement and heart rhythm. Typically, an apnea monitor is set to signal a breathing pause of 20 seconds or greater, or an episode of slowing of the heart rhythm, a rate that is determined according to the age of the child.

Apnea monitors do not replace the use of more extensive polysomnographic evaluation when sleep-related breathing disorders are suspected. Polysomnographic monitoring has the advantage of being able to detect upper airway obstructive events as well as determining whether alterations in ventilation occur during sleep or specific sleep stages. In addition, polysomnographic monitoring is able to detect other physiological variables that may be associated with a respiratory pause, for example, the electroencephalographic pattern in a child who has epileptic seizures as a cause of respiratory cessation. (See also CENTRAL SLEEP APNEA SYNDROME and OBSTRUCTIVE SLEEP APNEA SYNDROME.)

Argonne anti-jet-lag diet   Developed by Dr. Charles Ehret of Argonne's Division of Biological and Medical Research as part of his studies of biological rhythms. (The Argonne National Laboratory is a center of research in energy and fundamental sciences of the United States Department of Energy and is located in Argonne, Illinois.) The Argonne anti-jet-lag diet is based upon the finding that high carbohydrate food, such as pasta, fruit and some desserts, will produce an increased level of energy for about one hour, and subsequently will produce tiredness and sleepiness. Conversely, high protein foods, such as fish, eggs, dairy products and meat, will give a sustained increased level of energy, possibly by its metabolism to catecholamines such as adrenaline. In addition, caffeine-containing drinks, such as coffee, can advance or delay the sleep pattern, depending upon the time they are taken.

The Argonne anti-jet-lag diet consists of a pattern of feasting and fasting for four days prior to departure. The first day, breakfast and lunch consist of high protein meals and the evening meal consists largely of carbohydrates. This pattern of food intake is repeated on the third day. On the second and fourth days of the diet, fasting occurs so that only light meals of fruits, soups and selected solids are taken. Caffeinated beverages are allowed only between 3 and 5 P.M. Upon the day of departure, if the traveler is westbound, he is advised to drink caffeine beverages in the morning before departure. When traveling eastbound, caffeine beverages are taken between 6 and 12 P.M.

The first day in the new environment is one of fasting.

The Argonne anti-jet-lag diet may be useful for some people; however, many find its pattern of feasting and fasting impractical and it has not been effective for everyone who has rigidly adhered to the plan. (See also DIET AND SLEEP, TIME ZONE CHANGE [JET LAG] SYNDROME.)

arise time   Time on the clock after final wake up, at which an individual gets out of bed.

arousal   A change in the sleep state to a lighter stage of sleep. Typically, arousal will occur from a deep stage of non-REM sleep to a lighter non-REM sleep stage, or from REM sleep to stage one or wakefulness (see SLEEP STAGES). Arousals sometimes result in a full awakening and are often accompanied by body movement and an increase in heart rate.

Arousals occurring from stage three and four sleep may be accompanied by the characteristic features of AROUSAL DISORDERS, namely, SLEEP-WALKING, SLEEP TERRORS and CONFUSIONAL AROUSALS. In these disorders, arousal is followed by an incomplete waking and the persistence of electroencephalographic patterns of sleep.

arousal disorders   Disorders of normal AROUSAL. In 1968, Roger Broughton described four important common sleep disorders as abnormalities of the arousal process: SLEEP ENURESIS (bedwetting), somnambulism (SLEEPWALKING), SLEEP TERRORS and NIGHTMARES. At that time, it was believed that all four of these disorders shared common electrophysiological and clinical features.

Two of the disorders, somnambulism and sleep terror, most consistently demonstrate the classical feature of the arousal disorders. They occur during an arousal from slow wave sleep, rather than REM sleep. Since Broughton's original description, a third disorder, the nightmare, has been shown to occur more typically from REM sleep; and sleep enuresis, although occurring from slow wave sleep, can also occur out of other sleep stages.

In addition to the sleep stage association, the other major features of the four arousal disorders are: (1) the presence of mental confusion and disorientation during the episode; (2) automatic and repetitive motor behavior; (3) reduced reaction and insensitivity to external stimulation; (4) difficulty in coming to full wakefulness despite vigorous attempts to awaken the individual; (5) inability to recall the event the next morning (retrograde amnesia); and (6) very little dream recall associated with the event.

Although mentioned by Broughton in his original article, the disorder of CONFUSIONAL AROUSALS has recently been established as another arousal disorder.

arrhythmias   Heart rhythm irregularities. The most common cause of sleep-related arrhythmias is OBSTRUCTIVE SLEEP APNEA SYNDROME, which produces a pattern of slowing and speeding up of the heart (brady-tachycardia). This pattern may be picked up on a 24-hour electrocardiographic recording (for instance, during Holter monitoring). The presence of brady-tachycardia during sleep, and its absence during wakefulness, is a characteristic feature of obstructive sleep apnea syndrome. Other cardiac arrhythmias that can occur in association with the obstructive sleep apnea syndrome include episodes of sinus arrest, lasting up to 15 seconds in duration, and tachyarrhythmias, such as ventricular tachycardia. Cardiac arrhythmias due to obstructive sleep apnea are believed to be a cause of sudden death during sleep.

Other disorders that can produce cardiac irregularity during sleep include REM SLEEP-RELATED SINUS ARREST. This disorder is characterized by episodes of cardiac pause, lasting several seconds, that occur during REM sleep in otherwise healthy individuals. This disorder may require the implantation of a cardiac pacemaker in order to prevent complete cardiac arrest.

Another disorder that may be associated with cardiac irregularity is SUDDEN UNEXPLAINED NOCTURNAL DEATH SYNDROME (SUND) which is seen in Southeast Asian refugees. In this disorder, sudden death occurs during sleep and a cardiac cause is suspected. Ventricular tachycardia has been detected in the few patients who have been resuscitated.

Patients who have cardiac arrhythmias due solely to heart disease often have an improvement in the cardiac irregularity during sleep, particularly during non-REM sleep, when the heart rate slows and the rhythm becomes more stable. During REM sleep there can be an exacerbation of cardiac irregularity, particularly during the episode of phasic rapid eye movement activity. (See also SLEEP-RELATED BREATHING DISORDERS.)

artifact   Interfering electrical signals that occur during the recording of sleep. They may be caused by the person being studied or by environmental interference, sometimes from the sleep lab itself, and can obscure the information being recorded.

Too much artifact may make a sleep recording impossible to score and analyze and therefore render it useless.

Sixty hertz activity, often due to nearby electrical appliances or cables, is a common cause of artifact during sleep recordings.

asthma   See SLEEP-RELATED ASTHMA, SLEEP-RELATED BREATHING DISORDERS.

atonia   The absence of muscle activity. Skeletal muscle, even in the resting state, has a degree of muscle activity that maintains the tension in muscles (muscle tone). A reduction in muscle tone causes the muscle to relax and become weak and unable to maintain tension. Atonia is typically seen in a muscle that is removed from its neurological input, such as when a nerve is severed; it is also seen as a characteristic feature of REM SLEEP when all skeletal muscles, except for the inner ear muscles, the eye muscles and the respiratory muscles, have absent tone. In general, muscle tone is highest in wakefulness, reduces as sleep becomes deeper and is typically absent during REM sleep.

autogenic training   A behavioral technique used in the treatment of INSOMNIA. A form of self-hypnosis, autogenic training conditions patients to concentrate on sensations of heaviness and warmth in the limbs, thus inducing sleepiness. Although some studies have questioned how effective this technique is for all patients, it seems that at least some are helped by it. (See also BEHAVIORAL TREATMENT OF INSOMNIA, DISORDERS OF INITIATING AND MAINTAINING SLEEP, HYPNOSIS, PSYCHOPHYSIOLOGICAL INSOMNIA.)

automatic behavior   Unconscious psychological and physical actions. Such behavior includes repetitive movements typical of some forms of SLEEP-RELATED EPILEPSY. Automatic behavior can also occur with normal activities, such as driving, and is seen in patients with NARCOLEPSY and other forms of severe sleepiness. In automatic behavior, an individual may perform complex normal activities, yet have amnesia for these acts.

awakening   A change from non-REM or REM SLEEP to the awake state or WAKEFULNESS. Wakefulness is characterized by fast, low-voltage EEG activity with both alpha waves and beta waves. There is an increase in tonic EMG activity and rapid eye movements, and eye blinks occur. An awakening is always accompanied by a change in the level of consciousness to the alert state. (See also NREM-REM SLEEP CYCLE.)

B

barbiturates Medications used as hypnotic agents since the turn of the century; about 50 are available commercially. Since the 1960s, barbiturates have largely been replaced by the BENZODIAZEPINES because the latter have less potential for drug addiction and a reduced risk of death from overdose. Yet, despite disadvantages of barbiturates, they are effective hypnotic agents although rarely prescribed now. The most commonly prescribed barbiturates include amyobarbital (Amytal), pentobarbital (Nembutal) and secobarbital (Seconal).

Barbiturates depress the central nervous system and therefore can be very toxic in high doses, producing coma and even death. Clinically they produce a range of effects from mild sedation through sleep induction. Phenobarbital is commonly used as an effective anticonvulsive agent. Short-acting, intravenous barbiturates are used for general anesthesia.

Hypnotic barbiturates have profound effects upon sleep. They decrease SLEEP LATENCY, reduce the number of sleep stage shifts to WAKEFULNESS, and reduce stage one sleep (see SLEEP STAGES). The drug also increases the amount of fast EEG beta activity throughout the sleep recording. SLOW WAVE SLEEP is generally reduced in amount; however, phenobarbital sometimes increases stage four sleep in healthy individuals. The REM SLEEP latency is increased, and there is reduction in the total amount of REM sleep, the number of REM sleep cycles and the density of rapid eye movements during REM sleep.

Tolerance to the beneficial hypnotic effect of the medication generally occurs within two weeks of continuous use. There are variable effects of the rebound in slow wave and REM sleep after termination of barbiturate use.

basic rest-activity cycle (BRAC) In 1960, NATHANIEL KLEITMAN first suggested that a cycle of activity and rest occurs throughout a 24-hour period. His original suggestion was based upon recognizing a periodicity in the feeding intervals of infants. Kleitman had noticed that there were four cycles of feeding and rest during the day, and five at night. Similar cycles of behavior have been demonstrated in adults for many activities, such as eating, drinking and smoking. The NREM-REM SLEEP CYCLE of approximately 90 minutes in nocturnal sleep and the cycle of alertness as determined by pupillary measures are other examples.

The periodicity of the basic rest-activity cycle may vary among species and appears to be 23 minutes in cats, which correlates with the self-feeding cycle as well as the non-REM-REM sleep cycle. The longer cycle of 72 minutes has been determined in monkeys. The human basic rest-activity cycle is approximately 96 minutes in adults.

This basic rest-activity cycle is believed to be determined by a central nervous system mechanism. Studies in cats have shown that lesions in the basal forebrain of cats will alter the period of the sleep-wake cycle but do not alter the basic rest-activity cycle, suggesting that the underlying basic rest-activity cycle is independent of sleep and wakefulness.

beds   There was probably a time in the early Neolithic period when a transition occurred from sleeping on the ground to sleeping in a bed. The change to sleeping in a bedroom occurred around the time of the Sun King of France, Louis XIV, who developed a separate room for sleeping, which was in a very prominent position in his palace. Prior to that time, most people would sleep in a communal room.

The kings and queens of ancient days often had varied types of beds, ranging from flat tables with wooden headrests to cushions on the floor or beds encrusted with gold and jewels. In the Middle Ages, the typical bed consisted of pallets of straw; however, the wealthy developed ornate canopied beds with thick hangings to prevent drafts in otherwise austere castles.

Louis XIV would hold court while lying in his bed, which was placed in a key position in his palace so it was more like a public room. At that time, beds became more elaborate and were often regarded as prized items to be passed down through the family.

Nowadays, beds are used for a variety of activities, including writing, reading, watching television and sexual intimacy, as well as sleeping. Charles Darwin is reported to have written his *Origin of Species* while lying in bed, and Benjamin Franklin is reported to have had four beds in his bedroom so he could move to a fresh bed whenever he felt the need. Lawrence of Arabia is reported to have slept usually in a sleeping bag, and Charles Dickens rearranged the bed so that the head was always pointing to the north.

In recent years, the bed has undergone some modern changes. Mattresses have been improved with the use of inner springs. The more typical single-sized bed has given way to queen- or king-size beds. Water beds have been popular, particularly with young adults, and various forms are available, some with a single water-filled bag and others with numerous tubes of water contained within a padded mattress covering.

The accessories to the bed have also developed, with some beds having built-in electronic equipment so that a person can lie in bed and watch television, or listen to stereophonic music that can be adjusted by remote control.

It is evident that if someone needs to sleep, he or she can sleep on any surface. During wartime, soldiers have slept under the most arduous conditions in trenches, exposed to the weather and the noise of gunfire. In many primitive cultures, the bed consists of a matting placed on the floor of a room inside a dwelling or even on the ground exposed to the environment.

For most westerners, selecting a bed or a pillow is a matter of personal preference. However, certain physical concerns, such as height, should be taken into consideration; very tall or heavyset persons may need larger beds to comfortably accommodate their body size. The firmness or softness of a mattress is also a matter of taste. (See SLEEP SURFACE.)

Whether or not sheets are used on a bed, as well as the type of material (cotton, satin, combination fabrics), is another matter of personal taste, as well as whether both a bottom and top, or just a bottom, sheet are used.

Since persons adapt to their typical bed, a change in a bed may require a period of adjustment. Hence vacationers will complain they failed to get a good night's sleep, even in the most comfortable bed in the finest hotel, simply because the bed is unfamiliar. Similarly, infants changing from a crib to a bed for the first time may require a period of time to adjust to the new bed and mattress.

If someone has difficulties initiating sleep, it may be better to restrict the number of non-sleep-related activities that are associated with the bed. For example, children who have difficulty falling asleep may need to have distracting toys or books removed from their beds, or from the area immediately surrounding the bed.

Finding a comfortable position in bed for sleeping can be influenced by such factors as pregnancy or back problems. During pregnancy, it may be necessary to use pillows under the stomach and between the knees and thighs to enable a woman to sleep on her side, a more comfortable position for some than sleeping on the back. A larger bed may also help the pregnant woman to spread out more as her increasing size makes a smaller bed uncomfortable. Those with back problems might be in less agony if they avoid sleeping on their stomachs and sleep on a firm surface, and those with breathing problems might find their breathing is improved if they sleep on their sides. (See also SLEEP HYGIENE.)

bedtime   The time when an individual attempts to fall asleep, *not* the time when an individual gets into bed, which may not be the same. Typically, bedtime is associated with the time that the bedroom light is turned off in anticipation of sleep.

Especially for young children, bedtime rituals are thought to ease the transition from wakefulness to sleep. Activities to help the child wind down from wakefulness to sleep include soft music, such as lullabies, either prerecorded and played on a tape recorder, or sung by a parent, or reading or telling a story. Children or adults may find that taking a bath immediately before bedtime can produce relaxation and assist the ability to fall asleep.

The ideal bedtime is tied to the anticipated wake up time the next morning. Thus, on a weekday bedtime may be earlier than over the weekend. Consistency in the precise bedtime, however, helps to regulate sleep and wakefulness. Too wide a variation in bedtime hours—say, from 11 P.M.

for adults on a workday night to 1 or 2 A.M. on weekend nights, or for children from 8 P.M. on a school night to 11 P.M. on a weekend night—may make adjusting to the weekday bedtime hour difficult on Sunday night. The resulting difficulty in falling asleep on Sunday night is often called SUNDAY NIGHT INSOMNIA, and the difficulty awakening on Monday morning is called the MONDAY MORNING BLUES. Too much variation in bedtime or waketime may cause a form of insomnia called INADEQUATE SLEEP HYGIENE, if mild, or IRREGULAR SLEEP-WAKE PATTERN, if severe.

Bedtimes for a young child have to be set by the parent or caretaker, as these children are too young to understand the need to ensure an adequate duration of sleep. If the parent does not establish appropriate bedtimes and waketimes, LIMIT-SETTING SLEEP DISORDER may result.

If a child finds a particular bedtime ritual helpful in getting to sleep, such as clutching a special stuffed animal or a blanket, using a night-light in the room or listening to a particular kind of music, it may be helpful to bring those props along when sleeping away from home for any period of time. But if a particular bedtime ritual becomes a major endeavor and sleep is markedly disturbed without it, then a form of insomnia called SLEEP ONSET ASSOCIATION DISORDER may result.

bed-wetting   See SLEEP ENURESIS.

behavioral treatment of insomnia   The use of nonpharmacological techniques to improve nighttime sleep. Behavioral treatments can be useful for most patients who have INSOMNIA, even if it is due to a physical or organic cause. However, these treatments are most useful for the psychophysiological forms of insomnia or insomnia related to psychiatric disorders, particularly ANXIETY DISORDERS.

Behavioral treatments include SLEEP HYGIENE, specific sleep behavior programs, RELAXATION EXERCISES to reduce arousal, and techniques to reduce excessive rumination during sleep, including COGNITIVE FOCUSING, SYSTEMIC DESENSITIZATION, PARADOXICAL TECHNIQUES and SLEEP RESTRICTION THERAPY.

There is an increase in the use of behavioral techniques in the management of chronic insomnia as physicians become warier of hypnotic medications. In fact, hypnotic medications are now recommended only for transient use, particularly in patients who have situational or transient insomnia. Behavioral techniques get to the source of the sleep disturbance and prevent the continuation of poor practices that maintain the insomnia. Typically these techniques are utilized along with other treatments, particularly in patients with PSYCHIATRIC DISORDERS who may need specific medications, to treat the psychiatric disorders. (See also AUTOGENIC TRAINING, BIOFEEDBACK.)

benign neonatal sleep myoclonus   An abnormal form of jerking that occurs in newborn infants. This asynchronous jerking (MYOCLONUS) occurs primarily during quiet or SLOW WAVE SLEEP, in clusters of four or five at a time, and recurs approximately once every second throughout sleep. Each myoclonic episode lasts between 40 and 300 milliseconds and causes jerking of the arms or legs, particularly the distal muscle groups. More major movements can cause the whole body to move. Usually the jerks occur asynchronously in a pattern that varies among infants.

This jerking usually lasts for only a few days or, at the most, a few months. It always has a benign course, and its cause is unknown. No treatment is necessary as this disorder always spontaneously resolves. It can affect both male and female infants and usually occurs within the first week of life.

There is no evidence of any underlying biochemical or neurological abnormality.

Benign neonatal sleep myoclonus needs to be differentiated from neonatal epileptic SEIZURES that most commonly occur in association with biochemical or infective causes. Drug withdrawal can also be a cause of similar movements.

Other forms of jerking, such as infantile spasms, commonly occur after the first month of life and therefore can be easily differentiated from benign neonatal sleep myoclonus. Infantile spasms also have a specific electroencephalographic pattern termed hypsarrhythmia, which does not occur in benign neonatal sleep myoclonus.

benign snoring   See PRIMARY SNORING.

benzodiazepines   Benzodiazepines were first introduced in the 1960s, primarily for their anti-anxiety effect. The first agent to be introduced was chlordiazepoxide, which had little hypnotic effect but appeared to be an effective anti-anxiety agent. The benzodiazepines were preferred over the previously-used barbiturate sedative medications because of a decreased tendency to produce fatal central nervous system depression, drug abuse and toxic side effects. The term "benzodiazepine" refers to the group structure, which is composed of a benzene ring fused to a seven-membered diazepine ring. Approximately 25 benzodiazepines that are slight variations of this basic structure are currently in clinical use.

In general, the benzodiazepines tend to decrease SLEEP LATENCY and reduce the number of awakenings and the amount of wakefulness that occurs during the major sleep episode. The amount of stage one sleep is usually decreased and the time spent in non-REM stage two sleep is increased. The amount of stage three and four (slow wave) sleep is reduced as is the total amount of REM sleep. REM sleep latency is usually increased and the frequency of the rapid eye movements during REM sleep is reduced.

The effect of benzodiazepines on sleep gradually diminishes over a few nights of consecutive use. If the medication is abruptly stopped after several weeks of chronic use there may be a REBOUND INSOMNIA that typically lasts one or two nights. This effect can be minimized by instituting a gradual withdrawal of medication.

bereavement   It is not unusual for the death of a loved one to be the precipitating cause of SHORT-TERM INSOMNIA. If a spouse with whom one has shared a bed or a bedroom has died, a person may find it hard to fall asleep alone. This type of short-term insomnia, an ADJUSTMENT SLEEP DISORDER, usually resolves itself within a few weeks. Continued insomnia may produce conditioned associations and lead to a PSYCHOPHYSIOLOGICAL INSOMNIA. Bereavement is one indication for the use of short-term HYPNOTICS to prevent such a conditioned insomnia from developing. The bereavement may be helped by consulting a bereavement counseling center or a therapist.

Berger, Hans   The first person to measure and record brain electrical activity, Hans Berger (1873–1941) reported the first human ELECTRO-ENCEPHALOGRAM in 1929. Berger began to study electrical activity in animals in 1910 at a hospital in Germany. In 1924, he first studied electrical activity in the brains of humans, particularly of those who had skull defects where the needles could be placed directly on the surface of the brain. His first report of alpha waves, recorded with the patient's eyes closed, was presented in 1929. The presence of alpha waves did not find general recognition until 1933, when Berger's work was publicized by the physiologist Lord Adrian, who called the ALPHA RHYTHM the Berger rhythm.

Berger's discovery led to the subsequent recognition of differences in the electroencephalogram during wakefulness and sleep, and this forms the basis of the electroencephalographic determination of SLEEP STAGES.

Berger rhythm   See ALPHA RHYTHM.

beta rhythm   Electroencephalographic frequency of 13 to 35 hertz that is typically seen during alert wakefulness. This activity may be associated with the ingestion of a variety of different medications, such as BARBITU-RATES and BENZODIAZEPINES. Beta activity, when seen in association with high ELECTROMYOGRAM (EMG) activity and a low voltage mixed frequency ELECTROENCEPHALOGRAM (EEG), is indicative of wakefulness. With relaxed wakefulness, the EEG frequency slows, and if the eyes are closed, alpha activity of 13 hertz or lower is typically seen. (See also ALPHA RHYTHM.)

biofeedback   Biofeedback technique can assist in recognizing when muscle tension is high, which may reflect impaired ability to fall asleep. Biofeedback involves sensors that detect changes in muscle activity and convey this information by means of different sounds. The individual can use the sounds to assist in relaxing the muscles as a change in the muscle tension is detected by the alteration in the sound produced by the muscles. After biofeedback training, a person can relax the muscles without the need for feedback sound information from the sensors. The relaxation technique can then be performed in bed, prior to SLEEP ONSET to assist sleep. (See also SLEEP EXERCISES, STRESS.)

biological clocks   The periodic oscillation that occurs in a wide variety of biological systems; the frequency of the oscillations serves an internal timing system. Virtually all plants and animals have an internal timing system, or biological clock, and there may be several of these processes that control different aspects of the physiology of the biological systems. The biological clocks measure time and synchronize an organism's internal processes with daily environmental events. The site of the major biological clock in humans is believed to be the SUPRACHIASMATIC NUCLEUS. (See also CIRCADIAN RHYTHMS; CHRONOBIOLOGY.)

biorhythm   A recurrent pattern of change in a physiological variable, such as a CIRCADIAN RHYTHM. However, the term *biorhythm* more commonly has become associated with the astrological prediction of life events and is not scientifically based. Biorhythm is rarely used in CHRONOBIOLOGY; the term *biological rhythm* is preferred.

body clock   Another term for BIOLOGICAL CLOCKS and CIRCADIAN RHYTHMS, it is related to CHRONOBIOLOGY, the scientific study of biological rhythms. The everyday cycle of sleep and wakefulness is systematized by the biological or body clock. Practically all plants and animals have an internal timing system, or biological clock. The plant experiment conducted by Jean-Jacques d'Ortous de Mairan in 1729 was significant because it demonstrated the presence of biological rhythms even when the ENVIRONMENTAL TIME CUES of light and dark were missing.

body movements   Those movements detected during polysomnographic recording that indicate a specific physiological event, as indicated by an increase in amplitude of the ELECTROMYOGRAM that lasts one second or longer. Body movements are associated with muscle artifact that can be seen obscuring the ELECTROENCEPHALOGRAM or ELECTRO-OCULOGRAM recording. Brief body movements are a normal accompaniment of healthy sleep but are increased in number in disorders that cause lighter sleep, such as INSOMNIA. (See also MOVEMENT AROUSAL, MOVEMENT TIME.)

bodyrocking   One of three disorders—bodyrocking, HEADBANGING and HEAD ROLLING—that involve repetitive movement of the head and occasionally of the whole body. These disorders are now known under the collective name rhythmic movement disorder.

Bodyrocking may occur during times of rest, drowsiness or sleep, as well as during full wakefulness. It is usually performed on the hands and knees with the whole body rocking in an anterior/posterior direction, with the head being pushed into the pillow.

The disorder most commonly occurs in children below the age of four years, with the highest incidence at six months of age. Treatment is usually unnecessary when the condition occurs in infancy as it typically disappears within 18 months. Bodyrocking can persist into older childhood, adolescence and, rarely, adulthood. Behavioral or pharmacological treatment may then be required. (See also INFANT SLEEP DISORDERS.)

body temperature   See TEMPERATURE.

brain-wave rhythms   A lay term that is often used to describe electroencephalographic patterns. *EEG wave* is the preferred term. (See also ELECTROENCEPHALOGRAM.)

bruxism   A stereotyped movement disorder characterized by grinding or clenching of teeth that can occur during sleep or wakefulness. When bruxism occurs predominantly during sleep, it is termed SLEEP BRUXISM. Bruxism can be associated with discomfort of the jaw and may produce abnormal destruction of the cusps of the teeth.

C

caffeine   Probably one of the first medications used for the treatment of EXCESSIVE SLEEPINESS. Caffeine is used to increase the level of alertness and is taken in the form of drinks, most commonly tea, coffee or cola. A typical cup of coffee contains about 100 milligrams caffeine, a bottle of cola drink about 50 milligrams. Also, over-the-counter medications containing caffeine are available (Vivarin, 200 milligrams caffeine; No Doz, 100 milligrams caffeine).

Caffeine can disturb the quality of nighttime sleep if ingested prior to bedtime. Sleep onset and sleep maintenance difficulties are not uncommon due to the effects of caffeine; even some individuals who believe that they sleep well after a cup of coffee have been shown to have increased sleep disturbance with frequent awakenings and reduced total sleep time.

Caffeine is not recommended for the treatment of daytime tiredness or sleepiness. It has a general stimulant effect that can produce cardiac stimulation with palpitations and hypertension as well as increased nervousness, irritability and tremulousness. Other more effective STIMULANT MEDICATIONS, such as methylphenidate, pemoline or amphetamines, are available for the treatment of sleepiness in patients who have disorders of excessive sleepiness.

Withdrawal of caffeine may produce an increased feeling of tiredness and lethargy during the first few days, which may lead to resumption of the caffeine intake. Therefore, excessive caffeine intake may be the cause of symptoms of excessive sleepiness.

CAHS (Central Alveolar Hypoventilation Syndrome)   A breathing disorder that results in arterial oxygen desaturation during sleep. CAHS occurs in persons with normal mechanical properties of the lungs, such as intact ribs, muscles, and lung fields. During sleep in healthy individuals there is a normal slight reduction in TIDAL VOLUME (the amount of air usually taken into the lungs during a normal breath at rest); however, in patients with CAHS the tidal volume greatly decreases. The reduction in tidal volume leads to an increase in the carbon dioxide level in the blood as well as reduced blood oxygen saturation. This change in the arterial blood gases (carbon dioxide and oxygen) can produce arousals that increase respiratory drive. The arousals disturb sleep quality and therefore sleep may be characterized by a complaint of insomnia. If the arousals and awakenings are frequent enough, excessive sleepiness may develop. CAHS is due to an abnormality of the central nervous system control of lung ventilation. (See also REM SLEEP, OBSTRUCTIVE SLEEP APNEA SYNDROME, CENTRAL SLEEP APNEA SYNDROME and POLYSOMNOGRAPHY.)

carbon dioxide Gas produced as a result of body metabolism. This metabolic product is eliminated from the body through the lungs during a process of exchange with oxygen from the atmosphere. Alterations of ventilation can cause a retention of carbon dioxide in the body and a reduction of blood oxygen.

Carbon dioxide and oxygen are the two most important blood gases in the regulation of respiration. The SLEEP-RELATED BREATHING DISORDERS commonly will affect lung ventilation, thereby producing an increased carbon dioxide level (hypercapnia) and a lowering of oxygen (HYPOXEMIA). Some patients with OBSTRUCTIVE SLEEP APNEA SYNDROME may have an increased level of carbon dioxide detectable during wakefulness, which is in part due to a resetting of the regulation of ventilation. Most patients with obstructive sleep apnea syndrome have only a transient elevation of carbon dioxide in association with the apneic episodes.

Increased levels of carbon dioxide produce a body acidosis that may be irritating to the heart, producing cardiac ARRHYTHMIAS. An elevated carbon dioxide level also stimulates ventilation through its chemoreceptors, thereby causing a lowering of the level by means of a feedback mechanism.

cardiovascular symptoms, sleep-related See SLEEP-RELATED CARDIOVASCULAR SYMPTOMS.

cataplexy A sudden loss of muscle power in response to an emotional stimulus. Cataplexy is typically seen in persons suffering from NARCOLEPSY, which is characterized by EXCESSIVE SLEEPINESS during the day. Cataplexy will usually cause a reduction in muscle power, leading either to complete collapse or, more typically, a drooping of the head, weakness of the facial muscles, weakness of the arms or sagging at the knees. Cataplexy is most often induced by laughter, but anger, surprise, startle, pride, elation or sadness can also induce episodes.

Cataplexy is an ATONIA (loss of muscle tone) that is normal of REM sleep. However, cataplexy is produced by an emotional change and not due to sleepiness. If episodes of cataplexy are long in duration, typical REM sleep occurs, with the usual change of the EEG activity and associated rapid eye movements.

Individuals who have pronounced episodes of cataplexy may suffer injuries due to a sudden collapse to the ground. Episodes of cataplexy usually last a few seconds. If the emotional stimulus continues, a state of continuous cataplexy can occur, termed STATUS CATAPLECTICUS. Cataplexy can be effectively treated by the use of tricyclic ANTIDEPRESSANTS, such as imipramine or protriptyline or the SEROTONIN reuptake inhibitors such as fluoxetine.

central sleep apnea syndrome   Disorder marked by a cessation of ventilation during sleep, usually associated with oxygen desaturation with an absence of airflow that lasts 10 seconds or more in adults, 20 seconds or more in infants.

This syndrome is typically associated with the complaint of INSOMNIA, particularly in older adults, or a complaint of EXCESSIVE SLEEPINESS during the day. Typically, patients will awaken several times at night, often with the sensation of gasping or choking during sleep. Not uncommonly, episodes of apnea will be asymptomatic, and if the episodes are frequent enough to cause disruption of much of the sleep episode, then daytime sleepiness will result. In children, central apneas are usually accompanied by a change in their facial color, such as cyanosis or pallor, and there may also be marked changes of the muscle tone with generalized body limpness.

Central sleep apnea syndrome is most commonly seen in patients with neurological disorders that affect the control of respiration. Spinal cord lesions or lesions of the brain stem commonly will produce central sleep apnea. Ventilation can be normal during wakefulness; however, complete cessation of breathing can occur during sleep and the patient may be able to breathe only during arousals or wakefulness. This inability to breathe during sleep has been called ONDINE'S CURSE and, if left untreated, may have a fatal outcome.

Cheyne-Stokes respiration   A pattern of breathing described by John Cheyne and William Stokes in 1818 that is characterized by a regular crescendo and decrescendo fluctuation in respiratory rate and volume. This breathing pattern can occur during wakefulness, but it is most commonly is seen in drowsiness and can persist into non-REM sleep (see SLEEP STAGES). Cheyne-Stokes breathing usually does not occur during REM SLEEP.

chloral hydrate   See HYPNOTICS.

chronic insomnia   See LONG-TERM INSOMNIA.

chronic obstructive pulmonary disease   Also called chronic obstructive respiratory disease; this is a respiratory disorder characterized by a chronic impairment of airflow through the respiratory tract. This disorder can disrupt sleep due to the altered cardiorespiratory physiology. Persons with chronic obstructive pulmonary disease frequently will complain of disturbed sleep and INSOMNIA.

The sleep disturbance that occurs is typically one of difficulty in initiating sleep, and there are frequent awakenings at night, often with the sensation of shortness of breath and difficulty in breathing. There may be excessive coughing during sleep and the need to get out of bed in order to breathe more easily. Some of the sleep disturbance may be due to MEDICA-TIONS that are required to improve breathing, which often have a stimulant effect, thereby adding to the complaint of insomnia.

Typically during sleep, patients with chronic obstructive pulmonary disease will demonstrate a reduction in TIDAL VOLUME, with increasing HYPOX-EMIA or elevation of the carbon dioxide level in the bloodstream. This particular pattern is more common in patients called "blue bloaters," who have evidence of right-sided heart failure due to pulmonary hypertension and an increase in the blood hemocrit level. Patients who are blue bloaters usually suffer severe oxygen desaturation during sleep.

A second group called "pink puffers" characteristically has shortness of breath associated with increased lung volumes. The hypoxemia and elevation of carbon dioxide levels during sleep is not as severe as that seen in blue bloaters.

Chronic obstructive pulmonary disease can be due to a variety of disorders, such as respiratory infections or bronchopulmonary dysplasia; however, the most common cause in adults is chronic SMOKING.

POLYSOMNOGRAPHY demonstrates a prolonged SLEEP LATENCY and frequent awakenings during the major sleep episode. Some patients may be unable to lie flat during sleep because of severe shortness of breath and therefore polysomnography may need to be performed with the patient in a semi-recumbent position. There is typically a reduction of SLOW WAVE SLEEP as well as REM SLEEP with fragmentation of the sleep stages—particularly REM sleep, due to oxygen desaturation. Obstructive and central apneic events may occur concurrently with the sleep-related hypoxemia. Cardiac ARRY-THMIAS may be associated with the hypoxemia or may occur independently. A MULTIPLE SLEEP LATENCY TEST may demonstrate a reduced mean sleep latency, particularly in patients with frequent nocturnal sleep disruption or a complaint of EXCESSIVE SLEEPINESS during the day.

The sleep disturbance of a patient with chronic obstructive pulmonary disease needs to be differentiated from other causes of complaints of insomnia. Anxiety and DEPRESSION, or PSYCHOPHYSIOLOGICAL INSOMNIA, may coexist with the chronic obstructive pulmonary disease. Acute anxiety due to an exacerbation of lung disease may produce an ADJUSTMENT SLEEP DIS-ORDER.

The blue bloater form of chronic obstructive pulmonary disease is similar to CENTRAL ALVEOLAR HYPOVENTILATION SYNDROME. It may be difficult to differentiate the two disorders if the history of development of chronic obstructive pulmonary disease is unknown.

Treatment involves ensuring optimum treatment of the chronic obstructive pulmonary disease. Stimulant bronchodilator medications, used for the treatment of the lung disease, should be reduced to effective but not excessive doses. If OBSTRUCTIVE SLEEP APNEA SYNDROME or CENTRAL SLEEP APNEA SYNDROME is present, or even alveolar hypoventilation, the use of a CONTIN-UOUS POSITIVE AIRWAY PRESSURE device (CPAP), with or without the addition of low oxygen therapy, may be helpful. Such treatment is best performed under polysomnographic monitoring. Attention should be given to SLEEP HYGIENE measures, and other lifestyle changes should be strongly recommended, such as weight reduction and avoidance of smoking.

chronic obstructive respiratory disease   See CHRONIC OBSTRUCTIVE PULMONARY DISEASE.

chronobiology   The scientific study of biological rhythms. Biological rhythms can have markedly varying period lengths, from less than a second for heart rate to as long as a year for hibernational cycles in animals. In humans, the biological rhythms of approximately one day are those that are commonly referred to under the term CIRCADIAN RHYTHMS.

chronotherapy   Treatment developed by Charles Czeisler in 1981 to correct the displaced sleep period of patients with the circadian rhythm sleep disorder of DELAYED SLEEP PHASE SYNDROME. The treatment involves a progressive delay of a sleep period so the major sleep period is rotated around the clock to an improved SLEEP ONSET time. For example, prior to shifting the sleep period an individual who is unable to fall asleep before 3 A.M. would be instructed to maintain a regular sleep onset time at 3 A.M., sleeping for eight hours until 11 A.M., for a period of five days. After the five-day stabilization period, the patient would be instructed to go to bed three hours later, and arise three hours later each day until the sleep onset time reaches a more appropriate time at night. Depending upon the amount of time that the sleep period is displaced, the process of shifting the sleep periods takes about six to seven days. Once having reached a more desirable sleep onset time, the patient is instructed to maintain a regular bedtime and arise eight hours later so that the sleep period can become stabilized at the new sleep onset and awake times.

Some patients find they are able to maintain the improved timing of the sleep episode; however, others will find that they drift to a later period of time and may require a repeat course of chronotherapy in order to reestablish more appropriate sleep onset and wake times.

The same process of shifting the sleep by three hours has been applied successfully to one patient with ADVANCED SLEEP PHASE SYNDROME, who rotated the sleep period in an anticlockwise direction.

circadian rhythms   Franz Halberg in 1959 proposed this term to describe endogenous rhythms that had a period length of about 24 hours. The term was coined from the Latin *circa,* meaning "about," and *dies,* meaning "a day." Although most circadian rhythms are 24 hours in duration, the term was originally applied to the endogenous rhythms that run in humans at a slightly longer period of approximately 25 hours. ENVIRONMENTAL TIME CUES prevent the true period length of the underlying circadian rhythm from becoming manifest, so the circadian rhythm length is maintained at 24 hours. Without environmental time cues sleep onset would occur on average one hour later and we would awaken one hour later. Therefore, we would live on a 25-hour-long day. (See also ENDOGENOUS CIRCADIAN PACEMAKER, FREE RUNNING, TEMPORAL ISOLATION.)

circadian rhythm sleep disorders   Previously called sleep-wake schedule disorders, these are disorders of the timing of sleep within the 24-hour day. These disorders were originally grouped together in the first edition of the "Diagnostic Classification of Sleep and Arousal Disorders," published in 1979 in the journal SLEEP. The disorders were divided into two groups—transient and persistent.

The main disorders in the transient group include TIME ZONE CHANGE (JET LAG) SYNDROME and SHIFT-WORK SLEEP DISORDER. The five persistent circadian rhythm sleep disorders are: FREQUENTLY CHANGING SLEEP-WAKE SCHEDULE, DELAYED SLEEP PHASE SYNDROME, ADVANCED SLEEP PHASE SYNDROME, NON-24-HOUR SLEEP-WAKE SYNDROME and IRREGULAR SLEEP-WAKE PATTERN. In all of these disorders, there is an alteration in the timing of sleep in that it is either advanced, delayed or occurs irregularly during a 24-hour period. Some of these disorders are related to an irregularity or disruption of the normal ENVIRONMENTAL TIME CUES and are thereby thought to be of socio-environmental cause. Other circadian rhythm sleep disorders suggest a defect in the intrinsic mechanism of the circadian pacemaker or its mechanism of entrainment (ability to keep to a set pattern) and hence are thought to be of endogenous or organic cause. Recently, new types of chronobiological tests have become available, such as the constant routine, that can determine whether the abnormality in the circadian pacemaker is of endogenous etiology.

Some of the circadian rhythm sleep disorders, such as delayed sleep phase syndrome, have been subtyped into an intrinsic type, in which the circadian pacemaker or its mechanism is believed to be abnormal, and an extrinsic type, in which socioenvironmental factors appear to be responsible.

clinical polysomnographer   Specialist trained in the clinical interpretation of the results of the POLYSOMNOGRAMS of patients with a wide variety of sleep disorders. This term has now been superseded by the term "sleep specialist" (see SLEEP DISORDER SPECIALIST). Most clinical polysomnographers work in full-service SLEEP DISORDER CENTERS. Certification in clinical polysomnography was a requirement for the accreditation of sleep disorder centers by the American Sleep Disorders Association (now the American Academy of Sleep Medicine). The new examination for sleep specialists is run by the AMERICAN BOARD OF SLEEP MEDICINE.

(See also ACCREDITATION STANDARDS FOR SLEEP DISORDER CENTERS, POLYSOMNOGRAPHY.)

clomipramine   See ANTIDEPRESSANTS.

clonazepam   See BENZODIAZEPINES.

cocaine   Cocaine can have pronounced effects upon sleep due to its stimulation of the central nervous system; it produces restlessness and INSOMNIA. There is also some evidence to suggest that the chronic nasal ingestion of cocaine induces a nasal congestion that can exacerbate the OBSTRUCTIVE SLEEP APNEA SYNDROME.

codeine   Drug shown to improve alertness in patients with EXCESSIVE SLEEPINESS. It can achieve this without the side effects of central nervous system or peripheral stimulation. However, side effects such as constipation, and the potential for drug abuse, may occur.

In doses of 30 to 180 milligrams per day, codeine phosphate is effective in the treatment of NARCOLEPSY but is rarely used because other STIMULANT MEDICATIONS, such as pemoline, methylphenidate, dextroamphetamine, and MODAFINIL, are more effective. However, codeine may be useful for patients who are unable to tolerate these other central nervous system stimulants.

cognitive focusing   A technique used in the management of INSOMNIA that involves focusing on reassuring thoughts. Patients with insomnia typically awaken at night and are unable to return to sleep because they are haunted by recurring, unwanted and unpleasant thoughts. Cognitive focusing involves learning to focus on reassuring thoughts and pleasant images so that sleep is more likely to occur. (See also BEHAVIORAL TREATMENT OF INSOMNIA, DISORDERS OF INITIATING AND MAINTAINING SLEEP, HYPNOSIS, PSYCHOPHYSIOLOGICAL INSOMNIA.)

coma   A state of psychological unresponsiveness that can be differentiated from sleep and wakefulness. The primary difference from sleep is that there is no psychologically understandable response to an external stimulus, or to an inner need. Patients in acute coma may look as if they are asleep; however, this state never lasts more than two or four weeks, no matter how severe the brain injury. Patients in sleeplike coma then pass into a chronic state of unresponsiveness in which they appear to be awake but lack cognitive mental ability. This state has variously been termed *vegetative state, akinetic mutism, coma vigil* or the *apallic syndrome.* Coma can be the result of chemical toxicity that affects the whole central nervous system, or it may result from extensive damage to the cerebral hemispheres or the brain stem.

Normal sleep-wake patterns and cycling of REM and NREM sleep usually do not occur in patients with acute coma until they pass into the chronic vegetative state where the pattern of sleep and wakefulness usually returns. There are several forms of coma in which the electro-encephalographic pattern differs. The more typical form of acute coma and coma due to metabolic or pharmacological causes has a 1-to-5-hertz slow wave EEG pattern. A form of coma termed *alpha coma* has a pattern of nonreactive alpha activity that is not blocked by eye opening or other sensory stimuli. This particular form of coma is most often due to brain stem lesions at the level of the pons or to post-anoxic encephalopathy.

A form of coma called spindle coma occurs in approximately 6% of all comatose patients; it is characterized by the presence of 14 hertz SLEEP SPINDLES with vertex sharp waves and K complexes superimposed on a background of slower delta and theta activity. The sleep spindle activity resembles that seen in stage two sleep. This form of coma appears to result from interruption of the ascending reticulo-thalamo-cortical pathways.

Another coma pattern is called theta coma and is characterized by typical 4-to-7-hertz theta activity that is superimposed on a low voltage delta pattern of activity. This particular pattern is often indicative of a disruption of brain stem reticular pathways to the thalamus and is highly predictive of a poor outcome—typically, death.

With all forms of coma, the occurrence of a normal sleep-wake pattern, or presence of non-REM/REM cycling, is typically associated with an improved prognosis. (See also NON-REM-STAGE SLEEP, REM SLEEP, UNCONSCIOUSNESS.)

conditioned insomnia   An essential part of PSYCHOPHYSIOLOGICAL INSOMNIA that develops through a process of negative associations between the usual sleep environment and sleep patterns. A prior episode of poor quality sleep leads to the development of the negative associations, which produce the conditioned insomnia, a learned pattern of poor quality sleep. For instance, if a person has difficulty falling asleep in his or her bedroom, the person may come to believe sleep is difficult or impossible there. Also, a person who frequently reads or works in bed may have difficulty in accepting the bed as a sleeping place.

confusional arousals   Episodes of mental confusion that typically occur during arousals from sleep. These episodes most often occur with arousals from DEEP SLEEP in the first third of the night. The individual usually sits forward in bed and feels disoriented in time and space, with behavior that may be inappropriate, such as picking up a phone to speak into it in response to a ringing alarm clock. There may also be slowness in speech and thought. Responses to commands and questions are often slow and inappropriate. Episodes may last from several minutes to several hours.

Confusional arousals were first mentioned by Roger J. Broughton in 1968 in his classic article on the arousal disorders. Other terms that have been applied to confusional arousals are *sleep drunkenness, excessive sleep inertia* and *Schlaftrunkenheit* (in the German literature) and *l'ivresse du sommeil* (in the French literature).

The confusional arousals are thought to be related to an abnormality of the normal arousal mechanism during sleep. The abnormality may be a defect of the Ascending Reticular Activating System (ARAS).

Confusional arousals are most typical in childhood, often before puberty, less common in older children or adolescents and even rarer in adults.

Episodes may be precipitated by conditions that predispose the individual to excessive fatigue, such as SLEEP DEPRIVATION or an altered sleep-wake pattern. MEDICATIONS, particularly depressants of the central nervous system, can also induce episodes. Sometimes confusional arousals are seen in association with other sleep disorders, such as IDIOPATHIC HYPERSOMNIA or SLEEP APNEA. More typically, episodes of confusional arousal occur in individuals who are predisposed to have SLEEPWALKING or SLEEP TERRORS, with a strong familial tendency marking all three behaviors.

Polysomnographic recordings of confusional arousals generally show an arousal occurring from the slow wave non-REM sleep (see SLEEP STAGES) in the first third of the night; the recordings are characterized by delta activity with mixes of theta and poorly-reactive ALPHA RHYTHMS.

Confusional arousals are a generally benign phenomenon, although injuries may occur if the individual accidentally knocks into furniture or other objects near the bedside. Confusional arousals may be considered to be a minor manifestation of sleepwalking or sleep terrors. Sleep terrors are characterized by an intensely loud scream that heralds the episode, whereas sleepwalking is characterized by walking during the event. Other behaviors that may have some similarities with confusional arousals are sleep-related epileptic SEIZURES, particularly those of the partial complex type.

Treatment of confusional arousals is rarely necessary unless the episodes occur in conjunction with other arousal disorders, such as sleepwalking or sleep terrors. In certain circumstances, it may be helpful to use either BENZODIAZEPINES or tricyclic ANTIDEPRESSANTS, such as imipramine, in order to suppress episodes. However, more commonly the only action that need be taken for confusional arousals is to secure the bedroom and prevent injuries from objects or furniture near the bedside. (See also AROUSAL DISORDERS.)

congenital central alveolar hypoventilation syndrome (CCHS)   See CAHS (CENTRAL ALVEOLAR HYPOVENTILATION SYNDROME).

congestive heart failure   The inability of the heart to pump blood, with resulting elevation of systemic, venous and capillary pressure and the transudation of fluid into the tissues. Congestive heart failure can occur as a result of disorders that affect cardiac function.

OBSTRUCTIVE SLEEP APNEA SYNDROME can produce pulmonary hypertension and result in right-sided heart failure, with the development of liver congestion and ankle edema. Treatment of obstructive sleep apnea syndrome usually results in improved cardiac function, with correction of the congestion and edema.

Congestive heart failure can produce CHEYNE-STOKES RESPIRATION which is a crescendo-decrescendo pattern of ventilation that can produce awakenings due to fluctuations in blood gases. This pattern of breathing can lead to LONG-TERM INSOMNIA.

Patients who have impaired cardiac function that results in lung congestion can present symptoms such as ORTHOPNEA or PAROXYSMAL NOCTURNAL DYSPNEA when in a recumbent or reclining position during sleep. (See also SLEEP-RELATED BREATHING DISORDERS, SLEEP-RELATED CARDIOVASCULAR SYMPTOMS.)

continuous positive airway pressure (CPAP) An effective and commonly used treatment for OBSTRUCTIVE SLEEP APNEA SYNDROME. The system was first devised in 1981 by Colin Sullivan of Australia; today a number of commercially-developed systems are available for home use.

The CPAP device consists of an air pump housed in a small box about one cubic foot in size, which is placed at the patient's bedside. Tubing of approximately one inch in diameter conveys the air to a mask, which is placed over the patient's nose so that the mouth is free. The mask is attached to the head with elasticized straps. The patient puts on the CPAP mask, turns on the machine and sleeps with the mask in place during the night until awakening, when the mask is removed. This system has been demonstrated to relieve severe obstructive sleep apnea syndrome, with resumption of normal quality sleep at night and resolution of the cardiac features, as well as complete resolution of the associated daytime sleepiness.

The CPAP system provides an air splint to the upper airway thereby preventing its collapse. During the inspiratory phase of an obstructive apnea, the upper airway tissues collapse because of a negative inspiratory pressure, thereby producing upper airway obstruction. The continuous positive air pressure device provides a low flow of air with a pressure of between 2 and 20 centimeters of water, which prevents the negative suction effect on the tissues of the upper airway, thus preventing their collapse.

Most patients with obstructive sleep apnea syndrome are capable of using a CPAP system; however, some patients find the mask makes them feel claustrophobic, preventing its regular use. The development of chronic nasal irritation due to the air flow is also a major complication of the device. This irritation can be partially relieved by the use of extra humidification of the inspired air; however, occasionally nasal decongestant inhalers may be necessary. Despite optimum treatment of the nasal irritation, some patients will find relief only by discontinuing use of the CPAP system.

One of the major concerns regarding the use of nasal CPAP is that it is very dependent upon patient compliance with the treatment recommendations. Although for most patients the benefits are very apparent and reinforce the desire to use the system, some patients may not be motivated to utilize the system. This is of particular concern for patients with severe daytime sleepiness, who are employed in positions where sleepiness may put them or others at risk, such as bus drivers. Alternative treatments for obstructive sleep apnea may not be readily available, as the UVU-LOPALATOPHARYNGOPLASTY surgical procedure is not effective in approximately 50% of patients who have obstructive sleep apnea syndrome. The only effective surgical alternative is TRACHEOSTOMY, which is often rejected by the patient for cosmetic, social or medical reasons.

Despite the limitations of nasal CPAP treatment, this device has dramatically changed the management of obstructive sleep apnea syndrome and is a major advance in its treatment. (See also FIBEROPTIC ENDOSCOPY.)

convulsions   Generalized whole body movements that occur in association with epileptic activity. SLEEP-RELATED EPILEPSY is a primary cause of convulsions during sleep.

cortisol   A hormone released from the adrenal gland in response to stimulation by ACTH (adrenocorticotrophin hormone), which is released from the pituitary gland. The secretion of cortisol is reduced during sleep but is greatly increased around the time of awakening. It is important for the maintenance of body metabolism, and its absence leads to reduced energy and weight loss.

Cortisol is often measured in the blood to detect the specific phase of the CIRCADIAN RHYTHM. Shifts of the sleep pattern by 12 hours are usually not accompanied by acute shifts of the cortisol circadian rhythm, which takes up to two weeks to realign with the new time of sleep. The cortisol rhythm appears to be linked to the body temperature rhythm, which takes a similar amount of time to shift to coincide with the new time of sleep. (See also GROWTH HORMONE, MELATONIN, PROLACTIN, REVERSAL OF SLEEP.)

cot death   A term used, mainly in Britain, for SUDDEN INFANT DEATH SYNDROME (SIDS).

coughing   Coughing during sleep is due to an irritation of the upper airway and typically is associated with abrupt awakening, and difficulty in breathing. Patients with sleep-related breathing disorders are liable to have episodes of choking and coughing during sleep, particularly those with CHRONIC OBSTRUCTIVE PULMONARY DISEASE or SLEEP-RELATED ASTHMA.

Coughing can have many causes, such as inflammatory reactions to inhaled allergens, mechanical irritation due to dust particles, chemical irritation due to smoke or gas, and thermal irritation due to very hot or cold air. Treatment depends upon the cause of the coughing. Specific therapy should be directed to any underlying medical disorder, such as sleep-related asthma. A cough suppressant (antitussive) medication such as CODEINE can be of help. If secretions are thick and are the cause of coughing, an ultrasonic nebulizer will allow the secretions to be expectorated. Ipratropium, a bronchodilator with anticholinergic effects, is helpful for coughs due to asthma. (See also SLEEP-RELATED BREATHING DISORDERS.)

CPAP   See CONTINUOUS POSITIVE AIRWAY PRESSURE (CPAP).

cramps   Contractions of muscles that typically result in a painful sensation. The most common site for cramps during sleep is in the calf muscles. Cramps may be induced by metabolic changes, such as an alteration in the serum electrolytes.

Acute cramps can be partially relieved by stretching the muscle involved. Quinine sulfate is an effective medication for the prevention of muscle cramps. (See also NOCTURNAL LEG CRAMPS.)

crib death   Term that has been used, largely in the United States, for the SUDDEN INFANT DEATH SYNDROME.

Cylert   See STIMULANT MEDICATIONS.

D

Dalmane   See BENZODIAZEPINES.

daydreaming   The state of mind associated with withdrawal from environmental influences. Sleep does not occur but there may be DROWSINESS. Full alertness to the environment is reduced. Sleepiness can erroneously be mistaken for daydreaming, particularly in adolescents who tend to be sleep deprived and may not concentrate on schoolwork (see EXCESSIVE SLEEPINESS, SLEEP DEPRIVATION). If other features of sleepiness occur, such as eye closure, head drooping or even snoring, then there should be a consideration of a sleep disorder as a cause.

True dream phenomenon (see DREAMS) is a state associated with pronounced physiological changes, such as rapid eye movements and loss of muscle tone. Daydreaming does not represent daytime dreams and therefore should be differentiated from true dreaming sleep.

daytime sleepiness   See EXCESSIVE SLEEPINESS.

deaths during sleep   Several extensive epidemiological studies have demonstrated that death is most likely to occur over the usual nocturnal hours, with the greatest likelihood of death occurring between 4 A.M. and 7 A.M. The reason for this circadian variation in deaths is unknown; however, there are several disorders that are believed to increase the likelihood of death during sleep. SLEEP-RELATED BREATHING DISORDERS, including OBSTRUCTIVE SLEEP APNEA SYNDROME, have been reported to be associated with sudden death during sleep, and in patients with asthma there is a higher rate of death during the nocturnal hours compared to the daytime. (See SLEEP-RELATED ASTHMA.)

Patients with the obstructive sleep apnea syndrome have a high rate of sleep-related hypoxemia and cardiac arrhythmias related to the apneic episodes. The cardiac arrhythmias are believed to be the primary cause for the sudden unexpected death during sleep.

An American Cancer Society study conducted in 1964 (data was analyzed in 1979) of more than 1 million people found that men who slept four hours or less, or more than 10 hours, had a higher mortality rate than those who slept a normal six to eight hours. This association between sleep length and death may be related either to underlying medical illness, which produces sleep disturbance at night, or to disorders, such as sleep apnea, that usually produce a prolonged nighttime sleep episode.

There is also some evidence that people who take sleeping pills (HYPNOTICS) are more likely to have a nocturnal death. (See also MYOCARDIAL INFARCTION.)

deep sleep   Term describing stage three and stage four non-REM (NREM) sleep. This term was developed because of the increased threshold to awakening by various stimuli that occurs during these SLEEP STAGES. Rarely, in the older literature, the term was applied to REM sleep, but the term is most appropriately applied to stages three and four sleep.

delayed sleep phase   Term applied to a delay in falling asleep in relation to the usual time of sleep, according to the 24-hour clock; the sleep episode is consequently delayed in relation to underlying circadian patterns of other physiological variables (see CIRCADIAN RHYTHMS). The delay of the sleep phase can be temporary, such as typically seen with TIME ZONE CHANGE (JET LAG) SYNDROME, or can be a chronic state, such as seen in DELAYED SLEEP PHASE SYNDROME.

delayed sleep phase syndrome   One of the CIRCADIAN RHYTHM SLEEP DISORDERS. It is characterized by SLEEP ONSET and WAKE TIMES that are usually later than desired, with difficulty in initiating sleep onset. Once sleep onset does occur, sleep is of good quality, with few awakenings until the time of final awakening. This sleep pattern is mainly a difficulty in falling asleep at night, or a difficulty in awakening in the morning, which prevents fulfilling social or occupational obligations.

Delayed sleep phase syndrome was first described by Elliot D. Weitzman and Charles Czeisler in 1981. Their analysis of 450 patients who complained of INSOMNIA showed that 7% fulfilled the criteria for having delayed sleep phase syndrome.

Persons with delayed sleep phase syndrome have great difficulty falling asleep at a desired time. Attempts to fall asleep earlier are accompanied by prolonged periods of lying in bed awake until the time that they usually fall asleep. These patients are often prescribed MEDICATIONS to aid sleep, but sleeping medications are ineffective and only add to both the difficulty of awakening and the daytime sleepiness.

In typical cases of delayed sleep phase syndrome, the individual will be unable to initiate sleep onset until 2 A.M. or even as late as 6 A.M. In younger children, the sleep onset time may be earlier, but typically occurs two or more hours after the desired time to go to bed. Because there are attempts to get up at the desired time in the morning, which are only partially successful, the individual with delayed sleep phase syndrome is often sleep deprived and therefore suffers from symptoms of excessive daytime sleepiness, such as fatigue and tiredness. Episodes of sleep can occur inappropriately during the day whenever the individual is in a quiet situation, and this can cause school or work difficulties. Children are typically late to school, and adults are frequently late to their jobs.

On weekends, because there is usually no need to arise early in the morning, these individuals will sleep into the day, often sleeping till midday or even later. These long sleep episodes on the weekend help to make up for the chronic sleep deprivation that accumulates during the week.

The diagnosis of delayed sleep phase syndrome is made on the complaint of either an inability to fall asleep at the desired time, or the inability to awaken at the desired time in the morning. Sometimes the complaint of EXCESSIVE SLEEPINESS during the day will be given. The symptoms will be present for at least three months, and when not required to maintain a strict schedule, such as on weekends and while on vacations, individuals will have a normal sleep pattern in duration and quality, and will awaken spontaneously at a later time than desired.

Investigative studies have shown that the circadian pattern of body temperature is shifted to a later time so that the nadir (low point) does not occur at the more typical time of 5 A.M. but occurs after 8 or 9 A.M. (see CIRCADIAN RHYTHMS). Polysomnographic studies have shown that the sleep period is of short duration when the individual arises at the desired time and is characterized by reduced REM sleep. When the sleep period is allowed to proceed without interruption, such as is seen on the weekend, the sleep period is of normal duration, with normal amounts of each sleep stage.

Although alcohol and hypnotic abuse are commonly used in an attempt to correct the problem, true psychopathology is not typical. An atypical form of depression may be present in adolescents with this syndrome. The depression may be directly related to the social and functional difficulties induced by the abnormal sleep pattern.

In childhood, other disorders, such as LIMIT-SETTING SLEEP DISORDER, SLEEP-ONSET ASSOCIATION DISORDER or IDIOPATHIC HYPERSOMNIA, need to be differentiated from delayed sleep phase syndrome.

The prevalence of the disorder is unknown, but may be as common as 10% in the adolescent population. Adolescents seem particularly predisposed toward developing a delayed sleep pattern because of the natural tendency to delay sleep onset. The onset of the disorder is in late puberty or early adolescence, although major difficulties are not encountered until late adolescence or until the commencement of employment.

Although a male predominance of the delayed sleep phase syndrome is reported in the literature, this may be because of a referral pattern bias. This disorder does not appear to be inherited.

In many cases of delayed sleep phase syndrome, social and environmental factors in inducing the delay of the sleep pattern appear to be the predominant causes. However, some individuals have a circadian pacemaker system that is abnormal and unresponsive to the usual environmental time cues. The time cues are weak stabilizers of the natural physiological tendency to delay sleep onset. An abnormality of the pacemaker's phase response curve has been suggested as a cause.

Individuals who have delayed sleep phase syndrome should be differentiated from those who have a pattern of sequential delays of a sleep phase that occur continuously, the disorder known as the NON-24-HOUR SLEEP-WAKE SYNDROME.

Individuals who have irregularity of the sleep onset time, with the ability to advance the sleep onset time some days each week, are characterized as having INADEQUATE SLEEP HYGIENE rather than delayed sleep phase syndrome.

For the diagnosis, the sleep disturbance should be illustrated on a SLEEP LOG for a period of at least two weeks, and if there is any doubt about the diagnosis, appropriate polysomnographic monitoring should be performed.

Treatment depends on the severity of the disorder. Mild delayed sleep phase syndrome may be improved by strict attention to regular sleep onset and awake times. More severe disturbances may require incremental advances by 15 or 30 minutes per day until a more appropriate sleep onset time is reached. The most severe form of the disorder may require making advancements of the sleep pattern by enforcing a night of sleep deprivation to assist in the sleep advance process, or, more effectively, by the use of a technique termed CHRONOTHERAPY, which involves a three-hour delay in the sleep period on a daily basis until the sleep pattern is rotated around the clock and sleep onset occurs at a more appropriate time.

delta sleep   Term used to describe the stage of sleep when the ELECTROENCEPHALOGRAM (EEG) shows a high voltage, slow wave activity in the delta (up to four hertz) frequency. The term is synonymous with stage three and stage four sleep. Because of the slow frequency of activity seen on the EEG, this stage of sleep is also called SLOW WAVE SLEEP. (See also SLEEP STAGES.)

delta waves   A cycle of electroencephalographic activity with a frequency of less than four hertz (see ELECTROENCEPHALOGRAM [EEG]). For sleep stage scoring the minimum requirements for delta waves are that the amplitude of the waves must be greater than 75 microvolts, and the frequency must be less than two hertz in duration. Delta waves are seen during stages three and four sleep, and occasionally in stage two sleep. (The stage three/four sleep, also known as delta sleep, is regarded as the most important stage of sleep.) (See also DELTA SLEEP, SLEEP STAGES.)

Dement, William C.   Received both his M.D. with honors and a Ph.D. in neurophysiology from the University of Chicago. Dr. Dement (1928–   ) started the Sleep Laboratory at Stanford University in 1963, and he later founded, and now directs, the Sleep Disorders Center at Stanford University Medical Center in California and is professor of psychiatry at its medical school.

From 1952 to 1957, Dement, while in medical school, joined Eugene Aserinsky and Professor Nathaniel Kleitman; together they discovered and described rapid eye movement (REM) sleep.

dementia   A progressive and degenerative neurological disease that is associated with loss of memory and other intellectual functions. Patients with dementia commonly suffer sleep disturbances, typically due to behavioral disturbances during the sleep period; delirium, agitation, wandering and inappropriate talking often occur during nighttime hours. These disturbances in behavior begin in the evening, and therefore the term "sundown syndrome" has been used to describe patients with this form of sleep disturbance.

Patients suffering dementia commonly become major management problems for their families and often require institutionalization in a nursing home or hospital. The need for sedative medications (see HYPNOTICS) to suppress the behavior often contributes to the disturbance of sleep and wakefulness and can lead to further impairment of intellectual function. Patients may also suffer exaggerated NOCTURNAL CONFUSION, with the onset of acute medical illnesses, such as infections. The confusion can also be worsened by medications that are given for the infective illness.

The disturbance in sleep and wakefulness may be due to a loss of the brain center controlling the circadian pattern of sleep and wakefulness; disorders such as Alzheimer's disease and multiple cerebral infarction are typical causes of dementia. Polysomnographic studies have tended to show nonspecific sleep disruption with reduced sleep efficiency, and reduced stages of deep sleep (see SLEEP STAGES). Some patients can have respiratory disturbance during sleep, although this is not a typical feature of patients with dementia.

The diagnosis of dementia is made clinically and by tests such as brain imaging and electroencephalography. Reversible forms of dementia, for example, metabolic abnormalities and drug effects, must be considered. The treatment of sleep disturbance associated with dementia depends upon initiating good SLEEP HYGIENE and assuring that the dementia patient is fully active during the period of desired wakefulness and allowed to sleep in a quiet environment during the time of desired sleep. Hypnotic medications may have a paradoxical effect and increase activity in some patients. The longer-acting hypnotics may cause decreased behavior and alertness during the daytime, which will exacerbate the breakdown of the nighttime sleep pattern and therefore should be avoided. NEUROLEPTICS, such as haloperidol, and phenothiazines may be useful in some patients. (See also IRREGULAR SLEEP-WAKE PATTERN.)

depression   Emotional condition characterized by an episode of loss of interest or pleasure in most daytime activities that lasts two weeks or longer. Most patients with depression have sleep disturbance that is accompanied by INSOMNIA or, less commonly, by EXCESSIVE SLEEPINESS. Other associated symptoms include appetite disturbance, weight change, decreased energy, feelings of worthlessness and helplessness, excessive and inappropriate feelings of guilt, difficulty in concentrating and recurrent thoughts of death, with suicidal ideation or attempts.

The characteristic sleep disturbance seen in patients with depression is one of EARLY MORNING AROUSAL, although this does not invariably occur, and particularly not in adolescents, where a prolonged nocturnal sleep period is commonly seen. Other features of depression include a short REM sleep latency on all-night polysomnography as well as an increased REM density.

Depression is one feature of the MOOD DISORDERS. One form of depression recurs at intervals depending upon the seasons of the year and is termed SEASONAL AFFECTIVE DISORDER (SAD). Recently light therapy has been demonstrated to be an effective treatment for this disorder. Depression can also be treated by psychotherapy or ANTIDEPRESSANT medications that include the tricyclic antidepressants, serotonin reuptake inhibitors and MONOAMINE OXIDASE INHIBITORS.

dextroamphetamine   See STIMULANT MEDICATIONS.

diazepam   See BENZODIAZEPINES.

diet and sleep   Diet can have an important effect on the sleep-wake cycle; however, very few research studies have been performed in this area.

It is well recognized that stimulant drinks or foods, such as coffee or chocolate, can increase daytime alertness and reduce the ease of falling asleep at night. Patients with insomnia find that these agents typically cause them to have greater sleep difficulties and are usually advised to avoid the ingestion of CAFFEINE in any form.

The nighttime snack is believed to aid in sleep onset although the exact mechanism for this effect is unknown. It has been suggested that L-tryptophan (see HYPNOTICS), an important constitute of proteins, is useful in promoting sleep as it is known to be a precursor of SEROTONIN, a neurotransmitter believed to be involved in initiating and maintaining sleep. However, research studies on L-tryptophan have shown a mild effect, if any at all, in persons with insomnia. Furthermore, because of 30 cases in 1989 (including a few deaths) of eosinophilia-myalgia, a rare blood disorder possibly linked to supplements of L-tryptophan, the United States Center for Disease Control (CDC) requested that physicians temporarily stop prescribing L-tryptophan. The effect of the nighttime snack may not be due to its chemical constituents but through stimulation of the gastrointestinal neural pathways, producing a sensation of satiety and relaxation. Food drinks—containing milk products and cereal, such as Ovaltine and Horlicks—are useful in promoting sleep at night.

There is some evidence that the gastrointestinal effects of food ingestion may be mediated through a hormone called cholecystokinin (CCK), which is found in both the gastrointestinal tract and the brain. This hormone is released in response to food ingestion, and some studies have shown that the administration of CCK will promote sleep onset.

The effect of carbohydrates compared to proteins in sleep initiation has been disputed. Carbohydrates will allow L-tryptophan to be taken up more readily by the central nervous system and therefore may potentiate L-tryptophan's sleep-inducing effects. Proteins, through their breakdown into amino acids, are believed to increase the catecholamines, which are agents that increase energy. Therefore, based on this biochemical evidence, the suggestion has been that carbohydrates, which initially may induce energy, subsequently have an effect on promoting sleep, whereas proteins will be more liable to increase alertness. The effect of carbohydrates and proteins on alertness and sleepiness appears to vary from person to person. However, a pattern of carbohydrate and protein ingestion is reported to be useful for the treatment of jet lag and has been outlined in the ARGONNE ANTI-JET-LAG DIET, publicized by the Argonne National Laboratory. This diet involves an alternating pattern of feast and fast, and utilizes the stimulating effect of caffeine-containing drinks to alter the timing of sleep.

Large meals are best avoided immediately before sleep as they can produce increased gastrointestinal activity that may lead to disrupted nocturnal sleep. In addition, big meals just before sleep can exacerbate OBSTRUCTIVE SLEEP APNEA SYNDROME by preventing diaphragm action, and are often associated with SLEEP-RELATED GASTROESOPHAGEAL REFLUX. Meals containing spicy foods are also best avoided before sleep because of their stimulating effects.

Several sleep disorders are associated with the excessive ingestion of food or fluid during sleep at night. The NOCTURNAL EATING (DRINKING) SYNDROME is associated with awakenings at night in order to eat food. The desire to eat food becomes overwhelming and the person often cannot stop the behavior. For some people with this syndrome, the majority of the caloric intake is taken in the nighttime hours. Excessive drinking at night is more common in children who are given fluids during the nighttime hours, particularly infants who have frequent nighttime feedings. Sleep enuresis may occur in children, especially infants.

Patients with the Kleine-Levin form of RECURRENT HYPERSOMNIA often eat excessively (megaphagia) during the cyclical periods of excessive sleepiness. This syndrome is characterized by recurrent episodes of sleepiness that last for about two weeks and occur several times each year in association with behavioral disorders, such as hypersexuality and excessive eating.

DIMS   See DISORDERS OF INITIATING AND MAINTAINING SLEEP (DIMS).

disorders of excessive somnolence (DOES)   A category of the diagnostic classification of sleep and arousal disorders published in the journal *Sleep* in 1979. This group consists of disorders that primarily produce the complaint of inappropriate and undesirable sleepiness during waking hours. The sleepiness may produce impaired mental or work performance, induce a need for daytime NAPS, increase the total amount of sleep in a 24-hour day, increase the length of the major sleep episode or produce a difficulty in achieving full arousal upon awakening. The disorders of excessive somnolence should be differentiated from those disorders that produce tiredness and fatigue without an increased physiological drive for sleep, such as dysthymia, DEPRESSION or chronic illness.

There are 10 major groups among disorders of excessive somnolence that are induced by behavioral, psychological or medical causes, or may be induced by drugs or MEDICATIONS.

The most common cause of EXCESSIVE SLEEPINESS in the general population is insufficient sleep at night; however, other frequent causes of excessive somnolence include the effects of medications, which either disrupt nighttime sleep or induce sleepiness during the day, and psychiatric disorders, such as depression. However, the majority of patients that go to SLEEP DISORDER CENTERS with the complaint of excessive sleepiness have the OBSTRUCTIVE SLEEP APNEA SYNDROME. Respiratory impairment during sleep due to the obstructive sleep apnea syndrome, CENTRAL SLEEP APNEA SYNDROME or CHAS (CENTRAL ALVEOLAR HYPOVENTILATION SYNDROME) are major causes to be considered in any patient presenting with the complaint of excessive sleepiness. PERIODIC LIMB MOVEMENT DISORDER and, rarely, RESTLESS LEGS SYNDROME can also produce daytime sleepiness.

NARCOLEPSY is the most well-known pathological disorder inducing daytime sleepiness. This disorder can be differentiated from IDIOPATHIC HYPERSOMNIA, which has different clinical and polysomnographic features.

Recurrent episodes of sleepiness are seen in RECURRENT HYPERSOMNIA, such as the KLEINE-LEVIN SYNDROME, which is most typically seen in young adults in association with gluttony and hypersexuality. Another disorder that can produce intermittent excessive sleepiness is that related to the MENSTRUAL CYCLE.

Treatment of the disorders of excessive somnolence depends upon the underlying causes and can vary from behavioral techniques, such as extending the amount of time spent in bed at night, to the use of STIMULANT MEDICATIONS in the treatment of narcolepsy. Mechanical devices, such as CONTINUOUS POSITIVE AIRWAY PRESSURE devices, may be used in the treatment of obstructive sleep apnea syndrome.

disorders of initiating and maintaining sleep (DIMS)   A group of disorders characterized by the symptom of INSOMNIA. These sleep disorders may result in difficulty getting to sleep, frequent awakenings or arousals during the night, EARLY MORNING AROUSAL or a complaint of NONRESTORATIVE SLEEP.

The term "disorders of initiating and maintaining sleep" was first publicized in the diagnostic classification of sleep and arousal disorders, published in the journal *Sleep* in 1979. This is one of four categories of sleep disorder in the classification system, and it consists of a list of nine major groups of disorders. The cause of these sleep disorders varies greatly and may be due to behavioral, psychological, psychiatric, or medical factors or may be due to medication and drug effects.

In the population as a whole, the most common disorder among the disorders of initiating and maintaining sleep is that due to an acute stressful event, such as a family, marital, work or other stress. Because this form of insomnia is usually self-limited and lasts only a few days, patients with this type of insomnia usually do not consult sleep disorder specialists or sleep disorder centers.

The most common insomnia disorders that are seen in most sleep disorder centers are either PSYCHOPHYSIOLOGICAL INSOMNIA caused by negative conditioning factors or insomnia due to psychiatric disorders, such as ANXIETY or DEPRESSION. Respiratory impairment can contribute to insomnia by means of CENTRAL SLEEP APNEA SYNDROME or OBSTRUCTIVE SLEEP APNEA SYNDROME. Abnormal limb activities, such as those seen in the PERIODIC LIMB MOVEMENT DISORDER or RESTLESS LEGS SYNDROME, are also causes of difficulty in initiating and maintaining sleep.

One form of insomnia, IDIOPATHIC INSOMNIA, appears to have a primary central nervous system cause, possibly on a genetic basis or due to an acquired subtle abnormality, perhaps in neurotransmitter function.

The treatment of DIMS depends upon the underlying cause of the disorder. For all patients good SLEEP HYGIENE is an essential part of treatment. Specific treatments can range from behavioral treatments of insomnia such as STIMULUS CONTROL THERAPY or SLEEP RESTRICTION THERAPY, to the use of HYPNOTICS or ANTIDEPRESSANTS. Mechanical treatments, such as the use of continuous positive airway pressure devices, may be required for the treatment of obstructive sleep apnea syndrome.

disorders of the sleep-wake schedule   See CIRCADIAN RHYTHM SLEEP DISORDERS.

diurnal   Occurring during the day. Opposite of NOCTURNAL.

DOES   See DISORDERS OF EXCESSIVE SOMNOLENCE.

dopamine   A central nervous system neurotransmitter that has very important effects upon both the cardiovascular and central nervous systems. Dopamine is the immediate metabolic precursor of norepinephrine and epinephrine. It has stimulant effects upon the heart, causing an increase in heart rate and blood pressure. Dopamine appears to be involved in the maintenance of wakefulness; however, it may also have a role in REM SLEEP, possibly in its suppression.

Dopamine at low doses promotes sleep; but high doses delay sleep onset and increase wakefulness.

An alteration in dopamine metabolism appears to be present in patients with NARCOLEPSY; consequently, medications that stimulate the production of dopamine may be useful in the treatment of narcolepsy. The central nervous stimulants such as pemoline, methylphenidate and amphetamine have their effect upon narcolepsy through dopamine. L-Tyrosine (see STIMULANT MEDICATIONS), a precursor of dopamine, has been shown to have a beneficial effect on the clinical symptoms of narcolepsy.

dream anxiety attacks   Synonymous with NIGHTMARES, the term was first proposed in the diagnostic classification of sleep and arousal disorders, published in the journal *Sleep* in 1979, as a means of indicating dreams that occurred in relationship to anxiety at night.

dream content   Since classical Greece, DREAMS have been used to gain a better understanding, at first of the world and in the last century, of each individual. SIGMUND FREUD used dreams to try to better understand the conflicts of the patients in his psychoanalytic practice. His monumental work *The Interpretation of Dreams* (1900) spells out his complex ideas on the manifest and latent content of dreams.

Psychologist Carl Gustav Jung in his essay "Approaching the Unconscious" delves into the importance of dreams and dream symbolism. For Jung, dreams were a way to achieve psychological health and to work through daytime conflicts. Jung found Freud's use of free association with dreams too confining and instead he suggested ". . . to concentrate rather on the associations to the dream itself, believing that the latter expressed something specific that the unconscious was trying to say."

Dreams have contained the idea, or the entirety, of some literary works, composed partly or totally during a dream (see DREAMS AND CREATIVITY).

Researchers have discovered that the sex of the dreamer influences dream content. Women tend to have dreams with indoor settings, with less aggression than in male dreams. However, these differences may reflect the learned cultural traits of males and females rather than true gender differences.

Daytime experiences can influence dream content; disturbing dreams are often associated with daytime stress. (See also NIGHTMARES.)

dreams   Dreams have fascinated mankind since antiquity. For instance, the Bible contains many references to dreams, both in the Old and the New Testament. Aristotle, one of the first to observe that the brain can be very active during sleep, placed little importance upon the role of dreams and suggested that they were a means of eliminating excessive mental activity.

The scientific investigation of dreams began toward the end of the last century. The study by Mary Calkins of Wellesley College in 1893 accurately documented 205 dreams and confirmed the impression that most dreams were recalled from sleep that occurred in the latter third of the night.

The most significant advance in the interpretation of dreams occurred with SIGMUND FREUD's psychodynamic writings on dreams in his initial publication *The Interpretation of Dreams* in 1900. Wrote Freud: "*The Interpretation of Dreams* is the royal road to a knowledge of the part the unconscious plays in the mental life."

The first major development in the scientific investigation of dreams occurred in 1953 when specific physiological changes were documented during dreaming sleep and REM (rapid eye movement) sleep. This discovery, made by Eugene Aserinsky and NATHANIEL KLEITMAN at the University of Chicago, led to an intense investigation, by electrophysiological means, of the nature of dreams. It became clear that dreams were more vivid and more easily recalled from awakenings out of REM sleep than out of non-REM. Although dreams occur in non-REM sleep, they contain less clarity and tend to be short sequences of vaguely recalled thoughts. The rapid eye movements that occur during REM sleep were initially believed to be related to the dream content and led to the development of the scanning hypothesis. Observations of eye movements under closed or partially opened eyelids were recorded and the subject awoken and interrogated as to the possible eye movements that would have occurred during the dream. By this means, the sequence of eye movements was traced and in some cases was correlated with the actual eye movements observed in the sleeper. This hypothesis has been viewed with skepticism by many researchers in recent years.

The function of dreams has been explored by many researchers. The importance of dreams in the development of a mature central nervous system was originally proposed by Howard Phillip Roffwarg. The importance of REM sleep in consolidating learned material was emphasized by Edmond M. Dewan and Ramon Greenberg, and a similar theory has proposed that REM sleep is important in increasing protein synthesis in the central nervous system for the development of learning and memory. Some researchers have taken the opposite approach to explaining dreams in that they believe that dreams eliminate unwanted information from the central nervous system. Dreaming may be important in uncluttering the brain so that new information can be more easily retained in memory.

Many famous people have reported that dreaming was important in their development of great works of art (see DREAMS AND CREATIVITY).

Visual input is important for the development of typical dreaming. People who have been blind from birth do dream but their dreams contain less visual and more auditory content. People who have been rendered blind from an early age after the development of visual input tend to retain the ability to have visual dreams. The question of whether people dream in black and white or color was explored by Calvin Hall, and he determined that approximately 30% of dreams were reported to have vivid color content. The content of dreams is also influenced by the sex of the dreamer. Females tend to have dreams that are more likely to be set indoors and are less aggressive than the dreams of males. However, these differences may be related more to personality differences than to true sex difference.

Dream activity within the cerebral hemispheres is believed by some to occur primarily in the right hemisphere because of the association with the storage of visual memory. Right-hemisphere function in dreaming is supported by reports of patients with right-hemisphere lesions who have a loss of dream recall. However, lesions of the posterior region of the brain affecting either hemisphere are also associated with dream loss.

The ability to dream appears to be present from infancy, and some researchers, such as Howard Roffwarg, have hypothesized that REM sleep is important for normal brain development. Children as young as three years of age report dream content, although it is often difficult to assess whether the reported dream activity is elaborated upon. Young children tend to dream of unpleasant events, such as being chased, and by age four the dream content appears to include more animal dreams. By age five or six, the dreams include ghosts, physical injury and even death.

The content of dreams can be influenced by daytime experiences. Unpleasant dreams are usually associated with daytime psychological stress. Research has attempted to incorporate material into dreams, including using auditory, tactile or visual stimuli. Incorporation of auditory stimuli into dream content is rather poor, occurring in approximately 10% of attempts. If water is sprayed on the face of the dreamer, some content regarding water is found in about 40% of recalled dreams. Exposure to light flashes can be incorporated into dream content, but only about 20% of the time is it recalled. Experimentation by having patients wear colored glasses throughout the day so that they experience only the color red have led to an increase in the recall of red content in the dreams. Mental activity that occurs immediately prior to the onset of sleep is often incorporated into the dream content.

REM sleep is associated with a number of phasic events of which the eye movement is the most prominent. In animals, ponto-geniculate-occipital (PGO) spikes can be detected by electrodes placed over the cortex. These spikes occur at the onset of REM sleep and are thought to be important in the initiation of the REM sleep state. Various theories have been reported as to the importance of PGO spikes. Some researchers think they may be related to hallucinatory behavior whereas others believe that they may improve brain function by the elimination of unwanted memories.

It has been hypothesized that the human equivalent of PGO spikes is more common in patients with psychiatric disorders characterized by hallucinations, such as schizophrenia. The PGO spikes are generated in the pons of the brain stem, which is believed to be the site of origin for REM sleep. During REM sleep, activity is relayed from the brain stem to the cortex where it is associated with the dreaming. Simultaneously, REM activity passes down the brain stem to the medullary region where stimulation causes an inhibition of the spinal cord motoneurons, leading to the loss of muscle tone during REM sleep. Additional information on the neurophysiology of REM sleep was discovered with the recognition of the syndrome of REM sleep without atonia, which occurs in cats following pontine lesions. In this syndrome, the output from the pons to the medullary inhibitory centers is prevented so that the atonia associated with REM sleep does not occur. Cats with such lesions tend to "act out" their dreams. This suggests that the muscle atonia of REM sleep is a protective mechanism to prevent excessive motor activity during that sleep stage.

In recent years there has been an increased interest in a phenomenon known as LUCID DREAMS where the dreamer is aware of being asleep and of dreaming. It seems almost as if the dreamer is awake and asleep at the same time. Various techniques, such as posthypnotic suggestions and somatic sensory stimulation during REM sleep, have been reported to increase the likelihood of lucid dreaming. It has been suggested that the increased ability to have lucid dreams might be useful in stimulating creativity and might even be useful in controlling NIGHTMARES.

Nightmares are unpleasant dreams that occur in connection with the REM sleep stage. These episodes can be confused with SLEEP TERRORS, in which panic occurs out of slow wave sleep. The nightmare, also known as a dream anxiety attack, produces an abrupt awakening from sleep with recall of frightening dream content. The nightmare sufferer can usually recall in detail the dream content—typically, a threat to the dreamer's safety. Nightmares are more common in the latter third of the night because of the increased likelihood of REM sleep at that time.

NARCOLEPSY, a disorder of excessive sleepiness and characterized by sleep onset REM periods, is also associated with frequent and vivid dreaming, and there may be a slight increase in a tendency for nightmares. The sleep onset dreams of the narcoleptic are often unpleasant. A more extreme form of nightmare activity can occur at sleep onset—TERRIFYING HYPNAGOGIC HALLUCINATIONS; however, these can also occur in people without any obvious precipitating disorder.

The dreaming stage of sleep is associated with penile erections in males. Although sexual dream content is not usually associated with REM SLEEP-RELATED PENILE ERECTIONS, sexual dreams are common in adolescence. Sexual dreams increase the likelihood of a NOCTURNAL EMISSION (wet dream) in which ejaculation occurs in association with the penile erection. Nocturnal emissions are more likely to occur in males who have abstained from sexual activity for a long period of time and are also more common in adolescence.

The dream stage of sleep is a very important sleep stage because of its association with dramatic changes in physiology and the association with nightmares, erectile ability during sleep, REM sleep behavior disorder, narcolepsy, and because of its psychoanalytical significance. Investigation into dreams and their associated pathophysiology is a fertile area of investigation. (See also ALCOHOLISM, DREAM ANXIETY ATTACKS.)

dreams and creativity   History includes several examples of artists who have created works while dreaming, or have dreamed the solution to a creative problem they were coping with during the day. For instance, the English artist and poet William Blake stated that, while searching for a less expensive way to do engraving, he dreamed that his deceased brother came to him and suggested that Blake use copper engraving, a method he immediately began to explore. English poet Samuel Taylor Coleridge is reported to have dreamed part of his poem "Kubla Khan."

Other examples, cited in Patricia Garfield's book, *Creative Dreaming*, include Guiseppe Tartini, Italian violinist and composer; anthropologist Hermann V. Hilprecht; German chemist Friedrich A. Kekule, who discovered the molecular structure of benzene in a dream; and English author Robert Louis Stevenson (1850–1894), who wrote that he dreamed the essence of the Dr. Jekyll and Mr. Hyde story. Garfield includes a list of "what we can learn from creative dreamers," including the suggestion that if you have a creative dream, you should ". . . clearly visualize it and record it in some form as soon as possible: write it, paint it, play it, make it. Visualize it while you translate it into a concrete form." (See also DAYDREAMING, DREAM CONTENT and DREAMS.)

drowsiness   A state of wakefulness characterized by brief episodes of sleep, typically lasting only seconds. The individual is often not aware that sleep is actually occurring and perceives the state as one of tiredness and a strong desire for sleep.

During drowsiness, the ELECTROENCEPHALOGRAM (EEG) records an "alpha dropout" with reduced alpha activity giving way to low-voltage, mixed slow and fast activity. Slow waves in the range of 2 to 7 hertz occur, often mixed with fast activity of 15 to 25 hertz. As the drowsiness deepens, the electroencephalogram rhythm slows, with more frequent episodes of two to three hertz activity intermixed with brief episodes of return to alpha activity in response to arousing stimuli.

Occasionally, when a person experiences drowsiness, the EEG will show the presence of positive occipital sharp transients of sleep (POSTS) that occur in the occipital regions and are most commonly seen in adolescents and young adults. In addition, transient sharp waves, termed benign epileptiform transients of sleep (BETS), can also be seen.

Drowsiness is a relaxed state that can be considered an intermediary stage between wakefulness and light sleep. During drowsiness, the individual is able to comprehend environmental stimuli and will deny being asleep. Not uncommonly, individuals who are in stage one sleep, which is characterized by loss of alpha activity and reduced appreciation of environmental stimuli, will report that they were in a state of drowsiness and deny being asleep.

Drowsiness occurs naturally prior to sleep onset, but it can also be brought on by medications prescribed specifically for that purpose or as a side effect of a medication prescribed for another purpose, such as for motion sickness, hay fever or colds. Certain illicit substances, such as heroin or marijuana, may also induce drowsiness.

drowsy driving   Term applied to driving a car or truck when not fully alert. The danger of drowsy driving, also referred to as driver fatigue, is that it may lead to falling asleep at the wheel with resultant injuries or even fatalities to the driver, passengers and any other individuals who come into contact with the vehicle which would be out of control due to the sleeping driver. Causes of drowsy driving include sleep deprivation, shift work, certain medications that have sleepiness as a side effect, drinking alcoholic beverages, eating a large meal, especially one that has an excess of carbohydrates, and the soporific effect of highway driving, especially at night. Fifty-one percent of the 1,154 adults surveyed by telephone for the National Sleep Foundation's 2000 poll said that they had actually dozed off while driving drowsy during the previous year. Men were more likely than women to drive drowsy (63% versus 43%) and younger adults were more likely than older adults to drive drowsy (60% of 18-year olds versus 21% of those 65 years and older).

The most common way to deal with drowsy driving, according to the National Sleep Foundation 2000 poll, was to use caffeine (63%). Roughly one of five drivers (22%) said they pulled over to take a nap when they feared their exhaustion might cause them to fall asleep at the wheel.

In recent years, consumer and driver education and public awareness campaigns from the Automobile Association of America as well as sleep associations like the National Sleep Foundation have emerged to get the word out about the hazards of drowsy driving.

drugs   See ANTIDEPRESSANTS, BARBITURATES, BENZODIAZEPINES, HYPNOTICS, MONOAMINE OXIDASE INHIBITORS, NARCOTICS, RESPIRATORY STIMULANTS, STIMULANT MEDICATIONS.

dustman   See SANDMAN.

dyssomnia   A disorder of sleep or wakefulness that is associated with a complaint of difficulty of initiating or maintaining sleep or EXCESSIVE SLEEPINESS. Dyssomnia is used, as opposed to the term PARASOMNIA, which refers to a sleep disorder that occurs during sleep but does not primarily produce a complaint of insomnia or excessive sleepiness.

E

early morning arousal   Term used to denote final awakening that occurs following the major sleep episode at a time earlier than desired. The term is commonly used as synonymous with "premature morning awakening" and is usually associated with underlying DEPRESSION, although it may be caused by other medical or psychiatric disorders, such as DEMENTIA or mania. Early morning arousal may also be due to a CIRCADIAN RHYTHM SLEEP DISORDER, such as ADVANCED SLEEP PHASE SYNDROME, in which the sleep onset time is early and hence the wake time is also early. The early morning arousal is often preceded by numerous brief awakenings before the final awakening. (See also INSOMNIA.)

early morning awakening   See EARLY MORNING AROUSAL.

EDS   See EXCESSIVE SLEEPINESS.

EEG   See ELECTROENCEPHALOGRAM (EEG).

Elavil   See ANTIDEPRESSANTS.

electrical status epilepticus of sleep (ESES)   An abnormal ELECTROENCEPHALOGRAM pattern that occurs during NON-REM-STAGE SLEEP. This disorder is characterized by continuous, slow-spike-and-wave discharges that occur and persist throughout non-REM sleep. At least 85% of non-REM sleep is occupied by this abnormal pattern. Electrical status epilepticus of sleep does not produce direct clinical features of epilepsy and therefore its name is regarded as slightly inappropriate. It is really an electrical abnormality, rather than a true seizure disorder. However, children with electrical status epilepticus of sleep have significant cognitive and behavioral disorders that are believed to be directly related to the electroencephalographic pattern.

ESES is most often seen in childhood around eight years of age and affects males and females equally. It tends to disappear with increasing age and its duration, although difficult to know exactly, appears to be in terms of months or years. Some children who suffer from ESES also can have more typical epilepsy. Most often, the seizures are a generalized or focal seizure disorder that usually predates the discovery of the ESES.

This disorder appears to be rare although the exact prevalence is unknown. As it was first recognized in 1971 and has only been detected in childhood, it is not known whether a familial pattern exists. Pathological studies have failed to reveal any specific central nervous system abnormality to account for this disorder.

Children may have associated severe language impairment, with reduced mental ability, and impairment of memory and temporo-spatial orientation. There may be reduced attention span, hyperkinesis, aggressiveness and even psychotic states.

The disorder is diagnosed by demonstrating the characteristic electroencephalographic pattern that occurs for more than 85% of the non-REM sleep. This particular pattern does not occur during wakefulness. Sleep organization is generally preserved, with a normal proportion of non-REM and REM sleep. However, the electroencephalographic pattern tends to obscure the more typical features of slow wave sleep so that SLEEP SPINDLES, K-COMPLEXES and vertex transient waves are usually indistinguishable.

The abnormal slow wave activity needs to be distinguished from other epileptic disorders, such as benign epilepsy with rolandic spikes (BERS). The benign epilepsy of childhood has clinical seizures that are usually evident, and the electroencephalographic pattern is characterized by frequent spike activity. Although benign epilepsy of childhood commonly occurs during non-REM sleep, it never fills more than 85% of slow wave sleep.

Other seizure disorders, such as the Lennox-Gastaut syndrome, may need to be differentiated. However, this particular form of epilepsy has typical tonic seizures associated with the abnormal electroencephalographic pattern.

Another form of epilepsy associated with language difficulty is called the Landau-Kleffner syndrome. This form of epilepsy is associated with clinical features of epilepsy and a typical electroencephalographic pattern that is localized to one or both temporal lobes.

Electrical status epilepticus of sleep is treated by standard anticonvulsants that include phenytoin. SESE is an acronym for subclinical electrical status epilepticus of sleep, which is synonymous with electrical status epilepticus of sleep.

electroencephalogram (EEG)   Recording of the electrical activity of the brain. The term typically applies to measurements made by applying electrodes to the scalp. The electroencephalographic activity is composed of frequencies that are divided into four main groups: those that are below 3.5 per second (DELTA), 4 to 7.5 per second (THETA), 8 to 13 per second (ALPHA) and those above 13 per second (BETA). Sleep electroencephalographic frequencies are usually of the theta or delta range, except that of REM SLEEP which consists of mixed theta and alpha activities. The deepest stage of sleep, SLOW WAVE SLEEP, has EEG activity in the delta range.

EEG waves are also described in terms of their amplitudes. The amplitude of waves detected at the scalp is usually 10 to 100 microvolts (mv). Alpha activity is usually 10 to 20 mv. Beta activity is also low amplitude, rarely exceeding 30 mv. Theta waves can be higher, up to 50 mv, and delta waves are of the highest amplitude, up to 100 mv in children.

The recording is usually on paper, although it is now possible to record on magnetic tape and computer disk. Typically the electroencephalogram is measured along with the ELECTRO-OCULOGRAM and the ELECTROMYOGRAM for the recording of sleep stages and wakefulness. Electrodes for the measurement of the brain activity to document sleep are typically placed at the C3 or C4 positions according to the 10-20 system used throughout the world. Electroencephalograph electrodes can also record other electrical signals that come from the body, such as muscle activity or eye movements.

electromyogram (EMG)   The recording of muscle electrical potentials in order to document the level of muscle activity. The electromyogram is usually recorded by a polysomnograph machine, along with the ELECTROEN-CEPHALOGRAM and ELECTRO-OCULOGRAM, in order to stage sleep. The electrodes for the measurement of the electromyogram are typically placed over the tip of the jaw to record activity in the mentalis muscle. Sometimes electromyographic activity is also recorded from other muscle groups to determine other abnormal activity during sleep. For example, measurements of the masseter muscle activity are useful for determining the presence of BRUXISM (tooth grinding), and activity recorded from the anterior tibialis muscles can document the presence of PERIODIC LEG MOVEMENTS during sleep.

Electromyographic activity recorded in the polysomnogram typically will show an increased level of activation during wakefulness; this decreases as the subject passes through the non-REM sleep stages (see NON-REM-STAGE SLEEP) to the deeper stages of sleep, when the chin muscle activity is very low. In REM SLEEP, electromyographic activity is characterized by a silent background, but with brief phasic muscle activity from most muscle groups. Rarely, background electromyographic activity can be increased in REM sleep in association with REM SLEEP BEHAVIOR DISORDER.

electro-oculogram (EOG)   A recording of eye movements by means of changes in the electrical potentials between the retina and the cornea. There is a large potential difference, often over 200 microvolts, between the negatively-charged retina and the positively-charged cornea. Electrodes that are placed lateral to the outer canthus of the eyes record changes in the dipole with movements of the eyes. Measurement of eye movement activity is essential for staging sleep.

In stage one sleep, there are slow rolling eye movements, and the eyes become quiescent (not moving) in deeper stages of non-REM sleep. REM SLEEP is characterized by rapid eye movement. Rapid eye movements similar to those seen in REM sleep can be seen during wakefulness, and the measurement of other physiological variables, such as the EEG and EMG, help in the differentiation of REM sleep from wakefulness. (See also SLEEP STAGES.)

EMG   See ELECTROMYOGRAM (EMG).

endogenous circadian pacemaker   An internal mechanism that triggers the periodic processes that are involved in the human circadian timing system, this structure controls the timing of various rhythmical processes in the body, such as the sleep-wake cycle, that have a cycle of approximately 24 hours. The site of the pacemaker appears to be the SUPRACHIASMATIC NUCLEUS at the base of the third ventricle in the hypothalamus of the brain. The endogenous circadian pacemaker is also known as the X-oscillator, the type-1 oscillator, the "C" process and the endogenous rhythm.

endogenous rhythm   See ENDOGENOUS CIRCADIAN PACEMAKER.

endoscopy   A procedure whereby an observation can be made anywhere inside the body. In sleep disorders medicine, endoscopy commonly is performed in patients who have UPPER AIRWAY OBSTRUCTION in order to determine the site of that obstruction. A fiberoptic endoscope (see FIBEROPTIC ENDOSCOPY) is placed through the nose so that an observer can view the tissues of the nose and upper airway. This procedure can be performed not only on the awake patient but also on a patient who is asleep or under anesthesia.

enuresis, sleep-related   See SLEEP ENURESIS.

environmental sleep disorder   A sleep disorder that has its roots in a disturbing environmental condition that produces a complaint of INSOMNIA or EXCESSIVE SLEEPINESS. Light and environmental noise are typical causes. Usually the sleep disorder is resolved when the environmental disturbance is eliminated.

environmental time cues   Environmental factors that influence a pattern of behavior, such as the sleep-wake cycle, and help to maintain regular 24-hour periodicity. Maintenance of a 24-hour sleep-wake cycle is dependent upon environmental time cues occurring prior to the onset of the major sleep episode and also at the time of awakening. Such time cues include alarm clocks, light stimuli, social interaction and noise stimulus. In an environment free of environmental time cues, an individual may free run with a sleep-wake cycle that is longer than 24 hours, typically 25 hours, causing the individual to fall asleep one hour later and arise one hour later on a daily basis. This FREE RUNNING pattern of sleep and wakefulness causes the sleep-wake pattern to occur out of synchrony with that of most other people. The German term *zeitgeber* is synonymous with environmental time cues. (See also CHRONOBIOLOGY, CIRCADIAN RHYTHM SLEEP DISORDERS, NON-24-HOUR SLEEP-WAKE SYNDROME, NREM-REM SLEEP CYCLE.)

EOG   See ELECTRO-OCULOGRAM (EOG).

epilepsy   Epileptic seizures may disturb sleep and, if they occur frequently enough, may be a cause of daytime sleepiness. Sometimes the medications used for epilepsy, such as phenobarbitol, can contribute to daytime sleepiness. SLEEP DEPRIVATION is a known precipitant of epileptic seizures. Most seizures, if they occur during sleep, occur during the non-REM sleep stages. Rarely do seizures occur during REM sleep. A particular type of epilepsy called benign focal epilepsy of childhood (Rolandic epilepsy) has a marked tendency to occur during sleep. In some patients, SLEEP TERRORS or SLEEPWALKING episodes may need to be distinguished from epileptic seizures. (See also RAPID EYE MOVEMENT SLEEP.)

epoch   A measure of sleep activity used in order to stage sleep (see SLEEP STAGES); typically epochs are 20- to 30-second samples of sleep that have been recorded by POLYSOMNOGRAPHY. Epochs often reflect the recording speed of the polysomnograph, and refer to a single page of recording; polysomnograph recordings performed at 15 millimeters per second will typically produce a 20-second epoch on standard EEG paper, whereas recordings performed at 10 millimeters per second will produce 30-second epochs on standard EEG paper. A typical polysomnographic recording of sleep will produce approximately 1,000 epochs of sleep at the standard 10 millimeters per second recording rate.

Epworth Sleepiness Scale (ESS)   A questionnaire that is used to assess whether someone is suffering from excessive daytime sleepiness. It was developed by Murray W. Johns, M.D. at the Sleep Center at Epworth Hospital in Melbourne, Australia.

erections during sleep   Penile erections typically occur during sleep in all healthy males from infancy to old age. Erections are associated with REM SLEEP, not usually with sexual dreams. The erections occur during each of the episodes of REM sleep and can last up to 20 minutes. The presence of penile erections during sleep helps differentiate IMPOTENCE due to psychogenic causes from that due to physical causes, such as a neurological or vascular disorder. (See also IMPAIRED SLEEP-RELATED PENILE ERECTIONS, SLEEP-RELATED PAINFUL ERECTIONS.)

erratic hours   Term applied to varied SLEEP ONSET and WAKE TIMES. Alterations in the time of going to bed at night, and of awakening in the morning, are common precipitating factors in the development of INSOMNIA. Regularity in going to bed and awakening is a key element of good SLEEP HYGIENE.

Maintaining regular sleep onset and wake times is an important element of STIMULUS CONTROL THERAPY for insomnia, as well as SLEEP RESTRICTION THERAPY. (See also IRREGULAR SLEEP-WAKE PATTERN.)

ESES   See ELECTRICAL STATUS EPILEPTICUS OF SLEEP (ESES).

esophageal reflux   Term applied to the regurgitation of gastric contents into the esophagus. Esophageal reflux typically occurs in individuals who have some incompetence of the gastroesophageal sphincter between the esophagus and the stomach. This incompetence may be due to a hiatus hernia. Patients with OBSTRUCTIVE SLEEP APNEA SYNDROME are more likely to have esophageal reflux during the struggle to breathe that is associated with apneic events. This reflux may cause an awakening from sleep and produce gagging or COUGHING, sometimes associated with laryngospasm. (See SLEEP-RELATED GASTROESOPHAGEAL REFLUX, SLEEP-RELATED LARYNGOSPASM.)

evening person (night person)   An individual who prefers to go to bed later, and arise later, than is typical for the general population. Such persons have a delay in their sleep phase, and the pattern of body TEMPERATURE and other circadian rhythms is delayed. An evening person is sometimes referred to as a "night owl." (See also ADVANCED SLEEP PHASE SYNDROME, DELAYED SLEEP PHASE SYNDROME, MORNING PERSON, OWL AND LARK QUESTIONNAIRE.)

evening shift   Work shift from about 3 P.M. to 11 P.M. that is before the NIGHT SHIFT.

excessive daytime sleepiness   See EXCESSIVE SLEEPINESS.

excessive sleepiness   The inability to remain awake during the awake portion of an individual's sleep-wake cycle (see NREM-REM SLEEP CYCLE). Excessive sleepiness is synonymous with EXCESSIVE DAYTIME SLEEPINESS (or EDS) and somnolence but is the preferred term.

Excessive sleepiness may be present at night for an individual who has the major sleep period occurring during the day, for example, a shift worker. Excessive sleepiness may be reported subjectively or be quantified by means of electrophysiological measurements of sleep tendency. Tests that can quantify excessive sleepiness include the MULTIPLE SLEEP LATENCY TEST, the MAINTENANCE OF WAKEFULNESS TEST, PUPILLOMETRY and VIGILANCE TESTING. Subjective rating scales, such as the STANFORD SLEEPINESS SCALE (SSS) and the EPWORTH SLEEPINESS SCALE (ESS), are often used to determine a subject's level of sleepiness.

The causes of excessive sleepiness range from OBSTRUCTIVE SLEEP APNEA SYNDROME to NARCOLEPSY, TIME ZONE CHANGE (JET LAG) SYNDROME or INSOMNIA. The sleepiness can be caused by an ADJUSTMENT SLEEP DISORDER related to a temporary stressful event, such as illness or death in the family, midterm or final exams at school or anxiety about a particular crisis at work. The insomnia and the excessive sleepiness related to that insomnia clears up as soon as the interim situation is resolved.

Excessive sleepiness can also be chronic, such as that seen in children or adolescents suffering from DELAYED SLEEP PHASE SYNDROME so that every day, especially during the school week, they get too little sleep and are tired the next day.

Adults who suffer from INSUFFICIENT SLEEP SYNDROME may have a chronic problem with excessive sleepiness that has a negative impact on their health, career success or social relationships.

The consequences of excessive sleepiness may include mild to severe fatigue, crankiness, depression and reduced concentration, or even such catastrophic consequences as fatigue-related driving accidents (DROWSY DRIVING) as well as industrial or home ACCIDENTS.

exercise and sleep   Exercise can increase or reduce the quality of sleep, or have no effect at all. It is well recognized that intense exercise performed immediately before sleep will impair the ability to fall asleep. The increased autonomic system activation produced by the exercise increases AROUSAL and therefore sleep onset will be delayed. Good SLEEP HYGIENE includes avoiding intense exercise before going to bed at night.

However, a relaxing exercise, such as yoga, may be beneficial to sleep by reducing muscle tension. Mild relaxing exercises, such as those recommended by Edmund Jacobson, can be beneficial and are a well-recommended form of relaxation therapy (see JACOBSONIAN RELAXATION).

There are differing opinions on the role of daytime exercise in improving the quality of nighttime sleep. Initial reports have demonstrated that intense daytime exercise will increase the amount of SLOW WAVE SLEEP at night; however, this increase appears to occur only in trained athletes. Initially it was suggested that exercise by means of producing wear and tear on the tissues would lead to enhanced deep sleep as a restorative process. However, there is no evidence that deep sleep is restorative after exercise, and studies with invalids on complete bed rest show little difference in the amount of slow wave sleep present compared with more active populations.

The role of exercise in improving slow wave sleep in trained individuals is also controversial as there are some who believe that the increase is due to an increase in body TEMPERATURE. Trained athletes on sustained exercise are more liable to produce an increase in their core body temperature compared with unfit individuals. Other studies looking at the effects of body heating by artificial means have demonstrated that slow wave sleep can be increased in the absence of exercise. (See also SLEEP EXERCISES.)

exhaustion   A state of extreme mental or physical fatigue. Exhaustion is not synonymous with EXCESSIVE SLEEPINESS. Persons can become exhausted from mental strain and feel a tiredness and weakness that has nothing to do with an increased physiological drive for sleep. Similarly, a form of exhaustion can occur following exercise where fatigue occurs; however, acute sudden exercise can lead to a state of relaxation that will allow an underlying drive for sleep to become manifest. For example, someone who is slightly sleepy, due to an insufficient quality or amount of sleep, may sleep during the day following exercise as the exercise causes him or her to become relaxed and sleep occurs.

extrinsic sleep disorders   Sleep disorders that originate, develop or arise from causes outside of the body. Examples of extrinsic sleep disorders include environmental sleep disorder, ADJUSTMENT SLEEP DISORDER and ALTITUDE INSOMNIA. Removal of the external factor usually resolves the sleep disturbance unless another sleep problem develops in the interim. This group of disorders is one of three subcategories of dyssomnias in the American Sleep Disorder Association's INTERNATIONAL CLASSIFICATION OF SLEEP DISORDERS. (The other two subcategories are INTRINSIC SLEEP DISORDERS and CIRCADIAN RHYTHM SLEEP DISORDERS.)

eye movements   Typically recorded for the detection of sleep stages. Usually, awake persons will have rapid eye movements; these slow during DROWSINESS so that slow eye movements are a common feature of stage one sleep. The eyes become quiescent during SLOW WAVE SLEEP. The REM stage of sleep (see REM SLEEP) is characterized by rapid eye movements that are similar to those seen during wakefulness.

The eye movement activity, in conjunction with the ELECTROENCEPHALO-GRAM pattern and ELECTROMYOGRAM, is one of the three main physiological variables that are recorded during POLYSOMNOGRAPHY.

F

family bed   The practice of having an infant or child sleep in bed with its mother, father or both parents. Advocates of the family bed emphasize that it helps promote bonding among child and parents as well as promoting an adult-type sleep-wake cycle. In the early months or years, if a mother is breast-feeding, it can minimize the disruption to her sleep if she just turns to the nearby infant for a feeding, rather than going into another room. However, infants have died because the sleeping parent has accidentally smothered the child.

If a child enters a parent's bed in the middle of the night, the parent should carry, or walk, the child back to his or her own room. If the child has difficulty falling asleep, the parent could comfort the child till sleep occurs, or just sit in a nearby chair, rather than allowing a return to the parent's bed. (See also BEDS, INFANT SLEEP, INFANT SLEEP DISORDERS.)

fast sleep   See REM SLEEP.

fatal familial insomnia   A rare disorder, primarily seen in people of Italian descent, characterized by a severe insomnia associated with degeneration of the central nervous system; it is ultimately fatal. This disorder is associated with abnormalities of the autonomic neurological system that produce symptoms of insomnia, temperature changes, excessive salivation, excessive sweating and rapid heart and breathing rates.

Fatal familial insomnia has insomnia persistent throughout the course of the disorder. As the autonomic symptoms develop, sleep becomes more disrupted and there is usually development of other neurological features; dysarthria, tremors, muscle jerks (myoclonus) and dystonic posturing can occur. The patient has a deteriorating level of mental alertness and frequently lapses from wakefulness into sleep. Often there can be an "acting out" of dreams during sleep. The disorder leads to coma and finally to death.

Fatal familial insomnia is a prion disease which primarily occurs in adults between the fifth and sixth decades of life, affecting males and females equally. It appears to have a familial transmission as several members of one family with the disease have been reported.

Polysomnographic investigations in the early stages of this disease generally show severely disrupted sleep patterns with wakefulness intervening between short episodes of sleep. There is very disrupted REM SLEEP with maintenance of muscle tone and abnormal movements associated with DREAMS. Slow wave sleep diminishes and becomes absent during the course of the disease. The electroencephalogram gradually becomes less reactive to environmental stimuli and progressively decreases in amplitude until death.

Fatal familial insomnia needs to be differentiated from other forms of degenerative neurological disease such as Creutzfeldt-Jakob disease, which is characterized by a progressive deteriorating dementia and myoclonic jerks. Other forms of dementia, such as Alzheimer's disease, are relatively easily distinguished from fatal familial insomnia. The abnormal movements that occur during REM sleep are similar to those seen in REM SLEEP BEHAVIOR DISORDER, which does not have a progressively deteriorating course. Other sleep stages are generally intact in the REM sleep behavior disorder, whereas in fatal familial insomnia, loss of stage three and four sleep, and a severely disrupted sleep pattern, are characteristic.

No treatment is known to affect the course of the underlying disorder. (See also CEREBRAL DEGENERATIVE DISORDERS, DEMENTIA, NOCTURNAL PAROXYSMAL DYSTONIA.)

fatigue   A state of reduced efficiency due to prolonged or excessive exertion. Fatigue needs to be differentiated from EXCESSIVE SLEEPINESS, which is a state of increased drive for sleep. The term "fatigue" is often erroneously interpreted as meaning sleepy; however, individuals can be severely fatigued without the ability to fall asleep during a day of usual wakefulness. The state of EXHAUSTION is similar to fatigue and indicates primarily a mental rather than a muscular form of fatigue.

femoxetine   See ANTIDEPRESSANTS.

fiberoptic endoscopy   Otolaryngological procedure typically performed in sleep medicine for the evaluation of the upper airway. This procedure is commonly performed in patients with OBSTRUCTIVE SLEEP APNEA SYNDROME in order to determine the site of upper airway obstruction.

This procedure has been reported to be helpful in the evaluation of the site of upper airway obstruction and in predicating a patient's response to UVULOPALATOPHARYNGOPLASTY. Cephalometric radiographs are often employed along with fiberoptic endoscopy in the evaluation of the upper airway changes in patients with obstructive sleep apnea syndrome. (See also SURGERY AND SLEEP DISORDERS.)

fibromyositis syndrome   See FIBROSITIS SYNDROME.

fibrositis syndrome   Syndrome characterized by diffuse, nonspecific muscle aches and pains that are typically associated with complaints of unrefreshing sleep at night. The musculoskeletal symptoms are not due to any articular, nonarticular or metabolic disease.

The sleep disturbance is one of frequent arousals and brief awakenings and a feeling upon awakening in the morning of being unrefreshed. There may be discomfort in the muscles and joints during the night and morning stiffness upon awakening. Tiredness, fatigue and, rarely, sleepiness may be present during the daytime. An increased prevalence of periodic limb movements has also been described.

Polysomnographic investigations show a characteristic pattern of alpha sleep in which alpha activity occurs superimposed on other sleep stages. When this pattern occurs during slow wave sleep it is often termed ALPHA-DELTA ACTIVITY. The sleep stages are otherwise normal in percentage; however, there may be an increased number of brief awakenings and arousals. Patients usually lack evidence of pathological daytime sleepiness.

There is no clear cause or pathology found to explain the discomfort.

Treatment of the sleep disturbance is with the tricyclic ANTIDEPRESSANT medication amitriptyline. In addition, attention to good SLEEP HYGIENE is helpful. Typically the anti-inflammatory medications that are used for rheumatic disorders are not effective in the fibrositis syndrome.

Fibrositis syndrome has also been called rheumatic pain modulation disorder, fibromyositis syndrome or fibromyalgia.

final awakening   See ARISE TIME.

final wake-up   See ARISE TIME.

first night effect   A pattern of increased SLEEP LATENCY, and reduced TOTAL SLEEP TIME on the first night of a polysomnographic recording in the laboratory. The first night effect is believed to be due to several factors, including the discomfort to the subject of the recording electrodes, the new sleep environment and psychological effects, including anxiety regarding a polysomnographic recording. However, the subject adjusts to the above factors, and the disruptive effects on sleep typically are present only on the first night of recording. (See also POLYSOMNOGRAPHY, SLEEP-WAKE DISORDERS CENTER.)

fluoxetine   See ANTIDEPRESSANTS.

flurazepam   See BENZODIAZEPINES.

fluvoxamine   See ANTIDEPRESSANTS.

food allergy insomnia   A disorder of initiating and maintaining sleep that is caused by food allergy; typically occurring in infants and associated with irritability, frequent arousals, crying episodes and daytime lethargy. Other signs or features of an allergic response may be present, but they are usually not the predominant feature of the disorder. For example, skin irritation, gastrointestinal upset or respiratory difficulties may all occur.

Although this is a disorder that primarily affects children, it can also occur in adults who may develop an allergy to eggs or fish, with resultant insomnia. When the disorder occurs in children, it usually occurs in infancy and resolves spontaneously by the age of four years at the latest. There may well be a family history of allergic phenomena. The allergy most commonly is related to the ingestion of cow's milk and therefore may occur soon after the introduction of cow's milk to the diet.

Food allergy insomnia should be differentiated from infant colic in which sleep disturbance may be associated with acute crying spells that occur episodically (gastrointestinal symptoms may accompany the acute episodes). SLEEP-RELATED GASTROESOPHAGEAL REFLUX, INFANT SLEEP APNEA and infantile epileptic seizures need to be differentiated from food allergy insomnia.

Treatment involves removal of the offending allergen. Allergy tests may be necessary to determine the exact allergen, but once it is removed from the diet, the sleep disturbance usually resolves rapidly.

fragmentary myoclonus   Disorder characterized by clusters of brief muscle jerks that occur predominantly in NON-REM-STAGE SLEEP. These involuntary "twitch-like" contractions can occur in various skeletal muscles in an asynchronous and asymmetrical manner. Muscles of the limbs and face and trunk can all be involved. The brief muscle contractions can occur for prolonged periods throughout sleep. At times, the muscle jerks produce ELECTROENCEPHALOGRAM (EEG) evidence of an AROUSAL with a transient K-COMPLEX; however, there is usually no change in the EEG in association with the activity.

The muscle jerks are very brief, usually 75 to 150 milliseconds in duration, with an amplitude of about 50 to several hundred microvolts. The activity usually commences soon after sleep onset and continues throughout non-REM sleep, including SLOW WAVE SLEEP, and persists into REM SLEEP.

Fragmentary myoclonus is associated with EXCESSIVE SLEEPINESS. The activity has been described in other sleep disorders, including the SLEEP-RELATED BREATHING DISORDERS, NARCOLEPSY, PERIODIC LIMB MOVEMENT DISORDER and other causes of INSOMNIA.

In most situations, fragmentary myoclonus does not require treatment. However, if frequent EEG arousals are associated with the activity and excessive sleepiness is a feature, then suppression of the arousals by means of BENZODIAZEPINES may be helpful.

fragmentation   See NREM-REM SLEEP CYCLE.

free running   A chronobiological term that applies to a biological rhythm isolated from ENVIRONMENTAL TIME CUES such as light, food, temperature, social interactions and clock time. Under these conditions, the rhythm will continue with its own internal period length, which for CIRCADIAN RHYTHM is close to, but not exactly, 24 hours in duration.

frequently changing sleep-wake schedule　One of the sleep-wake schedule disorders of the *Diagnostic Classification of Sleep and Arousal Disorders,* which was published in the journal SLEEP in 1979. This term refers to sleep disorders that are due to persistent alteration of the sleep-wake schedule, such as those due to a changing work shift pattern or flight across time zones. The sleep-wake pattern is constantly disrupted. The terms SHIFT-WORK SLEEP DISORDER and TIME ZONE CHANGE (JET LAG) SYNDROME are preferred.

Freud, Sigmund　"Father of Psychoanalysis" (1856–1939) who viewed DREAMS as doors to the unconscious, the keys to understanding and eventually unblocking repressed sexual and aggressive forces that motivate and perhaps unconsciously control a person's behavior. In 1900, Freud published his groundbreaking treatise, *The Interpretation of Dreams,* which explained dreams as the fulfillment of certain unconscious impulses considered unacceptable on a conscious level.

Freud believed repressed sexual and aggressive desires are disguised in dreams in three ways: through symbolism, such as by using objects to represent sexual organs; by condensation, where one dream image represents several aspects of a person's life; and by displacement, in which an unacceptable wish is focused on something other than the real object of the wish.

He also believed DREAM CONTENT took two forms: the manifest content, or that part of the dream we remember, and the latent content, the true underlying meaning of the dream.

In their treatment, Freudian psychoanalysts use dream interpretation to help patients gain insight, and eventual control, over the unconscious forces causing conflicts and emotional disturbances.

G

gamma-hydroxybutyrate (GHB)   The precursor of the naturally occurring agent gamma-aminobutyric acid. This agent has been found to be
effective in controlling the auxiliary symptoms of NARCOLEPSY, primarily
the symptom of CATAPLEXY. Gamma- hydroxybutyrate has been shown to
have little effect in improving daytime sleepiness. It is known to increase
SLOW WAVE SLEEP, with little effect upon REM SLEEP. The medication is given
once or twice in two- or three-gram doses at night. As the medication has
a short duration of action, it is necessary to give a second dose halfway
through the sleep period. Gamma-hydroxybutyrate may be useful in the
treatment of cataplexy in patients who are unable to use the tricyclic ANTI-
DEPRESSANTS because of anticholinergic side effects. Very few side effects
have been recorded with gamma-hydroxybutyrate. However, the drug has
been abused, and when combined with benzodiazepines has been called
the "date rape" drug. One side effect reported is SLEEPWALKING, possibly due
to the effect of gamma-hydroxybutyrate in increasing the amount of slow
wave sleep. Gamma-hydroxybutyrate is available in Canada but unavailable in the United States except on a research basis for the treatment of
narcolepsy.

Gardner, Randy   San Diego high school senior who, in 1964, broke the
Guinness Book of World Records record by staying awake the longest—264
hours, or 11 days. Sleep researcher WILLIAM C. DEMENT observed Gardner
during his ordeal and concluded, "staying awake for 264 hours did not
cause any psychiatric problems whatsoever." In his book *The Promise of
Sleep* (1999), however, Dement wondered if Gardner may have been
sleepwalking for some of the time since, back in 1965, the recording
devices for monitoring sleep were much less sophisticated than today's
devices.

Gelineau, J. B. E.   Jean-Baptiste Edouard Gelineau (1828–1906) was a
French physician who is credited with first suggesting the term NARCOLEPSY
for a mysterious syndrome characterized by sudden sleeping, especially at
inappropriate times during the day. Gelineau, in his 1880 article published
in the *Gazette des Hopitaux,* proposed the word *narcolepsy* along with a
detailed description of a 38-year-old male wine barrel retailer who had
sleep attacks and accompanying falls. The falls are now known as CATA-
PLEXY but Gelineau called them "astasia."

genetics   The science of the biological unit of heredity that is transmitted
from one cell to another during the process of reproduction. Although a

number of sleep disorders, including SLEEPWALKING and SLEEP TERRORS, are believed to have a genetic origin, with a genetic predisposition passed on through the family, only NARCOLEPSY has been demonstrated to have a specific genetic factor, which is present in nearly every patient with the disease. The human leukocyte antigen DR2 is present in more than 90% of patients diagnosed with narcolepsy. The allele HLA DQB1-0602 is the most specific genetic factor also found in more than 90% of patients with narcolepsy. (See also HISTOCOMPATABILITY ANTIGEN TESTING.)

GHB   See GAMMA-HYDROXYBUTYRATE.

growth hormone   Secreted from the pituitary gland in relation to the onset of sleep, with maximal secretion occurring in the first third of the night. Although originally thought to be primarily related to the onset of stages three and four sleep, it is now believed to be more related to the time following the onset of sleep (see SLEEP STAGES). Growth hormone is tied to the sleep-wake cycle so that acute shifts of sleep by 12 hours will cause an acute shift of the growth hormone secretory pattern. There is minimal growth hormone secretion during the daytime, with small peaks of production that occur in relation to stress or exercise. A shift of the sleep pattern by several hours is immediately accompanied by a shift of growth hormone secretion. This shift is not accompanied by an immediate shift in some other hormone rhythms, such as cortisol. The cortisol circadian rhythm, although related to the sleep-wake cycle, can become disassociated from sleep following an acute shift of the timing of sleep. After one or two weeks, the cortisol pattern readjusts to the new time of sleep and therefore its relationship with growth hormone is reestablished.

Growth hormone is important for growth, particularly in childhood. Maximal levels are secreted around the time of puberty and are important in the maintenance of normal body size. Absence of growth hormone will lead to dwarfism and excessive production of growth hormone will lead to gigantism. However, the removal of the pituitary and loss of growth hormone secretion in adults appears to have few physical effects.

Although prolactin, which is inhibited by dopamine, is very much affected by medications, growth hormone secretion during sleep is largely unaffected. Medications that do influence the production of growth hormone during sleep include cholinergic inhibitory medications, such as methscopolamine, which causes a large increase in the sleep-related growth hormone release. (See also CORTISOL, DOPAMINE, PROLACTIN.)

H

Halcion   See BENZODIAZEPINES.

headaches   Pain or discomfort in the head that is experienced during wakefulness; however, some headache forms can occur during sleep or may be present upon awakening from sleep. MIGRAINE and chronic paroxysmal hemicrania have been demonstrated to have an association with REM SLEEP, and patients with the OBSTRUCTIVE SLEEP APNEA SYNDROME can have headaches upon awakening in the morning. (See also SLEEP-RELATED HEADACHES.)

headbanging (jactatio capitis nocturna)   Also known as rhythmic movement disorder. This behavior is included in a group of three disorders—headbanging, HEAD ROLLING and BODYROCKING—that have as their main characteristic a repetitive movement of the head and, occasionally, of the whole body. These disorders may occur during the time of rest, drowsiness, sleep or full wakefulness. The condition has been reported to occur during deep slow wave sleep, as well as in REM sleep. The episodes occur very frequently, on an almost nightly basis, and usually last for about 15 minutes. The frequency of the movement can vary, but it typically occurs at the rate of 45 episodes per minute and can be as fast as 120 episodes per minute.

The disorder was first described clinically in 1905, by Zappert, when he coined the Latin term *jactatio capitis nocturna,* which is still commonly used.

The head movements in the headbanging form of this disorder are in an anterior/posterior direction. Usually the head is banged into a pillow or a mattress. Occasionally the head movement can be into solid objects, such as a wall or the side of a crib.

When the head movements occur side to side, the condition is termed *head rolling.*

Bodyrocking is most often performed on the hands and knees. The whole body is rocked in an anterior/posterior direction, with the head being pushed into the pillow.

It has been reported that as many as 66% of children exhibit some sort of rhythmical activity at nine months of age, and the prevalence decreases to approximately 8% at four years of age. It is rare for the condition to occur for the first time after two years of age; however, it may persist through adolescence into adulthood.

Headbanging is reported to be more common in males than in females, and rarely has been reported to occur in families. The mentally retarded are more likely to exhibit the behavior. The disorder has to be distinguished from an epileptic disorder and from the fine head oscillations of spasmus nutans.

Polysomnograph studies of the activity usually demonstrate frequent episodes during sleep, most often in the lighter stages one and two sleep. Rarely has the condition been reported to occur only during REM sleep, which may indicate a variant of the disorder. Episodes can occur during deep slow wave sleep, although, again, this has rarely been reported. Daytime electroencephalography is usually normal between episodes.

The cause of the movements is unknown, but numerous theories have been proposed. There is little evidence to support a psychiatric or organic neurological disorder to account for the behavior. A neurophysiological basis for the activity is the most likely, related to normal development. It has been suggested that the activity may be a pleasurable sensation, and therefore a form of vestibular self-stimulation.

Treatment is usually unnecessary when the condition occurs in childhood, as it typically will disappear within 18 months, often at around four years of age. When the condition persists into adolescence or adulthood, behavioral or pharmacological approaches may be needed. Sedative medications have been beneficial, and some patients have had a favorable response to tricyclic ANTIDEPRESSANTS. Measures may have to be taken to prevent injury from the repetitive movements in young children.

head rolling   Repetitive movement of the head from side to side, which may occur during rest, drowsiness, sleep or wakefulness; more typical in children below the age of four than in older children or adults. (See also HEADBANGING.)

heart attack   See MYOCARDIAL INFARCTION.

heartburn   Discomfort experienced in the middle of the chest; associated with reflux of acid from the stomach into the esophagus. Heartburn commonly accompanies gastroesophageal reflux and can occur during sleep as a symptom of SLEEP-RELATED GASTROESOPHAGEAL REFLUX. Heartburn during sleep may be due to the OBSTRUCTIVE SLEEP APNEA SYNDROME during which increased abdominal pressure produces a reflux of acid into the esophagus.

hertz (Hz)   Term synonymous with cycles per second (cps); it refers to a rhythm frequency most commonly applied to the ELECTROENCEPHALOGRAM (EEG).

hibernation   A state produced in animals as a response to seasonal environmental changes. During winter, animals are at risk in the environment due to the cold and the lack of food. Hibernating animals are typically those who are unable to travel long distances to make a major environmental change.

During hibernation, a sleep-like state exists with a reduction of metabolic activity and respiratory and circulatory rates. Body temperature can gradually drop to near freezing point; this is associated with a change in the electroencephalographic pattern, typically one of SLOW WAVE SLEEP with reduced or almost absent REM SLEEP. During the hibernation, the animal typically withdraws to its usual sleeping environment and reserves of stored fat are used to maintain the metabolic rate at only 10% to 15% of its normal rate. During the depth of the hibernation, the slow wave pattern of non-REM sleep gives way to a flattening of the electroencephalographic pattern, with no resemblance to sleep or wakefulness.

With the rising environmental temperatures at the end of hibernation, the electroencephalographic patterns revert back to normal as the body temperature slowly returns to a level typical during warmer seasons. (See also ELECTROENCEPHALOGRAM.)

histamine   A naturally occurring substance that is released during injury to tissues. The word is derived from the Greek word for tissue, *histos*. Histamine appears to act via two distinct receptors, the H1 and H2 receptors. The antihistamines have their effects primarily through blocking the H1 receptors; medications that inhibit gastric secretion work through blocking the H2 receptors.

There is some evidence to suggest that histamine is involved in the control of arousal and wakefulness. Animal studies have demonstrated that histamine is increased in the brains of animals during darkness, and that inhibition of histamine synthesis reduces wakefulness.

histocompatibility antigen testing   A test of the genetic constituents that play a role in determining rejection of a tissue graft. The major histocompatability complex (MHC) is composed of a group of genes that are located on chromosome 6, and the products of these genes are present on cell surfaces. The MHC in humans is called the human leukocyte antigen (HLA). There are three classes of human leukocyte genes and products, which are called class I, II, III. The HLA class I and class II products are located on cell surfaces. HLA class I products are found on most cell surfaces and consist of the HLA types A, B, C and E. The HLA class II products are found on the surface of the immune cells, such as lymphocytes. The HLA class II products consist of DR, DQ and DP.

The HLA D region has been found to have a specific association with the sleep disorder NARCOLEPSY.

hypernycthemeral sleep-wake syndrome   Term synonymous with NON-24-HOUR SLEEP-WAKE SYNDROME. The term *hypernycthemeral* is derived from the Greek word for *hyper,* meaning "above," and *nycthemeron,* meaning "pertaining to both night and day." This term was first proposed by Kokkoris, Weitzman and colleagues in 1978.

hypernycthemeral syndrome   See NON-24-HOUR SLEEP-WAKE SYNDROME.

hypersomnia   See EXCESSIVE SLEEPINESS.

hypertension   An elevation of blood pressure typically seen in patients who have a diastolic blood pressure greater than 90 millimeters of mercury or a systolic blood pressure greater than 160 millimeters of mercury.

Hypertension has been reported in approximately 30% of patients with the OBSTRUCTIVE SLEEP APNEA SYNDROME. Studies of groups of hypertensive patients have demonstrated that between 25% and 30% have episodes of oxygen desaturation during sleep or an abnormal number of apneic episodes during sleep.

Treatment of the obstructive sleep apnea syndrome is typically associated with a lowering of blood pressure or improved blood pressure control.

Some medications used to treat hypertension can affect the sleep wake cycle. Beta blockers, such as propranol, can produce sleep disturbance that is characterized by INSOMNIA; and there is evidence that beta blockers may even worsen the obstructive sleep apnea syndrome. Other antihypertensive medications, such as clonidine, can produce excessive sleepiness.

Because of the high association between hypertension and the obstructive sleep apnea syndrome, patients with hypertension should be questioned as to the presence of snoring, obesity, disturbed sleep and the occurrence of apneic episodes during sleep to see if they have that disorder.

hyperthyroidism   A disorder associated with excessive production of thyroid hormone from the thyroid gland in the neck. This is usually caused by enlargement or overactivity of the thyroid gland and produces characteristic symptoms of insomnia, weight loss, irritability, diarrhea, weakness, palpitations and tremulousness. Some patients with hyperthyroidism have a diffuse enlargement of the thyroid gland associated with antibodies that stimulate the thyroid gland. This disorder, which is termed Graves' disease, characteristically produces eye protrusion due to accumulation of excessive tissue behind the eyes.

The sleep disturbance associated with hyperthyroidism is typically one of difficulty in initiating and maintaining sleep. Sleep may be more restless and frequent arousals may be seen during polysomnographic testing. However, some patients have an increase in SLOW WAVE SLEEP.

Hyperthyroidism is treated by medications that suppress the activity of the thyroid gland, such as carbimazol, or by radioactive iodine, which destroys a portion of the thyroid gland. Surgical treatment may also be indicated. With treatment of the hyperthyroidism, the sleep disturbance usually resolves.

Following treatment for hyperthyroidism, sometimes the thyroid gland is rendered incapable of producing an adequate amount of thyroid hormone, thereby producing a deficiency in thyroid hormone. As a result, HYPOTHY-

ROIDISM may occur many years after chemical treatment of hyperthyroidism. Hypothyroidism is associated with the development of excessive lethargy and sleepiness. Muscle changes associated with the lack of thyroid hormone can produce impaired respiration during sleep, with the development of CENTRAL SLEEP APNEA SYNDROME or hypoventilation during sleep.

hypnagogic   Term applied to events occurring immediately prior to, or during, sleep onset; usually applied to dream activity during sleep onset, which is termed HYPNAGOGIC HALLUCINATIONS. Events that occur at the end of the sleep episode, in the transition from sleep to wakefulness, are called HYPNOPOMPIC.

hypnagogic hallucinations   Visual images that occur at sleep onset; most typically associated with REM SLEEP. Hypnagogic hallucinations are a characteristic feature of the sleep onset REM period that occurs in patients with NARCOLEPSY. Occasionally the imagery may be extremely frightening, and such situations have been termed TERRIFYING HYPNAGOGIC HALLUCINATIONS. Images that occur upon awakening or at wake times are called HYPNOPOMPIC hallucinations.

hypnic jerks   See SLEEP STARTS.

hypnogenic paroxysmal dystonia   The original term used for the disorder now called NOCTURNAL PAROXYSMAL DYSTONIA.

hypnolepsy   A term used for EXCESSIVE SLEEPINESS that resembles NARCOLEPSY. Hypnolepsy occurs as a result of a central nervous system lesion. The term is rarely used in current medical literature.

hypnology   Term not widely used that refers to the science of the phenomena of sleep. It is derived from the Greek words *hypno,* meaning "sleep," and *ology,* meaning "study of."

hypnopedia   This term refers to LEARNING DURING SLEEP.

hypnopompic   Characteristic of events that occur in the transition phase from sleep to wakefulness, most commonly at the end of the main sleep episode. Occasionally, vivid hallucinations will be perceived at this time, particularly in patients with NARCOLEPSY. The term *hynopompic* is also commonly used to apply to seizures that occur at the time of awakening, or immediately thereafter. (See also HYPNAGOGIC HALLUCINATIONS.)

hypnos   The ancient Greek god of sleep. Many words, such as *hypnosis, hypnology* and *hypnopedia,* have been derived form this Greek word.

hypnosis   A mental state induced in individuals, who have increased suggestibility, by means of focusing attention and eliminating distracting environmental stimuli. An individual in the state of hypnosis does not usually go into sleep, although the relaxation can allow normal physiological sleep to occur. Typically, hypnosis produces a slowing of the encephalographic pattern; however, typical stage two features, such as SLEEP SPINDLES or the characteristic delta waves of SLOW WAVE SLEEP, do not occur.

Some of the features of hypnosis are very similar to sleep-related phenomena, such as the AUTOMATIC BEHAVIOR in SLEEPWALKING that typically would be seen in deep slow-wave sleep. These features are associated with the awake electroencephalographic pattern in hypnosis.

Hypnosis has been reported to be effective in treating some sleep disorders, such as sleepwalking or SLEEP TERRORS; however, other investigators have failed to find it a useful treatment.

hypnotic-dependent sleep disorder   A sleep disturbance characterized by the intolerance for, or withdrawal of, HYPNOTICS. The sleep disturbance may be due to the chronic ingestion of hypnotic medications or their acute withdrawal. During chronic ingestion, the hypnotic effect tends to wear off and the underlying INSOMNIA may persist despite use of the medication. In some patients, there may be an increase in the metabolism of the hypnotic agent so that after an initial hypnotic effect in the first part of the night, there may be an increase in sleep disruption. After chronic ingestion of hypnotics, complete cessation of their ingestion leads to one or more nights of increased sleep fragmentation, which often results in the reinstitution of hypnotic therapy.

The medications most commonly associated with hypnotic-dependent sleep disorder are the BENZODIAZEPINES and BARBITURATES. However, other hypnotic agents may also produce this disorder.

Treatment of hypnotic-dependent sleep disorder rests upon gradual reduction and withdrawal of the hypnotic agent, sometimes with the substitution of a medication with hypnotic properties but less dependency effects. For example, a tricyclic ANTIDEPRESSANT medication might be substituted. Encouragement of good SLEEP HYGIENE is essential during the withdrawal process. Patients need to be reassured and counseled about a temporary reoccurrence of insomnia during the withdrawal of the medication. (See also REBOUND INSOMNIA.)

hypnotics   Also known as sleeping pills, sedative medications and sedative-hypnotic medications, hypnotics are medications that induce drowsiness and facilitate the onset and maintenance of sleep. Typically, hypnotics will induce sleep similar to natural sleep in that normal REM/NREM sleep cycling occurs, and the person is able to be easily aroused from sleep.

Various potions have been used to induce sleep since antiquity; ALCOHOL was one of the most commonly used substances. Bromides were used as hypnotics in the middle of the 19th century, but chloral hydrate is the only hypnotic agent still in regular use that was introduced before the turn of the century.

During the first half of the 20th century, the most commonly used hypnotic medications were the approximately 50 derivatives of the BAR-BITURATES. The barbiturates were widely used for their central nervous system depressant effects and employed as antiepileptic agents, antianxiety medications, muscle relaxants and hypnotics. They were also effective in inducing anesthesia and are currently still used for their anesthetic effect.

Because of the unwanted sedative and sleep-inducing effects of the barbiturates, other non-sedative anticonvulsants were discovered in the 1930s and 1940s. Subsequently, the BENZODIAZEPINE hypnotics were introduced into clinical medicine in the 1960s. More than 3,000 benzodiazepine derivatives have been synthesized and about 25 are in current clinical use. The benzodiazepines have the advantage of being effective sedatives and hypnotics with little potential for serious side effects; in particular, they have low potential for producing serious central nervous system depression. The most common benzodiazepine hypnotics in the United States include flurazepam (Dalmane), temazepam (Restoril), triazolam (Halcion) and zolpidem (Ambien).

Although the barbiturates now comprise less than 10% of all prescription hypnotics, they are still very effective hypnotics. Because of their abuse potential, possible interaction with alcohol, the possibility of lethal overdose and their effect of inducing liver enzymes that can increase the metabolism of many medications, the barbiturates are of limited usefulness as everyday hypnotics. The barbiturates that have most commonly been used as hypnotics are secobarbital (Seconal), amobarbital (Amytal) and pentobarbital (Nembutal).

Other nonbarbiturate, nonbenzodiazepine hypnotic agents are also available and come from a variety of pharmacological groups. One of the most commonly prescribed agents is chloral hydrate (Noctec), which is a relatively mild hypnotic but is useful in the elderly because of its low potential for adverse reactions.

A variety of nonprescription hypnotic medications are available as over-the-counter medications. Many of these medications are antihistamines that have sedative side effects, such as doxylamine, phenyltoloxamine and pyrilamine. These agents are not very effective in the treatment of INSOMNIA, can lead to the development of tolerance and prominent residual daytime central nervous system depression, and are not recommended for general hypnotic use.

In recent years, there has been the realization that insomnia is not a primary diagnosis but rather a symptom of many underlying causes. Many of the causes of insomnia can be treated without the use of a hypnotic agent. The use of hypnotics for LONG-TERM INSOMNIA is to be avoided because of the potential problems of tolerance and the potential for drug abuse. Chronic insomnia can be managed by behavioral means, psychotherapy or non-hypnotic medications. The most appropriate use of hypnotic medications appears to be in the treatment of transient or SHORT-TERM INSOMNIA, such as JET LAG, where their use is for a few days only. The selection of a hypnotic is ideally made according to its duration of action so that people with daytime tiredness and fatigue are best treated by means of a short-acting hypnotic. Patients with mild features of anxiety are best treated by an intermediate-acting hypnotic, whereas patients with more severe anxiety are best treated by a long-acting hypnotic.

hypocretin (orexin)   A peptide first identified in 1998. Produced by pre-hypocretin mRNA, hypocretin exists as two related peptides: hypocretin-1 (orexin A) and hypocretin-2 (orexin B). These neuropeptides are produced in neurons of the hypothalamus and affect two receptors: hypocretin receptor-1 and hypocretin receptor-2. The hypocretins are localized in the synaptic vesicles and possess neuroexcitatory effects.

An abnormal hypocretin receptor gene has been shown to be responsible for canine narcolepsy. Abnormalities of either the hypocretin receptor gene or of the production of hypocretins may be responsible for human NARCOLEPSY. Hypocretin cells are reduced or absent in patients with narcolepsy.

hypopnea   An episode of shallow breathing during sleep that lasts 10 seconds or longer; associated with a reduction in airflow of 50% or more and a fall in the oxygen saturation level. The presence of some airflow distinguishes this event from apneic episodes. Hypopneas are usually seen in persons who have SLEEP-RELATED BREATHING DISORDERS, such as CENTRAL SLEEP APNEA SYNDROME or OBSTRUCTIVE SLEEP APNEA SYNDROME. (See also APNEA, APNEA-HYPOPNEA INDEX.)

hypothalamus   A region at the base of the brain believed to have an important role in the maintenance of sleep and wakefulness. Original investigations by Constantin von Economo on patients suffering from encephalitis lethargica in the second decade of this century showed that the anterior hypothalamus was commonly responsible for INSOMNIA, whereas lesions of the posterior hypothalamus were associated with excessive sleepiness. The hypothalamus is also involved in many other autonomic processes including thermoregulation and control of food and fluid intake.

The hypothalamus has connections with the retino-hypothalamic tract, which leads from the retina to the optic chiasm, and synapses in the SUPRACHIASMATIC NUCLEI for the control of CIRCADIAN RHYTHMS. Isolation of the suprachiasmatic nuclei of the hypothalamus will disrupt circadian rhythmicity although the temperature rhythm will continue. Transplantation of fetal suprachiasmatic nuclei cells into other animals who have had the suprachiasmatic nucleus destroyed will return circadian rhythmicity.

Other experiments of either stimulating or lesioning cells of the hypothalamic region have demonstrated effects on sleep or sleepiness; however, the exact role of the hypothalamic centers in the control of sleep and wakefulness is unknown.

hypothyroidism   A disorder characterized by a loss of production of thyroid hormone from the thyroid gland; caused by an intrinsic abnormality of the thyroid gland, or by reduced stimulation of the thyroid gland due to the loss of the brain thyroid-stimulating hormone. Thyroid deficiency can produce respiratory muscle failure with resulting OBSTRUCTIVE SLEEP APNEA SYNDROME or ALVEOLAR HYPOVENTILATION, which when severe may require the institution of mechanical ventilation. Hypothyroidism impairs the ventilation responses to HYPOXIA or hypercapnia and, in addition, leads to increased weight gain and deposition of mucopolysaccharides in the tissues of the upper airway.

Severe hypothyroidism can also produce tiredness, fatigue and sleepiness because of the reduced body metabolism. The diagnosis is made by the demonstration of a low free-thyroxine level in the blood, typically in association with an elevated, thyroid-stimulating hormone level. A thyroid scan is usually necessary to provide information on the function and anatomy of the thyroid gland. If the thyroid-stimulating hormone level is abnormally low, a brain CT scan, or MRI scan, is necessary to assess pituitary function.

The presence of sleep-related disorders, such as obstructive sleep apnea syndrome, can be confirmed by polysomnographic monitoring and the degree of daytime sleepiness by MULTIPLE SLEEP LATENCY TESTING.

The symptoms of hypothyroidism can be quite subtle, and it is therefore an important diagnosis to consider in any patient who has the obstructive sleep apnea syndrome. Thyroid levels should be checked in all patients, especially before surgical management of the syndrome.

Treatment of hypothyroidism involves replacement of thyroid hormone, typically with between 50 and 200 micrograms of thyroxine per day. The symptoms of daytime sleepiness and the features of SLEEP-RELATED BREATHING DISORDERS rapidly improve with replacement therapy. As hypothyroidism leads to a general increase in body weight, treatment often leads to weight reduction.

Severe hypothyroidism results in myxedema, which is characterized by generalized mucopolysaccharide accumulation throughout the body, resulting in thickening of the facial features and doughy induration of the skin. Respiratory depression is common in myxedema as are sleep-related breathing disorders, and the patient can lapse into myxedema coma, which is a hypothermic, stuporous state. Myxedema coma is frequently fatal. (See also POLYSOMNOGRAPHY, UPPER AIRWAY OBSTRUCTION.)

hypoventilation   See ALVEOLAR HYPOVENTILATION.

hypoxemia   A low level of oxygen in the blood. Hypoxemia during sleep typically occurs in patients with SLEEP-RELATED BREATHING DISORDERS such as the OBSTRUCTIVE SLEEP APNEA SYNDROME. The hypoxemia is usually detected by an oximeter, which measures the oxygen saturation of the hemoglobin. Hypoxemia can have important effects upon the body, particularly the cardiovascular system, as chronic hypoxemia can produce pulmonary hypertension that in turn can produce right-sided heart failure. Hypoxemia can also cause cardiac irritation, leading to cardiac irregularity or cardiac ischemia.

   Assisted ventilation during sleep may be required for patients who have hypoxemia, by means of either CONTINUOUS POSITIVE AIRWAY PRESSURE (CPAP) or artificial ventilation devices. Oxygen therapy, respiratory stimulant medications or relief of UPPER AIRWAY OBSTRUCTION by surgery are other means employed to relieve hypoxemia in some patients.

hypoxia   A reduction of oxygen supply to tissues below the level necessary to maintain normal cellular metabolism. Hypoxia can be produced either by a reduction in the oxygen level of the inspired air, such as that seen at high altitudes or due to UPPER AIRWAY OBSTRUCTION, or by means of an abnormality of the lung whereby oxygen is unable to adequately diffuse into the blood. Lung disease is a common cause of tissue hypoxia due to the deficient oxygenation of the blood (hypoxemia).

   Hypoxia due to low inspired levels of oxygen can produce periodic breathing, which causes an alternating pattern of hyperventilation and hypoventilation that is a characteristic feature of ALTITUDE INSOMNIA (acute mountain sickness). Upper airway obstruction, which occurs in the OBSTRUCTIVE SLEEP APNEA SYNDROME, can be associated with a reduction in lung oxygen levels, thereby producing hypoxemia with resultant arousal and ventilatory stimulation.

   Chronic lung disease, such as that seen in CHRONIC OBSTRUCTIVE PULMONARY DISEASE, particularly emphysema, is associated with impaired blood gas transfer and hypoxemia. Patients with chronic obstructive pulmonary disease can develop worsening hypoxemia during sleep, especially during REM sleep.

   As a result of hypoxia, sleep becomes fragmented, with an increased number of arousals and awakenings related to the hypoxemia. The direct effects of hypoxemia can be detrimental on the cardiovascular as well as other body systems. (See also CHEYNE-STOKES RESPIRATION.)

Hz   See HERTZ.

I

idiopathic hypersomnia   Disorder associated with EXCESSIVE SLEEPINESS; believed to be of central nervous system cause. This disorder has similarities to narcolepsy but lacks the associated REM phenomena. Features such as CATAPLEXY, SLEEP PARALYSIS and HYPNAGOGIC HALLUCINATIONS do not occur in patients with idiopathic hypersomnia.

Idiopathic hypersomnia has its onset during adolescence and early adulthood and is characterized by gradually increasing daytime sleepiness. Typically, patients with idiopathic hypersomnia will take frequent NAPS, usually of one to two hours in duration. The major sleep episode may be of normal or longer than normal duration.

Polysomnographic studies (see POLYSOMNOGRAPHY) demonstrate a normal or prolonged total sleep time without evidence of sleep disruption. Daytime MULTIPLE SLEEP LATENCY TESTING demonstrates a mean sleep latency that is consistent with pathological sleepiness but is characterized by the absence of naps with REM sleep. Typically, patients with idiopathic hypersomnia will develop deep sleep stages, such as stage three or four sleep during nap opportunities.

Central nervous system tests, including brain imaging and encephalography, are usually normal.

Treatment is similar to that for improving alertness in patients with narcolepsy. It involves the use of STIMULANT MEDICATIONS, such as pemoline (Cylert), methylphenidate (Ritalin) or dextroamphetamine (Dexedrine). Treatment is initiated with pemoline and may be changed to methylphenidate or dextroamphetamine if pemoline does not give an adequate response. Usually treatment is lifelong; there is no evidence for remission of the underlying sleepiness.

idiopathic insomnia   A lifelong form of insomnia that is believed to have a neurochemical basis; originally termed *childhood onset insomnia*. This insomnia is believed to be due to an inability to achieve a sustained high quality of sleep. Idiopathic insomnia is typically characterized by a prolonged SLEEP LATENCY, frequent awakenings at night and sometimes an EARLY MORNING AROUSAL. It is possible that people with idiopathic insomnia are those who comprise the lower 5% of the normal distribution of ability to have a normal quality sleep period. Elements of ANXIETY and hyperarousal may be present in such individuals, but there is no gross psychopathology warranting a diagnosis of ANXIETY DISORDER nor any evidence to suggest a diagnosis of DEPRESSION.

Idiopathic insomnia needs to be differentiated from PSYCHOPHYSIOLOGICAL INSOMNIA, which involves learned negative associations with sleep.

Idiopathic insomnia is more likely to be stable over time, with poor quality sleep occurring in all sleep environments; the insomnia does not have the intermittent exacerbations that are seen with psychophysiological insomnia. Psychophysiological insomnia also rarely occurs from childhood. Individuals who are SHORT SLEEPERS typically awake refreshed in the morning and lack a complaint of poor quality sleep or of frequent awakenings as do those with idiopathic insomnia.

INADEQUATE SLEEP HYGIENE may be confused with idiopathic insomnia, although the intermittent nature of inadequate sleep hygiene contrasts with the more fixed complaint of idiopathic insomnia.

Polysomnographic studies of individuals with idiopathic insomnia have demonstrated severe sleep disruption, which is characterized by a long sleep latency and frequent arousals with early morning awakening. Sleep efficiencies are usually greatly reduced and there may be specific sleep stage abnormalities, such as reduction of spindle activity in stage two sleep or reduced rapid eye movements during REM SLEEP. As with psychophysiological insomnia, a reversed first night effect may be seen in which individuals sleep much better in the sleep laboratory on the first night because of the change in their habitual environment.

Idiopathic insomnia is typically lifelong and appears to be genetically transmitted. There is some suggestion that babies born during a difficult labor may be predisposed to developing this disorder. Its prevalence is unknown. There is some evidence to suggest an alteration in serotonin metabolism with inadequate production of serotonin.

Treatment of idiopathic insomnia is generally unsatisfactory. Attention to SLEEP HYGIENE and BEHAVIORAL TREATMENT OF INSOMNIA, such as STIMULUS CONTROL THERAPY and SLEEP RESTRICTION THERAPY, are useful.

imipramine   See ANTIDEPRESSANTS.

impaired sleep-related penile erections   The inability to achieve a penile erection during sleep. (This term is preferred to *sleep-related penile tumescence.*) All males, from infancy to old age, have penile erections that occur during REM SLEEP. The inability to achieve an adequate erection during sleep at night may help differentiate an organic from a psychogenic cause of impotence. MEDICATIONS and sleep disorders that disrupt REM sleep may also cause impaired sleep-related penile erections. The measurement of penile circumference and rigidity during sleep is an important test for differentiating organic impotence.

If impaired sleep-related penile erections are present, other investigations, including penile blood pressure, penile neurodiagnostic tests and hormonal tests may be indicated in order to determine the cause of the impaired erectile ability. Occasionally, sleep disorders, such as OBSTRUCTIVE SLEEP APNEA SYNDROME, are associated with impaired sleep-related penile erections, which are improved by treatment of the sleep apnea syndrome.

The medication Viagra is effective at improving erectile ability if taken one hour before sleep, in those who have erectile difficulties.

In many patients with organic impotence, the only means of treatment is by the surgical implantation of an artificial penile prosthesis. Patients with normal erectile ability during sleep, but with a complaint of impotence, may best be treated by means of sex, marital or psychiatric therapy. (See also ALCOHOLISM, SLEEP-RELATED PAINFUL ERECTIONS.)

impotence   The inability to attain an adequate penile erection for sexual intercourse. Impotence may be due to psychological or psychiatric disorders, such as DEPRESSION or ANXIETY DISORDERS. Physical causes of impaired erectile ability commonly include vascular disorders, such as peripheral vascular disease of HYPERTENSION, or neurological disorders, such as peripheral neuropathies or spinal cord lesions (such as those due to a spinal cord injury). It is also a common manifestation of diabetes, probably because of a combination of vascular and neurological abnormalities associated with that disorder. Impotence also can occur in the OBSTRUCTIVE SLEEP APNEA SYNDROME, where it appears to have a higher prevalence than in the general population. Treatment of the obstructive sleep apnea syndrome leads to improve erectile ability.

(See also IMPAIRED SLEEP-RELATED PENILE ERECTIONS, NOCTURNAL PENILE TUMESCENCE TEST, SLEEP-RELATED PENILE ERECTION.)

inadequate sleep hygiene   Disturbance that results from practices that can have a negative effect on the sleep pattern. Improved SLEEP HYGIENE involves enhancing factors that will allow sleep to become more organized. Substances such as CAFFEINE, NICOTINE from cigarette SMOKING and other stimulants are likely to cause sleep onset difficulties or the inability to sustain quality sleep. ALCOHOL can also cause AROUSAL, but more commonly produces sedation followed by an arousal during the withdrawal phase.

Vigorous exercise before bedtime, intense mental stimulation late at night or late night social activities clearly increase arousal and reduce sleep quality. Spending an excessive amount of time in bed, irregular sleep onset and wake times or daily NAPS can all disturb the normal circadian pattern of sleep and wakefulness, leading to a breakdown in the sleep organization.

Inadequate sleep hygiene can lead to a persistent sleep disturbance, which develops into a PSYCHOPHYSIOLOGICAL INSOMNIA because of the learned negative associations due to the sleep disruption. Inadequate sleep hygiene can also accompany sleep disorders of other types. For example, INSOMNIA due to DEPRESSION may be complicated by spending an excessive time in bed and varying sleep onset and wake times. The start of the sleep disturbance typically occurs between young adulthood and old age; however, it can occur in adolescence.

Sleep studies document prolonged sleep latency, frequent nocturnal awakenings, early morning arousal and reduced sleep efficiency.

Treatment of inadequate sleep hygiene is to eliminate the negative behaviors, which usually leads to rapid resolution of the sleep disturbance.

infant sleep   Infant sleep is first recognized at a conceptual age of about 32 weeks. At this time, the infant state can be differentiated into WAKE-FULNESS, QUIET SLEEP and ACTIVE SLEEP.

At the time of birth, the infant demonstrates a sleep pattern totaling 16 to 18 hours of sleep during the 24 hours. Sleep is achieved in short episodes of three to four hours, with brief awakenings. Sleep is evenly distributed over the day, and gradually the amount of sleep at night compared to during the daytime increases, so that a clear night-day differentiation is evident by three months of age.

The sleep episodes of the infant are characterized by approximately 50% of REM and 50% of non-REM sleep. Infants will go from wakefulness directly into REM sleep, a feature that is not seen in older children or adults unless some pathology is present. The NREM-REM SLEEP CYCLE is slower than that seen in adults, occurring approximately every 60 minutes.

The EEG pattern begins to resemble the sleep of adults by three months of age. SLEEP SPINDLE activity begins at this time and within the next few months K-COMPLEXES can be seen. The total amount of sleep gradually falls so that by six months the infant is sleeping approximately 15 hours per day. As the sleep-wake pattern becomes more consolidated at night, the latency into REM sleep becomes biphasic so that the shortest REM latencies are usually seen between 4 and 8 A.M. whereas the longer latencies are typically seen between midday and 4 P.M. Longer REM latencies become more apparent following longer periods of wakefulness, and the prevalence of REM sleep during the daytime gradually reduces over the first year of life.

Because REM and non-REM sleep cannot be thoroughly distinguished at this stage, the terms *active sleep* and *quiet sleep* are used. Active sleep is characterized by body movement activity with occasional vocalizations, whereas quiet sleep consists of cessation of body movements as well as the EEG features consistent with non-REM sleep. The characteristic EEG pattern of active sleep is a low voltage, irregular pattern with 5 to 8 Hz theta and 1 to 5 Hz delta activity.

Quiet sleep is characterized by high voltage, slow wave activity in the delta range. There is also the trace alternant pattern of high voltage slow waves mixed with rapid low voltage activity that occurs in bursts alternating with periods of low voltage "flat" periods. The eye movement activity is increased during active sleep and absent during slow wave sleep. The muscle tone activity is elevated during quiet sleep and relatively low during active sleep.

Some sleep is not able to be differentiated into active and quiet and is often called indeterminant sleep. This type of sleep decreases as the infant develops. (See also ONTOGENY OF SLEEP.)

infant sleep apnea   A variety of respiratory disturbances that can occur in infants, predominantly during sleep. Infants who stop breathing during sleep often raise a fear of the SUDDEN INFANT DEATH SYNDROME (SIDS), in which otherwise healthy infants die suddenly during sleep. However, brief apneic pauses are common in infants; even for infants who have longer respiratory pauses, there is little evidence to substantiate that this is predictive of SIDS. Children who have very prolonged apneic pauses, greater than 20 seconds in duration, particularly premature infants, will have approximately a 5% greater risk of SIDS than otherwise healthy children. However, the observation of an infant who stops breathing and has some change in color, either by cyanosis or pallor, and who is often very limp at the time, is a frightening occurrence for a mother or father. Although the majority of such witnessed episodes are not associated with any significant cardiorespiratory events during infancy, there are a number of disorders in which respiration may be greatly compromised during sleep.

Infants who suffer other medical illnesses at the time of birth, either infection, trauma or hemorrhages, are more likely to develop respiratory irregularity that will be most prominent during sleep; in such circumstances some children may require aggressive intervention in order to maintain adequate VENTILATION. A number of sleep-related respiratory disturbances can occur in infants, such as the OBSTRUCTIVE SLEEP APNEA SYNDROME, CENTRAL SLEEP APNEA SYNDROME, CENTRAL ALVEOLAR HYPOVENTILATION SYNDROME and apnea of prematurity. The obstructive sleep apnea syndrome is characterized by UPPER AIRWAY OBSTRUCTION that occurs predominantly during sleep, particularly during REM sleep, and is associated with a reduction in oxygen levels in the blood as well as increases in carbon dioxide values. Apneic episodes of similar duration can occur in the central sleep apnea syndrome, but in this disorder upper airway obstruction is not the primary event, although there is a decrease in central nervous system respiratory drive. This form of apnea is more common in infants who have central nervous system lesions. Some infants do not have apneic pauses but will have prolonged episodes of reduced ventilation during sleep, with associated oxygen desaturation and increases in carbon dioxide levels. This form of respiratory disturbance, termed *central alveolar hypoventilation syndrome–congenital type*, may require assisted ventilation until the infant is able to sustain ventilation spontaneously after maturation of the respiratory system.

infant sleep disorders   INFANT SLEEP is very different from the sleep of young children or adults. It has a high percentage of REM sleep that fills

50% of the total sleep time, and sleep occurs in brief episodes throughout the 24-hour day. Approximately two-thirds of the day is spent in sleep.

During the first three months of life, the child's sleep appears to occur with a cyclical pattern that is slightly greater than 24 hours; therefore, the major sleep episode occurs slightly later on each successive day. This pattern, which is known as FREE RUNNING, is due to the underlying tendency of our biological circadian rhythms to have a period length slightly longer than 24 hours. This tendency in the infant is usually not a concern so long as the typical ENVIRONMENTAL TIME CUES are instituted to maintain the major sleep episode over the nighttime hours. If these environmental time cues, such as quieter nights and daytime stimulation, are not instituted, a delayed sleep pattern will develop. As a result, the major sleep episode occurs at a slightly later time and so the sleep episode will rotate around the clock. This is called the NON-24-HOUR SLEEP-WAKE SYNDROME and occurs in infants only if appropriate environmental cues are not instituted.

Colic is perhaps the most widely recognized cause of awakenings and crying at night in infants within the first four months of age. Usually colic occurs within the first three weeks of age and reduces in frequency so that about 50% of infants with colic will not have attacks after two months of age, and most infants will have outgrown colic by four months of age. The cause of colic is unknown and, although it is suspected of being due to stomach cramps, there is no scientific evidence to indicate that colic is of gastrointestinal cause. Current belief is that it is due to an immature central nervous system. There are some irregularities of behavior with increased arousal and sensitivity to environmental stimuli that cause the awakenings. Colic can lead to the development of more chronic sleep disturb-ances in the older infant if it is not appropriately managed in the first few months of life. The institution of good SLEEP HYGIENE and providing the appropriate sleep times is essential to ensure that more persistent sleep disturbances do not occur.

A benign form of abnormal movements can occur in newborn infants and is called BENIGN NEONATAL SLEEP MYOCLONUS. This disorder is associated with jerking movements of limbs, and even of the face or trunk, but is not associated with underlying epilepsy, and usually resolves within the first few weeks of life.

Usually the time between the second and sixth months of life is associated with a consolidated nighttime sleep episode and several daytime NAPS and is a relatively peaceful time for the mother. It is during this time that the major changes in the structure of the infant's sleep are occurring and so it is a critical time for the infant. Patterns of cortisol and growth hormone production are developing and become established by six months of age.

During the first six months of life, the respiratory system undergoes development. It is one of the most fragile body systems and is susceptible to variations that can be noted by the mother. Most healthy infants will have episodes of cessation of breathing that occur and last up to 20 seconds in duration. These episodes may concern a mother but may be a part of normal development and decrease in frequency as the child develops. Premature infants are more likely to have these apneas. A syndrome called apnea of prematurity can exist where prolonged episodes may be associated with changes in oxygenation of the blood, and therefore a child may briefly turn blue or pale in color. Within the first few months of life, these episodes spontaneously decrease as a more healthy infant pattern of ventilation develops. Healthy premature infants with persistence of prolonged episodes of apnea may be predisposed to the SUDDEN INFANT DEATH SYNDROME, a disorder that is of concern to most mothers because it is sudden, unexpected and occurs in otherwise healthy infants.

At six months of age, the infant's sleep pattern becomes lighter and the number of awakenings can increase. It is at this time that the infant is becoming more aware of the world, and the frequent awakenings and difficulty in initiating sleep may cause the parents concern and anxiety. It is important during this time that positive sleep hygiene practices are put into place, particularly the institution of limits on the time that the child is put down for sleep and the time that the child is allowed to sleep undisturbed. An appropriate amount of daytime stimulation is necessary so that the development of a full period of wakefulness can gradually occur. Physical illnesses, such as ear or other infections, can cause the sleep pattern to be interrupted, but as long as the appropriate cues and positive associations with sleep are instituted, the disturbance is usually only temporary.

One form of insomnia, related to an allergy to cow's milk, is called FOOD ALLERGY INSOMNIA and can produce irritability in the infant, resulting in frequent arousals and crying. Very often there are other manifestations of the allergy, such as skin difficulties and gastrointestinal upset. The close association of the onset of the insomnia with the change from breast-feeding to cow's milk is the first indication that this form of sleep disturbance might be present. Elimination of cow's milk in the diet brings about a resolution of the insomnia.

The main forms of pathological sleep disturbance in the infant include ventilatory abnormalities, such as the obstructive sleep apnea syndrome, or neurological disorders, such as epilepsy. The SLEEP-RELATED BREATHING DISORDERS are evidenced by difficulty in breathing during sleep or prolonged episodes of cessation of breathing. Apneic episodes of greater than 20 seconds in duration are an indication of pathology, and may be due either to upper airway obstruction or a central cause. Typical obstructive sleep apnea syndrome is less likely to occur in the infant than in the older child who has enlarged tonsils. When upper airway obstruction occurs, it usually occurs in both wakefulness and sleep. Excessive sleepiness is not evident in the infant, and the main features of upper airway obstruction are difficulty in breathing and the change in coloration or heart rate.

Upper airway obstruction is more common in infants with craniofacial abnormalities, such as those due to a small jaw or an enlarged tongue. Central apnea may be due to neurological disorders that may be have occurred during the time of a difficult delivery, such as an intracerebral hemorrhage. Central nervous system lesions can affect the control of breathing and lead to frequent episodes of breathing cessation during sleep, commonly called the CENTRAL SLEEP APNEA SYNDROME.

Many illnesses of an infective, biochemical or anatomical nature can predispose the infant to central apnea. For most infants, treatment of the underlying medical disorder will lead to resolution of the apneic episodes. However, some infants with primary respiratory difficulty may need to have artificial ventilation until the respiratory symptom has improved so that spontaneous control is possible. There has not been demonstrated a clear association between infants with apneic episodes of less than 20 seconds in duration and the subsequent development of sudden infant death syndrome.

Central nervous system disorders, such as epilepsy, can cause abnormal movements in infants during sleep. These episodes are often the result of central nervous system lesions, such as an intracerebral tumor. Metabolic abnormalities due to a change in the blood electrolytes are a common cause of seizures in the newborn infant, and with correction of the biochemical changes the seizure manifestations resolve. Sometimes epilepsy can be the cause of apneic episodes.

initiating and maintaining sleep   See DISORDERS OF INITIATING AND MAINTAINING SLEEP (DIMS).

insomnia   Term derived from the Latin words *in,* meaning "no," and *somnus,* meaning "sleep." Insomnia strictly means the inability to sleep.

Insomnia is applied to people who have a complaint of unrefreshing sleep, or difficulty in initiating or maintaining sleep. Although the term has been used to refer to a disorder in which sleep disturbance can be objectively documented, it is more generally used for any disorder associated with a complaint of disturbed or unrefreshing sleep.

Although many different classifications of insomnia have been developed, the differential diagnosis developed in the *International Classification of Sleep Disorders* has been clinically very useful. However, insomnia can be divided into slightly different groups associated with the following causes: behavioral or psychophysiological causes; psychiatric causes; environmental causes; drug-dependent factors; those associated with respiratory or movement disorders; those associated with alterations in the timing of the sleep-wake pattern or associated with the parasomnias or neurological disorders; those without any objective sleep disturbance; idiopathic insomnia; and a miscellaneous group of other causes of insomnia.

Insomnia Associated with Behavioral or Psychophysiological Causes

Insomnia associated with behavioral or psychophysiological causes includes ADJUSTMENT SLEEP DISORDER, PSYCHOPHYSIOLOGICAL INSOMNIA, INADEQUATE SLEEP HYGIENE, LIMIT-SETTING SLEEP DISORDER, SLEEP-ONSET ASSOCIATION DISORDER, NOCTURNAL EATING (DRINKING) SYNDROME.

These disorders often respond to the institution of SLEEP HYGIENE or BEHAVIORAL TREATMENT OF INSOMNIA.

Insomnia Associated with Psychiatric Disorders

Includes the mood disorders, such as depression or manic-depressive disease, PSYCHOSES, anxiety disorders, including PANIC DISORDERS, and ALCOHOLISM. Specific treatment of the psychiatric state is required; good sleep hygiene and behavioral treatments of insomnia can assist the resolution of the sleep complaint.

Environmental Factors

Particularly noise, temperature, or abnormal light exposure; may be important in the production of some forms of insomnia. The ingestion of some foods can produce a FOOD ALLERGY INSOMNIA, and toxins can produce a TOXIN-INDUCED SLEEP DISORDER.

Medications and Insomnia

Medications can be associated with the development of insomnia, with the chronic use of hypnotics leading to HYPNOTIC-DEPENDENT SLEEP DISORDER, which may exacerbate upon withdrawal of the hypnotic agent. The chronic use of stimulants, such as CAFFEINE, or weight-reduction medications, such as amphetamines, can produce a STIMULANT-DEPENDENT SLEEP DISORDER. The chronic use of alcohol for sleep purposes can lead to an ALCOHOL-DEPENDENT SLEEP DISORDER. Gradual withdrawal of the offending agent under clinical supervision, with maintenance of good sleep hygiene, is usually all that is required for the treatment of these forms of insomnia.

Sleep-Related Breathing Disorders

Can be associated with the complaint of insomnia, particularly in the elderly. OBSTRUCTIVE SLEEP APNEA SYNDROME, CENTRAL SLEEP APNEA SYNDROME and CENTRAL ALVEOLAR HYPOVENTILATION SYNDROME can all produce awakenings at night, with little evidence of daytime impairment of respiratory function. Polysomnographic investigation is usually necessary to understand the severity and extent of these disorders to determine appropriate treatment.

Other respiratory disorders, such as CHRONIC OBSTRUCTIVE PULMONARY DISEASE and SLEEP-RELATED ASTHMA, can have direct sleep effects. Insomnia may also be exacerbated by the RESPIRATORY STIMULANTS, such as the xanthines, that are used to treat these disorders.

Altitude Insomnia

Occurring at high altitudes and caused by the low level of inspired oxygen tension, which produces a periodic pattern of breathing often associated with insomnia. It usually resolves upon return to a lower altitude.

Insomnia and Abnormal Movement Disorders

Insomnia may be associated with abnormal movement disorders during sleep. Typical SLEEP STARTS, or hypnic jerks, can cause a sleep-onset insomnia, as can the RESTLESS LEGS SYNDROME, which is associated with disagreeable sensations in the legs. Rarely, nocturnal CRAMPS may cause sudden awakenings during sleep, leading to the complaint of insomnia.

The PERIODIC LIMB MOVEMENT DISORDER is a movement disorder that occurs solely during sleep. The patient may not be aware of it, but it is typically seen by a bed partner. It is associated with periodic movements of the limbs and disturbed quality of sleep, often leading to the complaint of insomnia or unrestful sleep.

The REM SLEEP BEHAVIOR DISORDER is associated with excessive movement and abnormal behavior during sleep. Insomnia also occurs in NOCTURNAL PAROXYSMAL DYSTONIA and RHYTHMIC MOVEMENT DISORDER, when it persists into adolescence or adulthood.

Insomnia Related to the Timing of Sleep

With the development of the science of CHRONOBIOLOGY, there has been the recognition that disorders of the timing of sleep are also associated with disturbed sleep quality. This is most evident to the general population through its awareness of TIME ZONE CHANGE (JET LAG) SYNDROME and SHIFT-WORK SLEEP DISORDER. A delay in the onset of sleep can produce a sleep onset insomnia in adolescence termed DELAYED SLEEP PHASE SYNDROME. In this disorder, the sleep pattern is delayed with regard to typical sleep times. Similarly, the opposite sleep pattern, the ADVANCED SLEEP PHASE SYNDROME, can cause an EARLY MORNING AROUSAL and a complaint of insomnia. Sleep occurs at an earlier time than desired. This particular sleep pattern is more common in the elderly, who find it difficult to stay awake late at night and yet awaken early in the morning, while it is still dark.

Behavioral or neurological disorders can produce an irregular sleep pattern characterized by frequently interrupted sleep episodes throughout the 24-hour day—the IRREGULAR SLEEP-WAKE PATTERN. Rarely, the NON-24-HOUR SLEEP-WAKE SYNDROME can occur; here, the sleep pattern continues to rotate around the clock, with a period length of 25, and not 24, hours.

Neurological Disorders and Insomnia

Neurological disorders are common causes of the inability to maintain sleep, and those most commonly seen, particularly in the elderly, include PARKINSONISM and DEMENTIA. Degenerative disorders and epilepsy are two other neurological disorders that commonly present with the complaint of disturbed sleep. Appropriate treatment of these neurological disorders includes attention to good sleep hygiene, with or without the use of hypnotic agents. FATAL FAMILIAL INSOMNIA, a rare form of insomnia, has a progressive deteriorating course that eventually leads to death. There is no known treatment.

Insomnia Associated with Parasomnias

Insomnia can be caused by PARASOMNIAS that do not typically produce complaints of insomnia or EXCESSIVE SLEEPINESS. CONFUSIONAL AROUSALS, SLEEP TERRORS, NIGHTMARES and SLEEP HYPERHIDROSIS (sweating) may cause awakenings that lead to insomnia.

Insomnia with No Objective Sleep Disturbance

A form of insomnia due to a misperception or misinterpretation of sleep. SLEEP STATE MISPERCEPTION, previously known as pseudoinsomnia, occurs when patients find sleep totally unrefreshing, when they deny having been asleep, despite having had a full night of good quality sleep. This unusual disorder is poorly understood and is often resistant to attempts at treatment.

Awakening at night with a sensation of an inability to breathe, termed the SLEEP CHOKING SYNDROME, can occur, yet polysomnographically documented sleep is entirely normal. This disorder might be an unusual manifestation of an anxiety or panic disorder.

Some people have a physiological requirement for less sleep than most and can be classed as SHORT SLEEPERS. However, the desire for longer sleep may lead to the complaint of insomnia. Reassurance that the short sleep is physiologically appropriate may be all that is required.

Idiopathic Insomnia

Some patients appear to have a lifelong inability to sustain good quality sleep, and the term IDIOPATHIC INSOMNIA (or childhood-onset insomnia) has been applied. This sleep disorder is believed to be due to a genetic or acquired abnormality in the sleep maintenance systems of the brain so that normal good quality sleep is never obtained. These patients are particularly susceptible to minor stressful or environmental stimuli, which cause an exacerbation of the insomnia. Lifelong attention to good sleep hygiene is necessary for such patients.

Other Causes of Insomnia

There are many other causes of insomnia, the majority of which are related to underlying medical disorders. Other causes of sleep disturbance that can lead to a complaint of insomnia include SLEEP-RELATED GASTROESOPHAGEAL REFLUX, FIBROSITIS SYNDROME, MENSTRUAL-ASSOCIATED SLEEP DISORDER, PREGNANCY-RELATED SLEEP DISORDER, TERRIFYING HYPNAGOGIC HALLUCINATIONS, SLEEP-RELATED ABNORMAL SWALLOWING SYNDROME and SLEEP-RELATED LARYNGOSPASM.

All of the above-mentioned sleep disorders need to be considered in the differential diagnosis of the patient presenting with insomnia. A detailed clinical and psychological history will often point to the cause of the insomnia without the need for objective polysomnographic evaluation (see POLYSOMNOGRAPHY); however, many of the above disorders need polysomnographic documentation. Typically, the patient will be evaluated for the quality of sleep, as well as for abnormal physiological events during sleep. One or two nights of recording in a SLEEP DISORDER CENTER is usually necessary. This information, along with the historical information taken at the initial evaluation, usually leads to a precise diagnosis so an accurate treatment plan can be outlined.

Treatment

See Chapter 3: Insomnia and Chapter 10: The Interplay Between Psychology and Sleep.

insufficient sleep syndrome   Disorder characterized by EXCESSIVE SLEEPINESS during the day due to an inadequate amount of sleep at night; typically follows episodes of sleep deprivation that have reoccurred over weeks or months. Often the inadequate nocturnal sleep is unappreciated by the patient, who presents the complaint of excessive sleepiness of unknown cause. Examination of a SLEEP LOG may demonstrate the characteristic features: shorter than normal major sleep episode with a short latency to sleep onset; and an early morning awakening, usually by an alarm or other disturbance. Polysomnographic monitoring may be necessary if the cause of daytime sleepiness is unclear or if other disorders of excessive sleepiness are considered.

Typically, insufficient sleep syndrome is a disorder seen in adolescents or young adulthood; however, it can occur at any age.

This disorder must to be differentiated from IDIOPATHIC HYPERSOMNIA, which is characterized by a normal or prolonged sleep episode at night, and from NARCOLEPSY, which is typically associated with REM sleep phenomena such as CATAPLEXY, SLEEP PARALYSIS and HYPNAGOGIC HALLUCINATIONS.

Treatment rests upon a regular extension of TOTAL SLEEP TIME to ensure that the individual's sleep duration meets his or her physiological needs. The amount of sleep time required varies among individuals; for some it may need to be as long as nine hours on a regular basis. (See also DISORDERS OF EXCESSIVE SOMNOLENCE.)

internal arousal insomnia   Term used for a state of heightened arousal that impairs the ability to fall asleep or to stay asleep. This form of heightened arousal is typically seen in insomnia disorders such as PSYCHOPHYSIOLOGICAL INSOMNIA, ANXIETY DISORDERS or agitated DEPRESSION. At the desired sleep time, patients become more alert with an increase in mental activity, because a flood of thoughts prevents them from "turning off" their minds. (See also INSOMNIA, MOOD DISORDERS.)

International Classification of Sleep Disorders   In 1985, the Association of Sleep Disorder Centers initiated the process of revising the original *Diagnostic Classification of Sleep and Arousal Disorders*. The original classification was published in 1979 in the journal SLEEP. This classification has been very widely used throughout the world; however, with the recent advances in SLEEP DISORDERS MEDICINE it was believed that a revision was required.

A committee was headed by Michael Thorpy, M.D., and consisted of 18 clinical sleep disorder specialists who set about the process of revising the classification.

The classification scheme differs from that of 1979 in that it breaks the sleep disorders into four groups: the dyssomnias; the parasomnias; medical and psychiatric sleep disorders; and the proposed sleep disorders.

The development of the international classification of sleep disorders involved the cooperation of individuals in sleep societies from around the world and led to the recommendation that the name "International Classification of Sleep Disorders" be applied to the new system. The new classification was published in 1990 by the American Sleep Disorders Association, a member society of the Association of Professional Sleep Societies. A minor revision of the classification was carried out in 1998. (See also CIRCADIAN RHYTHM SLEEP DISORDERS, DYSSOMNIA, PARASOMNIAS, PROPOSED SLEEP DISORDERS, REM PARASOMNIAS, SLEEP-WAKE TRANSITION DISORDERS.)

interpretation of dreams   The most significant advance in the interpretation of DREAMS occurred with SIGMUND FREUD's psychodynamic writings on dreams in his initial publication *The Interpretation of Dreams*, published in 1900. Freud wrote: "*The Interpretation of Dreams* is the royal road to a knowledge of the part the unconscious plays in the mental life."

Dreams were regarded by Freud as protecting mental health by allowing sleep to continue while mental conflict was being expressed and managed without producing sleep disruption.

Freud also regarded dreams as being symbols of internal conflicts and a representation of deep-seated, unfulfilled desires, particularly of a sexual nature.

Although Freud's interpretation of dreams is still widely held, modern science has added neurophysiological information that refutes some of Freud's hypotheses. (See also REM SLEEP.)

intrinsic sleep disorders   Medical or psychological sleep disorders that originate or develop from within the body, or arise from causes within the body. Examples of intrinsic sleep disorders include PSYCHOPHYSIOLOGICAL INSOMNIA, NARCOLEPSY and OBSTRUCTIVE SLEEP APNEA SYNDROME. EXTRINSIC SLEEP DISORDERS, originating from causes outside of the body, the CIRCADIAN RHYTHM SLEEP DISORDERS and intrinsic sleep disorders are three groups within the category of the DYSSOMNIAS, disorders that produce difficulty in initiating or maintaining sleep, excessive sleepiness or both. (See also INTERNATIONAL CLASSIFICATION OF SLEEP DISORDERS, PSYCHIATRIC DISORDERS.)

irregular sleep-wake pattern   A sleep pattern without the usual circadian cycle of sleep and wakefulness. Episodes of sleep and wakefulness of variable duration occur throughout the 24-hour day, with sleep occurring unpredictably at any time of the day. However, in any 24-hour period, total sleep duration is normal.

This sleep pattern is commonly seen in individuals who are institutionalized, where there is a loss of the normal ENVIRONMENTAL TIME CUES to help maintain a regular sleep-wake cycle. In addition, such patients usually have neurological disorders that predispose them to an inability to maintain a normal sleep-wake cycle. But this pattern can also occur in non-institutionalized individuals who do not have strong environmental stimuli to ensure a regular sleep-wake cycle, such as persons who work or sleep on irregular schedules.

This chronobiological sleep disturbance differs from the ADVANCED SLEEP PHASE SYNDROME, DELAYED SLEEP PHASE SYNDROME and NON-24-HOUR SLEEP-WAKE SYNDROME in that these other disorders have regular sleep-wake cycles, although they may be temporarily displaced in relationship to a 24-hour clock time. Furthermore, patients with disorders producing EXCESSIVE SLEEPINESS during the day may show a similar pattern of frequent sleep episodes, but most disorders of excessive daytime sleepiness occur in the presence of a relatively intact nocturnal sleep period. However, NARCOLEPSY, which typically produces frequent daytime sleep episodes, can be associated with a disrupted nocturnal sleep pattern, particularly when the disorder is severe. Irregular sleep-wake pattern also has to be differentiated from irregular cycles due to either shift work (see SHIFT-WORK SLEEP DISORDER) or time zone changes (see TIME ZONE CHANGE [JET LAG] SYNDROME).

In irregular sleep-wake pattern, daytime sleepiness and complaints of INSOMNIA are common. Full alertness is usually decreased, and memory and other cognitive functions are often impaired. Because of the unpredictability of sleep episodes occurring throughout the 24-hour day, many individuals with this pattern tend to remain in an environment where they can be close to a bed. Elderly patients may become more housebound and less likely to expose themselves to environmental stimuli that, ironically, could help them to maintain a more regular sleep-wake pattern.

This sleep pattern may be induced by the use of medications that provoke daytime sedation, such as tranquilizers, or stimulants that can increase arousal at night.

This particular sleep disorder is relatively rare, although the prevalence in individuals with central nervous system dysfunction is thought to be greater than in other groups (although the exact prevalence is unknown).

The pattern may occur at any age, although it is much more prevalent in the elderly. It does not appear to have any particular gender predominance.

Polysomnographic studies have demonstrated short (two-to-three-hour) episodes of sleep or wakefulness that occur at random throughout the 24-hour day. Sleep cycle monitoring is usually required for 48 hours or longer to substantiate this diagnosis. An alternative means of documenting this sleep-wake pattern is by using ACTIVITY MONITORS, which are movement detectors sensitive to the presence of sleep or wake episodes. Prolonged monitoring over days or weeks can be an effective way of documenting this sleep disorder. Because of the disruption of the sleep-wake cycle, the NREM-REM SLEEP CYCLE is often disrupted, and the ELECTROEN-CEPHALOGRAM may show a reduction in SLEEP SPINDLES and K-COMPLEX activity, as well as reduced SLOW WAVE SLEEP. REM SLEEP may also be disrupted.

Treatment of irregular sleep-wake pattern involves trying to maintain a regular major sleep episode at night and a full period of wakefulness during the day. In the institutionalized elderly, treatment includes providing stimulating activities during the day and preventing daytime sleep episodes. Appropriate environmental measures need to be in place to ensure a suitable nocturnal sleeping environment. Assistance in maintaining a good sleep episode at night might be brought about by the use of HYPNOTICS or, conversely, in order to assist alertness during the day, stimulant medications may be used. However, these medications are often of little assistance, and attention to the sleep-wake scheduling is usually most effective. Patients who have a central nervous system disease may lack the ability to maintain both a regular sleep episode at night and full awakeness during the daytime; therefore, attempts at correcting the irregular sleep-wake pattern may be unsuccessful.

J

Jacobsonian relaxation   Term for relaxation methods proposed by Edmund Jacobson for promoting restful sleep. The relaxation methods involve sequential relaxation of muscle groups of the limbs and trunk in order to reduce heightened arousal and muscle tension. This form of relaxation is commonly recommended for patients who have INSOMNIA, either of psychophysiological cause or insomnia due to ANXIETY DISORDERS. (See also SLEEP EXERCISES.)

jactatio capitis nocturna   This term is synonymous with HEADBANGING or RHYTHMIC MOVEMENT DISORDER. The term was first proposed in 1905 by Julius Zappert who provided the first clinical description of headbanging when he described six children with the disorder.

jet lag   Term applied to symptoms experienced following rapid travel across multiple time zones. The term derives from jet air travel, which enables travelers to cross time zones much more quickly than by other, slower forms of transportation, such as by boat, where adaptation to the change in time occurs. The symptoms of jet lag include sleep disruption, gastrointestinal disturbances, reduced vigilance and attention span, and a general feeling of malaise. The severity of the symptoms depends upon the number of time zones crossed and usually occurs with a change of more than one or two hours. The symptoms gradually abate as adaptation to the new time zone occurs over the ensuing days. There is evidence to suggest that individuals may differ in their ability to adapt to the time zone changes. The ability to adapt is also dependent on the direction of travel, either eastward or westward: Studies of circadian rhythmicity suggest that adaptation occurs at a rate of 88 minutes per day after westbound travel, and only 66 minutes per day after eastbound travel. (See also ARGONNE ANTI-JET-LAG DIET, CIRCADIAN RHYTHM SLEEP DISORDERS, TIME ZONE CHANGE [JET LAG] SYNDROME.)

K

K-alpha   A type of microarousal consisting of a K-COMPLEX followed by several seconds of ALPHA RHYTHM.

K-complex   A high-voltage ELECTROENCEPHALOGRAM wave that consists of a sharp negative component followed by a slower positive component. K-complexes typically have a duration exceeding .5 second, occur during non-REM sleep, and are required for the definition of stage two sleep (see SLEEP STAGES). They can be detected by electrodes placed over a wide area of the scalp, but they are most clearly detected in the fronto-central regions. Frequently, K-complexes are associated with SLEEP SPINDLES.

K-complexes need to be distinguished from vertex sharp waves, which are usually short in duration (less than 0.3 second), low in amplitude and usually restricted to the vertex area of the skull. K-complexes are thought to be manifestations of central nervous system-evoked stimuli, and can be elicited during sleep by external stimuli, such as a loud noise.

Kleine-Levin syndrome   Syndrome characterized by RECURRENT HYPERSOMNIA, gluttony and hypersexuality. This disorder was first described in part by Willi Kleine in 1925, and subsequently by Max Levin in 1929. Michael Critchley, in 1942, coined the term *Kleine-Levin Syndrome.* (See also DIET AND SLEEP).

Kleitman, Nathaniel   Dr. Kleitman (1895–1999) is called "the father of modern sleep research"; in 1952, at the University of Chicago, along with Eugene Aserinsky and, later, WILLIAM DEMENT, Kleitman discovered the REM phase of sleep. Dr. Kleitman, who retired in 1960, stated for this encyclopedia: "After rediscovering the REM phase of sleep, with E. Aserinsky and W. Dement, my most significant contribution was to demonstrate the operation of a BASIC REST-ACTIVITY CYCLE during wakefulness as well as in sleep, where it is represented by REM-non-REM repetition—thus demystifying the function of REM sleep (reported in *Sleep,* 5[1982], 311–317)."

Dr. Kleitman received the APSS Pioneer Award for his work in sleep research, as well as the 1966 Distinguished Service Award of the Thomas W. Salmon Committee on Psychiatry and Mental Hygiene of the New York Academy of Medicine. The American Academy of Sleep Medicine's annual award for outstanding contributions to sleep medicine was named after Kleitman and is called the Kleitman Award. Dr. Kleitman died in 1999 at the age of 104. (See also REM SLEEP, SLEEP DEPRIVATION.)

Klonopin   See BENZODIAZEPINES.

kyphoscoliosis   Curvature of the spine in the thoracic region that causes a backward and lateral curvature of the spinal column. The space available for the lungs is reduced and patients therefore are unable to adequately inflate the lungs, producing a restrictive lung disorder. The breathing pattern during sleep in patients with kyphoscoliosis may resemble a CHEYNE-STOKES RESPIRATION pattern—with or without central apneic episodes, solely with central sleep apnea, or even with obstructive sleep apnea. The breathing disturbance is greatest in REM sleep and is usually associated with blood oxygen desaturation.

laboratory for sleep-related breathing disorders   A medical facility providing diagnostic and treatment services for patients with SLEEP-RELATED BREATHING DISORDERS. The laboratory is under the directorship of a physician specializing in sleep-related breathing disorders, such as a pulmonary physician, and provides overnight polysomnographic services. Some laboratories also perform daytime MULTIPLE SLEEP LATENCY TESTS for EXCESSIVE SLEEPINESS.

Laboratories for sleep-related breathing disorders can be accredited by the American Academy of Sleep Medicine if they fulfill the standards and guidelines set by the association. However, these facilities are not required to have an accredited clinical polysomnographer on staff or the facilities for the diagnosis of other sleep disorders, such as INSOMNIA and excessive sleepiness. (SLEEP DISORDER CENTERS, comprehensive centers for patients with all forms of sleep disorders, provide appropriate services for such patients.)

lark   An early-to-bed-and-early-to-rise person. This term is used as the opposite of the EVENING PERSON or night owl, who is typically a person who goes to bed late at night and arises late in the day. (See also ADVANCED SLEEP PHASE SYNDROME, OWL AND LARK QUESTIONNAIRE.)

laryngospasm   Term applied to acute and transient obstruction at the laryngeal level of the respiratory tract, most commonly due to vocal cord spasm. Laryngospasm is synonymous with the term *glottic spasm*. Laryngospasm can occur during wakefulness or sleep and may be induced by irritation of the vocal cords, anesthesia or psychogenic mechanisms.

Gastroesophageal reflux (see SLEEP-RELATED GASTROESOPHAGEAL REFLUX) can cause laryngospasm due to irritation of the vocal cords by gastric acid. Episodes of laryngospasm can be precipitated by gastroesophageal reflux in the OBSTRUCTIVE SLEEP APNEA SYNDROME. However, episodes of laryngospasm can occur during sleep independent of gastroesophageal reflux or the obstructive sleep apnea syndrome. In such patients, a psychogenic cause is suspected. Some patients can produce laryngospasm voluntarily, sometimes even to the point of producing loss of consciousness.

SLEEP-RELATED LARYNGOSPASM has some features in common with other forms of sleep-related ANXIETY DISORDERS, such as PANIC DISORDER. It is associated with panic and fear, which occurs out of sleep, and lasts only a few seconds before subsiding. However, in sleep-related laryngospasm, the stridor (high-pitched sound during inspiration of air) is a characteristic feature.

Laryngospasm due to gastroesophageal reflux is treated by the standard means of controlling gastroesophageal reflux, such as sleeping in a semi-upright position or taking medications such as Prilosec. Surgery on the lower esophageal sphincter may be required to prevent reflux. If obstructive sleep apnea is the cause of laryngospasm, then treatment is directed toward relief of the obstructive sleep apnea. Patients with the sleep-related laryngospasm of the idiopathic form, presumably psychogenic, have episodes so infrequently that specific therapeutic interventions have not been explored.

laser uvulopalatoplasty   A surgical procedure that involves the removal of the uvula and a change in the shape of the soft palate. The procedure is performed for the relief of SNORING. It may also slightly reduce mild OBSTRUCTIVE SLEEP APNEA SYNDROME. The procedure is performed under local anesthesia in the physician's office and lasts about 20 minutes. It may need to be repeated several times until a satisfactory reduction in snoring is achieved. The main complication of the procedure is pain, which can be likened to a very bad sore throat that lasts for up to 10 days after the procedure.

latency to sleep   See SLEEP LATENCY.

L-dopa   An antiparkinsonian medication that has been demonstrated to be effective in reducing the severity of episodes of RESTLESS LEGS SYNDROME and PERIODIC LEG MOVEMENTS during sleep. (See also BENZODIAZEPINES, PERIODIC LIMB MOVEMENT DISORDER, RESTLESSNESS.)

learning during sleep   Some years ago, it was a vogue to try to develop ways of learning while asleep. But playing tape recordings through earphones that were plugged into sleeping subjects met with poor success. It is currently believed that exposure to auditory stimuli during sleep does not assist in learning. However, there is some evidence that learning during wakefulness immediately before sleep is often associated with better memory retention of information after several hours of sleep compared with learning following a similar number of hours of wakefulness. But, the difference is relatively small and is not thought to be of great benefit.

Material exposed to an awakened sleeper will be remembered more following awakenings from REM SLEEP than from awakenings out of SLOW WAVE SLEEP. However, there is no evidence to suggest that learning following an awakening from REM sleep poses any benefits over learning during usual wakefulness. Also, the element of sleep deprivation conveyed by awakening out of REM sleep may be detrimental to learning. EXCESSIVE SLEEPINESS can produce memory difficulties that may be due to the inability to retain information as a result of frequent microsleep episodes. (See also MICROSLEEP.)

light sleep   See SLEEP STAGES.

light therapy   Light has been shown to be effective in treating a number of psychiatric and sleep disorders. The effect of light is most evident in the treatment of SEASONAL AFFECTIVE DISORDER (SAD), which most commonly occurs in the mid- to late fall as the nights grow longer. The increased tendency for DEPRESSION is believed to be in part related to the reduced light exposure at that particular time of year. Those with SAD have other features of depression, such as increased weight gain, fatigue, loss of concentration and greater time spent in bed. Exposure to light of more than 2,000 lux for two or more hours in the morning, from, say, 6 to 8 A.M., can improve mood and decrease the seasonal affective disorder.

The individual with SAD may notice an improved daytime mood; however, there may be a mid-afternoon reduction in mood associated with the circadian variation in daytime alertness. Another exposure of light at that time, shorter than the first treatment, may improve the symptoms and reduce the need for a mid-afternoon nap.

Patients with DELAYED SLEEP PHASE SYNDROME can benefit from exposure to bright light toward the end of the habitual major sleep episode. The light exposure assists in producing a phase advance of the sleep period.

Bright light exposure may also be useful for treating sleep disorders due to shift work (see SHIFT-WORK SLEEP DISORDER) or jet lag (see TIME ZONE CHANGE [JET LAG] SYNDROME) as well as other causes of EXCESSIVE SLEEPINESS or INSOMNIA.

Although bright light systems are commercially available, natural bright light can also be utilized. In the course of good SLEEP HYGIENE, those prone to sleep disturbances should be exposed to natural light soon after awakening in the morning. Conversely, reduction of light exposure in the hours prior to bedtime can be useful in improving sleep onset.

The effect of light is believed to be mediated through the retino-hypo-thalamic pathway to the hypothalamus. In addition, light is known to affect the secretion of melatonin by the pineal gland, which may be important in the regulation of circadian rhythmicity. (See also CIRCADIAN RHYTHMS, MELATONIN, MOOD DISORDERS, PINEAL GLAND.)

limit-setting sleep disorder   A childhood sleep disorder characterized by inadequate limits on bedtime. A child who consistently refuses or stalls going to bed will delay bedtime—leading to resultant, insufficient TOTAL SLEEP TIME. When parents or caregivers institute limits, sleep normally occurs at the appropriate time. By adolescence, children are able to institute their own limits and this disorder does not occur. This disorder may be present in individuals who, for neurological or physiological reasons, are unable to institute their own bedtime.

In childhood, limit-setting sleep disorder generally begins once a child is at an age of being able to climb out of the crib, or is placed in a bed. The stallings are frequently associated with the need to either get something to eat or something to drink, to watch television or to play a game or to have a story read. These behaviors may progress to reporting unfounded fears regarding sleep, such as monsters in the bedroom.

The bedtime problem may be exacerbated by oversolicitous parents and is more likely to occur when both parents are working. They readily give in to the child's desire to spend extra time with the parents. Children with physical or mental handicaps may induce feelings of parental guilt, promoting inadequate limit-setting.

Parents may inadvertently contribute to limit- setting sleep disorder by allowing their school-age children to take a nap at any time during the day, which makes it more difficult to go to sleep at an appropriate hour at night. Furthermore, if parents have inconsistent evening schedules, or a child would miss seeing a working parent if he does go to bed at the designated hour, the parents may be unwittingly contributing to limit-setting sleep disorder. Allowing a drastically different bedtime on the weekends, versus weekday school nights, may also contribute to limit-setting sleep disorder.

The course of this sleep disorder varies upon whether caregivers institute and adhere to appropriate limits, or the child develops a sense of maturity related to school and other activities, which reinforces the need to set one's own limits. This type of sleep disorder may be more common in children who have a natural tendency to be "owls," either because of a genetic tendency or through learned behaviors due to parents tending to delay their own bedtime.

Limit-setting sleep disorder leads to inadequate sleep at night, with resulting irritability, fatigue, decreased attention, reduced school performances and tensions in interfamily social relationships.

Children with limit-setting sleep disorder generally show few abnormalities on polysomnography because appropriate limits are usually instituted in the course of performing sleep studies.

Treatment of limit-setting sleep disorder involves instituting, adhering to and enforcing appropriate bedtimes and wake times. A regular routine before sleep, as well as a consistent bedtime and wake time, will help to eliminate limit-setting sleep disorder.

This disorder needs to be differentiated from SLEEP ONSET ASSOCIATION DISORDER in which a bedtime object becomes necessary for good quality sleep and its withdrawal throws off the sleep pattern. Children who have the DELAYED SLEEP PHASE SYNDROME may have sleep onset difficulties. Limit-setting sleep disorder may develop into the disorder of INADEQUATE SLEEP HYGIENE if a child fails to assume responsibility for his own sleep hygiene and sleep pattern when it is appropriate to do so.

long sleeper   Term for someone who has a habitual sleep episode longer than the average for someone of the same age group. The quality of the sleep episode and the timing of sleep is normal. A long sleeper has a usual sleep duration of 10 hours or greater. Someone with a physiological need for a long sleep episode may regularly reduce the total sleep time by one or more hours, thereby leading to a state of chronic SLEEP DEPRIVATION, which may be compensated for on the weekends with longer sleep episodes.

Long sleepers have EXCESSIVE SLEEPINESS during the day if they get less sleep than they require. Full daytime alertness with a long sleep episode is necessary to confirm the diagnosis.

The sleep pattern of the long sleeper has usually been present since childhood and persists throughout life. Polysomnographic studies have demonstrated normal amounts of the deeper stages three and four sleep, but increased amounts of REM sleep and stage two sleep. The MULTIPLE SLEEP LATENCY TEST demonstrates normal daytime alertness without pathological sleepiness.

A diagnosis of a long sleeper is determined by the documentation of daily prolonged sleep episodes over a two- to four-week period.

Treatment is usually not required and individuals need to be reassured that their long sleep episode reflects one end of a continuum or pattern of normal sleep durations. Long sleepers may need to be counseled to maintain a regular full sleep episode at night to avoid sleep deprivation with resulting daytime sleepiness. Stimulant medications should not be given.

long-term insomnia   Term proposed by the consensus development conference convened by the National Institute of Mental Health and the Office of Medical Applications of Research of the National Institutes of Health in November of 1983. The summary statement of the conference broke down insomnia into TRANSIENT, SHORT-TERM and LONG-TERM. Long-term insomnia was defined as insomnia that lasted more than three weeks. The conference suggested that nondrug strategies, such as SLEEP HYGIENE or BEHAVIORAL TREATMENT OF INSOMNIA, be the initial approach to treating this type of insomnia. In addition, a short trial of a sleep-promoting medication (see HYPNOTICS) could also be indicated. "Long-term insomnia" is not a specific diagnostic entity but rather refers solely to duration. A large number of sleep disorders, such as PSYCHOPHYSIOLOGICAL INSOMNIA or insomnia due to psychiatric disorders, can produce insomnia, and can produce long-term insomnia. (See also ADJUSTMENT SLEEP DISORDER, DISORDERS OF INITIATING AND MAINTAINING SLEEP, PSYCHIATRIC DISORDERS.)

lucid dreams   DREAMS in which the dreamer is actually aware of dreaming, as though the dreamer is almost conscious—although he or she is in a state of REM SLEEP. Lucid dreams are more likely to happen in the later REM sleep episodes of the night, and they happen only infrequently. Some individuals seem to be particularly susceptible to having lucid dreams. Attempts to increase lucid dreams have been partially successful by means of certain training procedures, including posthypnotic suggestion and somatosensory stimulation. However, auditory information, when presented to the dreamer, does not appear to induce lucid dreaming.

M

maintenance of wakefulness test (MWT)   A test of the ability to maintain alertness during the daytime. The maintenance of wakefulness test is carried out in a manner similar to the MULTIPLE SLEEP LATENCY TEST (MSLT) in that there are five nap opportunities, two hours apart, each 20 minutes in duration. However, the difference between these two tests is that in the MWT, the patient is encouraged to try to stay awake, whereas in the MSLT, the patient is encouraged to relax and fall asleep.

In the maintenance of wakefulness test, the patient is seated in a semireclining position in a darkened room. The latency from lights out to sleep onset is recorded (see SLEEP LATENCY). Electrodes are placed on the head in order to electrophysiologically determine sleep onset.

For an individual who usually sleeps from 11 P.M. to 7 A.M., the five nap opportunities are carried out at 10 A.M., 12 noon, 2 P.M., 4 P.M. and 6 P.M. The average sleep latency over the five naps is recorded. Average latencies of 10 minutes or longer indicate normal daytime alertness, and latencies of less than 10 minutes indicate pathological sleepiness.

The maintenance of wakefulness test is most useful in determining treatment response to STIMULANT MEDICATIONS, such as Cylert or Ritalin, to determine whether treatment of EXCESSIVE SLEEPINESS has been effective.

Although the maintenance of wakefulness test has less diagnostic usefulness than the multiple sleep latency test, it is sometimes performed along with the MSLT in order to determine whether a patient with a disorder of excessive sleepiness has the ability to remain awake. This assessment can be useful for determining an individual's ability to drive a vehicle or operate dangerous machinery.

mandibular advancement surgery   Surgery occasionally performed for individuals with OBSTRUCTIVE SLEEP APNEA SYNDROME produced by a retroplaced lower jaw. This procedure consists of a sliding osteotomy that is a splitting of the mandible so that the anterior half can be moved forward. It is primarily performed on patients who have retrognathia (a jaw that is placed posteriorly), which produces either facial abnormalities or severe obstructive sleep apnea.

This procedure usually requires long orthodontic preparation, which may include temporarily advancing the jaw by means of rubber bands attached to teeth clips. Repeated polysomnographic evaluation is usually necessary, with the jaw temporarily advanced to determine the likelihood of surgical success. Postoperatively, patients have the teeth wired together until the healing is complete.

Mandibular advancement surgery has few acute or long-term complications, and its main disadvantage is the prolonged preoperative assessment and postoperative recovery periods.

maxillo-facial (maxillofacial) surgery   In SLEEP DISORDERS MEDICINE, maxillo-facial surgery is performed to prevent UPPER AIRWAY OBSTRUCTION during
sleep in patients with the OBSTRUCTIVE SLEEP APNEA SYNDROME. Surgery may
involve moving the jaw forward by means of a surgical procedure called
MANDIBULAR ADVANCEMENT SURGERY. This surgery involves splitting of the
mandible to produce a sliding osteotomy so that the anterior portion of the
jaw can be advanced. Alternatively, a small portion of the tip of the jaw,
which contains the attachments of the tongue muscle, can be advanced to
bring the tongue muscle forward. Sometimes the maxilla needs to be
advanced to obtain appropriate dental relationships in conjunction with
the mandibular advancement surgery. HYOID MYOTOMY is sometimes performed in conjunction with the anterior advancement of the tip of the
jaw. This procedure allows the muscles of the tongue to be advanced anteriorly to prevent obstruction at the base of the tongue during sleep. (See
also SURGERY AND SLEEP DISORDERS.)

mazindol   See STIMULANT MEDICATIONS.

medications   Most medications can have an effect on sleep either by disturbing the quality of nighttime sleep or by producing impaired alertness
or drowsiness during the daytime. The HYPNOTICS, including the BARBITU-
RATES and BENZODIAZEPINES, have a profound effect on inducing sleepiness
and therefore are given at night to improve the quality of nighttime sleep.
If given during the daytime, these medications are less effective in inducing sleep, although they will allow underlying sleepiness to occur.
   In general, the effect of hypnotic medications on nighttime sleep is
short-lasting, and they are not recommended for chronic INSOMNIA. There
may also be daytime side effects, such as impaired alertness, a particular
concern in the elderly, especially with long-acting hypnotic medications.
Some medications, such as the short-acting benzodiazepines, have been
reported to increase the level of alertness during the daytime but can also
induce feelings of ANXIETY and tension.
   The other group of medications that have profound effects upon the
sleep-wake cycle are the STIMULANT MEDICATIONS, including the amphetamines and their derivatives used for the treatment of disorders of EXCESSIVE
SLEEPINESS. RESPIRATORY STIMULANTS, such as the xanthines, are used for the
treatment of CHRONIC OBSTRUCTIVE PULMONARY DISEASE. When administered
at night, they can impair the ability to fall asleep.
   The stimulant medications, when given during the daytime, increase
the level of arousal, causing patients with disorders such as narcolepsy to
be less likely to have undesired sleeping episodes. However, these medications have only a small effect on preventing sleepiness, so that someone with a disorder of excessive sleepiness will find it relatively easy to fall
asleep if put in a situation conducive to sleep. When the stimulant medications are taken too close to nighttime sleep, they will impair the ability

to stay awake at night and lead to frequent interruptions and awakenings of nighttime sleep. A new medication, MODAFINIL, is called a "wake-promoting agent" as it improves alertness by decreasing sleepiness. It is not a stimulant and therefore has little in the way of side effects.

Medications used for other medical disorders, such as the treatment of PSYCHIATRIC DISORDERS, also impair the ability to stay awake. The NEUROLEPTICS, which include medications such as the phenothiazines, and the minor tranquilizers, such as the benzodiazepines, will enhance sleep onset in some people and may lead to impaired alertness during the daytime. Some of these medications are used for their hypnotic properties in the treatment of patients with abnormal behavior during sleep, for example, haloperidol and chlorpromazine. As with other medications with hypnotic properties, tolerance to their beneficial effects may develop in time.

Medications used for weight reduction purposes are often amphetamine derivatives, and therefore these medications can have an ability to impair the quality of nighttime sleep or reduce the tendency for daytime sleepiness. Medications such as mazindol and diethylpropion have been used for the treatment of excessive sleepiness due to disorders such as narcolepsy, even though their primary use is for the treatment of obesity.

Most other groups of medications have effects on the sleep-wake cycle that are predominantly side effects or adverse reactions. Antihistamines are typically associated with the production of DROWSINESS or sleepiness, and sometimes this side effect has been used for sleep-inducing purposes. One of the most commonly used hypnotic medications in childhood is chlorpheniramine. Promethazine, a phenothiazine derivative used for its antihistamine effects in the treatment of upper respiratory tract infections, also has sedative effects.

The use of antihistamines as hypnotics is not considered appropriate because more specific hypnotics are available, if necessary (though rarely required in childhood).

Anticonvulsant and analgesic agents can have sedative properties that impair daytime alertness, such as the benzodiazepines or barbiturates, which can cause increased sedation at night or in the daytime. Similar effects can occur with the analgesics, which can impair VENTILATION during sleep. The opioid analgesics, such as MORPHINE, and the sedative anticonvulsives are therefore contraindicated in patients with breathing disorders, such as the obstructive sleep apnea syndrome.

Cardiac medications, particularly the beta- blockers (drugs commonly used to treat hypertension or cardiac irregularities), can have detrimental effects upon the quality of nighttime sleep by increasing the number of arousals and awakenings. Medications such as propranolol and metoprolol are particularly associated with disturbed sleep at night. Sometimes the beta-blocker medications will increase dreaming at night and lead to more frequent nightmares. Excessive sleepiness during the daytime may occur either because of the impaired quality of sleep at night or as a direct effect of the medication during the daytime. The hypertensive medication clonidine, which has the effect of stimulating adrenoreceptors, can produce sleepiness.

Another group of medications that can have a profound effect on sleep and wakefulness are the ANTIDEPRESSANTS, particularly the tricyclic antidepressant medications, such as amitriptyline. These medications are commonly used for their sedating effects in improving the nighttime sleep of patients with depression. When administered during the daytime, they can produce unwanted sedation. When given at night, the tricyclic antidepressants suppress REM sleep; their abrupt withdrawal can lead to a REM sleep rebound with associated NIGHTMARES.

Because many medications can disturb nighttime sleep and daytime alertness, the role of medication should be considered in any patient presenting with symptoms related to sleep and alertness. SLEEP HYGIENE practices, along with alteration in the timing or dosage of medications, may have a very beneficial effect on the sleep complaints.

medroxyprogesterone   See RESPIRATORY STIMULANTS.

melatonin   A neurohormone that is found primarily in the PINEAL GLAND at the back of the brain. The pineal gland releases melatonin at night, in darkness, and its level in the blood reaches a peak between 1 A.M. and 5 A.M. The secretion of melatonin is inhibited by light through pathways that extend from the retina through the SUPRACHIASMATIC NUCLEUS to the pineal gland. The secretion of melatonin changes over life and appears to be maximal around the time of puberty, at which time it appears to be important in the development of sexual maturation.

The neurotransmitter serotonin is converted into melatonin in the pineal gland; therefore, medications that effect the synthesis of serotonin will also effect melatonin synthesis. Beta-blocker medications used in the treatment of cardiac disorders will suppress melatonin levels, whereas agents that stimulate serotonin production, such as 5-hydroxytryptophan (5-HT), will increase secretion.

Melatonin appears to be important in giving seasonal time cues. In animals, its administration can be used to affect the breeding season by inducing breeding behavior at an earlier time. Melatonin may also be able to alter circadian rhythmicity, as it appears to be able to synchronize the rest-activity cycle of animals. Attempts at manipulating the sleep-wake cycle by the administration of melatonin in humans have produced variable results.

menopause   Gradual reduction in ovarian function occurs in late to middle age in women associated with symptoms of emotional variability, depression and autonomic disturbances, such as hot flashes and night sweats. There is atrophy of estrogen-dependent tissues, such as breast tis sue and the vaginal lining. Sleep becomes more fragmented, with awakenings often related to hot flashes or night sweats. These symptoms are partially relieved by estrogen replacement treatment. (See also MENSTRUAL-ASSOCIATED SLEEP DISORDER, MENSTRUAL CYCLE.)

menstrual-associated sleep disorder   A disorder of unknown cause characterized by INSOMNIA or EXCESSIVE SLEEPINESS related to the menses or menopause. This disorder exists in three main forms: insomnia or hypersomnia, related to the MENSTRUAL CYCLE; and insomnia related to the MENOPAUSE. Insomnia, when it occurs in relation to the menses, usually occurs during the week prior to the onset of the menses. The insomnia is characterized by an inability to fall asleep, frequent awakenings at night and the inability to maintain sleep. Hypersomnia can also occur intermittently, but not necessarily during the week prior to the onset of the menses. There is no evidence of sleepiness at any other time of the menstrual cycle.

Insomnia related to the menopause is characterized by other features of the menopause, such as hot flashes and night sweats. The insomnia is primarily a maintenance insomnia with frequent awakenings rather than a sleep onset insomnia.

Polysomnographic monitoring has demonstrated fragmented sleep with prolonged awakenings and reduced SLEEP EFFICIENCY in the premenstrual insomnia form. Polysomnography during premenstrual hypersomnia demonstrates a normal major sleep episode. MULTIPLE SLEEP LATENCY TESTING can demonstrate increased sleepiness during the symptomatic time. Spontaneous awakenings with features of night sweats or temperature variation are seen in menopausal insomnia.

Menstrual-associated sleep disorder needs to be differentiated from PSYCHIATRIC DISORDERS producing insomnia or hypersomnia. In particular, the premenstrual syndrome, which is associated with marked emotional liability, may produce an insomnia in addition to other symptoms, such as excessive fluid gain, emotional symptoms of irritability, ANXIETY or DEPRESSION.

The menstrual-associated sleep disorder may be improved by the use of replacement hormone medications, such as progesterone or estrogen. Estrogen replacement also improves insomnia in some menopausal women. Attention to good SLEEP HYGIENE is helpful, and occasionally a short course of a hypnotic medication given premenstrually may be useful. (See also DISORDERS OF EXCESSIVE SOMNOLENCE, DISORDERS OF INITIATING AND MAINTAINING SLEEP, HYPNOTICS.)

menstrual cycle   Studies of sleep during the menstrual cycle have shown that during the premenstrual time, when progesterone and estrogen levels are high, there is a decrease in SLOW WAVE SLEEP. The amount of wake time during the major sleep episode is also increased during the premenstrual week. However, the change in healthy females is relatively small. There are slight differences in the amount of REM sleep throughout the menstrual cycle. (See also MENOPAUSE, MENSTRUAL-ASSOCIATED SLEEP DISORDER.)

methylphenidate hydrochloride   See STIMULANT MEDICATIONS.

microsleep   An episode of sleep lasting only a few seconds that occurs during wakefulness. Microsleep episodes are associated with disorders of EXCESSIVE SLEEPINESS during the day and may impair the ability to form new memory, and hence are a cause of AUTOMATIC BEHAVIOR. They most typically occur in patients with NARCOLEPSY; however, they can also be seen in patients with other disorders of excessive sleepiness.

migraine   Vascular headaches that are usually unilateral but can also be bilateral. These headaches can occur during sleep and, if so, are often associated with REM SLEEP. Migraine headaches are often characterized by a throbbing sensation that can awaken an individual from sleep—with the usual migrainous prodrome of visual aura with flashes of light followed by the development of the headache, most commonly in the fronto-temporal region of the head. Anorexia (loss of appetite), nausea, vomiting and photophobia (eyes sensitive to bright light) may develop in association with the migraine headaches. There may also be other neurological features, such as paresthesiae or muscular weakness. (See also SLEEP-RELATED HEADACHES.)

Mirapex   See PRAMIPEXOLE.

modafinil (Provigil)   A unique compound for the treatment of NARCOLEPSY. It has become the first-line treatment for narcolepsy in the United States since being made available early in 1999.

Animal studies suggest that modafinil may act in part through gamma-aminobutyric acidergic (GABA) systems and does not interact with central alpha 1-adrenergic, beta-adrenergic, serotonergic, opioid or cholinergic systems. Recent research has indicated that modafinil inhibits the tubero-mammillary nucleus (TMN). The TMN is an important nucleus that causes arousal by means of histamine.

Modafinil's pharmacologic profile is distinctly different from amphetamine and methylphenidate (see STIMULANT MEDICATIONS). The compound has low abuse potential in humans. It is less effective at relieving sleepiness than amphetamine but has a better safety profile. It is well tolerated. The most frequent adverse event reported is headache, which is usually mild and transient. Other effects include dry mouth and nausea.

Mogodon   See BENZODIAZEPINES.

Monday morning blues   The feelings experienced at or soon after awakening on a Monday morning; characterized by difficulty in awakening, tiredness, fatigue and grogginess. The symptoms are due to an insufficient amount of sleep that occurs because the sleep pattern has been shifted to a later phase over the prior Friday and Saturday nights. (Many people prefer to go to bed later on a Friday and Saturday night compared to their usual time of going to bed during the workdays or school days of the week.) The sleep pattern shift on the weekend causes difficulty in initiating sleep at an earlier time on Sunday night, resulting in a later-than-desired sleep-onset time. This is compounded by the fact that the time of arising on Monday is typically earlier than that which occurred on the prior Saturday and Sunday mornings. As a result, the total sleep duration prior to awakening on Monday morning is less than is required for full alertness.

Ensuring regular sleep hours seven days a week will prevent the Monday morning blues. Otherwise, a brief Monday afternoon nap will lessen some of the sleepiness.

The natural tendency to delay the timing of the sleep pattern, and the difficulty in making an adequate advancement, is due to the chronobiological PHASE DELAY of the sleep pattern. There is less physiological capability to make phase advances of the sleep episode. (See also DELAYED SLEEP PHASE SYNDROME, FREE RUNNING, SUNDAY NIGHT INSOMNIA.)

monoamine oxidase inhibitors   A group of drugs that have the ability to block the breakdown of the metabolism of naturally occurring monoamines. These medications are primarily used when the tricyclic ANTIDEPRESSANTS are ineffective in treating depression. However, the monoamine oxidase inhibitors are limited in their usefulness because there are often severe and unpredictable interactions between the monoamine oxidase inhibitors and many drugs and foods. In particular, foods containing tyramine, such as cheese, are liable to produce a hypertension crisis. The monoamine oxidase inhibitors can also produce excessive central nervous system stimulation, with the production of INSOMNIA or excessive sweating. Severe hypotension can occur. Other side effects, such as dizziness, headache, difficulty in urination, weakness, dry mouth, constipation and skin rashes, are common.

mood disorders   PSYCHIATRIC DISORDERS characterized by a partial or a full manic or hypomanic episode, or by one or more episodes of DEPRESSION. A common feature of mood disorders is sleep disturbance characterized primarily by INSOMNIA but also by EXCESSIVE SLEEPINESS. Mood disorders comprise a variety of disorders, including bipolar disorder, cyclothymia, major depressive disorders or dysthymia.

Patients with bipolar disorder have episodes of mania or hypomania. The patient has a degree of inflated self-esteem, is more talkative than usual, has a flight of ideas, is more distractible, has an increase in goal-directed activity, and has a heightened involvement in pleasure activity. In addition to episodes of mania, there are often episodes of depression. However, during the manic episode the sleep disturbance is characterized by a reduced sleep duration, often requiring only three or four hours of sleep, and at times going without sleep for several days in a row. In contrast, at times of depression, excessive time may be spent in bed, with feelings of fatigue, tiredness and sleepiness that occur throughout the daytime.

Patients with cyclothymia have numerous episodes of mania that are less intense (hypomania) and alternate with numerous episodes of depressive symptoms. The sleep pattern of those with cyclothymia may fluctuate between a night with one short sleep duration and one with much longer sleep durations.

Those with major depression have one or more episodes of depressed mood, with loss of interest in pleasurable activities, that lasts at least two weeks. During this time, sleep is commonly disturbed, with insomnia as the typical complaint. There is difficulty in initiating and maintaining sleep, with a characteristic EARLY MORNING AROUSAL. Sometimes patients with major depression also complain of excessive sleepiness or tiredness during the daytime and may spend prolonged periods in bed. Excessively long sleep durations are more commonly seen in adolescents with major depression. This severe depression is seen in individuals who have dysthymia in whom the depressed mood is constantly present, with features of poor appetite, low energy, low self-esteem, feelings of hopelessness and poor concentration. Sleep disturbance in such dysthymic patients is similar to that seen in individuals with major depressive disorders and is characterized by insomnia but occasionally by the complaint of excessive daytime sleepiness.

Polysomnographic features of patients with major depressive disorder particularly show changes in REM SLEEP. Typically, sleep latency is increased and there may be frequent awakenings and an early morning awakening; however, there is often reduced slow wave sleep and an increased amount of REM sleep. The first REM period of the major sleep episode often occurs earlier than normal, with a short first non-REM sleep period. The density of rapid eye movements, particularly in the first REM period, is increased. Patients with depression may show a sleep onset REM period, and there may be more sleep disruption with low REM sleep percentages, particularly in older patients.

Patients with bipolar depression may have an improved sleep efficiency, with a longer total sleep time than that seen in patients with a more typical major depression. However, bipolar patients typically will complain of feeling unrefreshed upon awakening. There may also be complaints of excessive daytime sleepiness, especially during the depression phases. During the manic phases, REM sleep, as well as stage three/four sleep, may be greatly reduced, as may the total sleep time.

Polysomnographic features, particularly those of REM sleep, may be useful in confirming a diagnosis of depressive disorder and may be helpful in differentiating a diagnosis of depression from DEMENTIA in elderly patients.

The treatment of the mood disorder is primarily by the use of psychoactive medications, particularly the ANTIDEPRESSANTS, including the tricyclic antidepressants, the serotonin reuptake inhibitors and the MONOAMINE OXIDASE INHIBITORS. In addition, electroconvulsive therapy and psychotherapy may be helpful in some patients. Patients with bipolar disorder may be helped with the use of mood stabilizing medications such as lithium carbonate. In addition to medication directed to the underlying mood disorder, the sleep disturbance can be helped by means of attention to SLEEP HYGIENE and behavioral treatments, such as STIMULUS CONTROL THERAPY and SLEEP RESTRICTION THERAPY. Because DELAYED SLEEP PHASE SYNDROME may be associated with atypical depression, treatment by means of CHRONOTHERAPY may be useful in patients who have a sleep phase delay.

Other sleep disorders that produce a complaint of insomnia or excessive sleepiness must be considered in any patient with a mood disorder who complains of sleep disturbance. SLEEP-RELATED BREATHING DISORDERS and PERIODIC LIMB MOVEMENT DISORDER may produce tiredness and fatigue, which may be confused with depression. The effects of medications and drugs such as ALCOHOL should also be considered to be a complicating factor in the sleep disturbance. Patients who have NARCOLEPSY not uncommonly will have depression secondary to the excessive sleepiness. If not recognized as due to the narcolepsy, excessive sleepiness may erroneously be ascribed solely to depression. Patients with other disorders of excessive sleepiness, such as IDIOPATHIC HYPERSOMNIA, can easily be misdiagnosed as having depression as the cause of their daytime sleepiness. Other sleep disorders are common causes of sleep symptoms similar to that seen in depression and, when appropriate, polysomnographic monitoring may be indicated to help arrive at an accurate diagnosis.

morning person   Term applied to persons who go to bed early and awaken earlier than what is typical for the general population. Morning persons awaken early because their sleep pattern is advanced—the pattern of body temperature and other circadian rhythms are ahead of most other people's. A morning person conforms to the "early to bed, early to rise" maxim.

Morpheus   The Greek god of dreams. The word MORPHINE was derived from Morpheus. (See also HYPNOS, SOMNUS.)

morphine   A derivative of the opium poppy, *Papaver somniferum*, which in 1806 was one of the first substances to be isolated from opium. It was named after MORPHEUS, the Greek god of dreams. Morphine has been used in medicine primarily as an analgesic to relieve PAIN but also as a treatment for acute congestive heart failure. It has sedative and respiratory depressant effects that limit its use in medicine. Morphine is also a drug that is abused for its euphoric properties, often being administered by intravenous injection in drug addicts.

Morphine has sedative effects that are associated with increasing SLOW WAVE SLEEP, often at the expense of REM SLEEP. Following morphine's administration, mental impairment commonly occurs and is characterized by learning and memory difficulties, as well as impaired psychomotor function and mood changes.

Morphine may be dangerous to patients with impaired ventilation. The combination of morphine with other sedative medications is particularly dangerous and can lead to respiratory arrest. (See also SLEEP-RELATED BREATHING DISORDERS.)

mountain sickness   See ALTITUDE INSOMNIA.

movement arousal   A lightening of sleep associated with a body movement; typically defined as an increase in EMG (ELECTROMYOGRAM) activity in association with a change in pattern seen in another recorded channel of either the EEG (ELECTROENCEPHALOGRAM) or ELECTRO-OCULOGRAM.

movement time   When a subject moves during a polysomnographic recording, the tracing pen will move widely, obscuring the recording of sleep stages. Movement time must last at least 15 seconds to be scored as movement time. Movement time is usually not counted with either sleep or wake time but is scored as a separate state, unless sleep can be scored for more than half of the epoch. In that case, the record is scored according to the prevailing sleep stage. If wake time precedes or follows the movement activity, then movement time is scored as wake time.

multiple sleep latency testing (MSLT)   First developed in 1978 by Mary Carskadon as a means of determining levels of daytime sleepiness. This test measures an individual's ability to fall asleep when given five nap opportunities throughout an average day. Naps would typically occur at 10 A.M., 12 noon, 2 P.M., 4 P.M. and 6 P.M. for an individual on an average 11 P.M. to 7 A.M. sleep schedule. Electrodes are attached to the head for the measurement of the ELECTROENCEPHALOGRAM, ELECTRO-OCULOGRAM and ELECTROMYOGRAM in order to determine the onset and type of sleep. The patient is asked to lie down in a darkened room and the time from lights out to the start of stage one sleep is the sleep latency on a particular nap. The patient is usually given a 20-minute opportunity to fall asleep. If sleep does not occur during this time, the test is terminated until the next nap opportunity. If sleep occurs, the individual is given a 10-minute opportunity to continue sleeping in order to determine the type of sleep that occurs. If sleep does not occur, then the latency is scored as lasting 20 minutes, and at the end of the five nap opportunities, the mean SLEEP LATENCY is determined. A mean sleep latency of greater than 10 minutes over the five naps is regarded as being normal. Values of less than 10 minutes indicate pathological sleepiness, and those less than five minutes indicate severe daytime sleepiness. The presence of two or more sleep-onset REM periods on a multiple sleep latency test following a night of documented normal sleep is indicative of NARCOLEPSY.

muscle tone   Term applies to resting muscle activity that is measured by means of the ELECTROMYOGRAM. Muscle tone is usually present during wakefulness but decreases during non-REM sleep stages. During REM sleep, muscle tone activity is almost absent.

myocardial infarction   Commonly known as a heart attack; occurs when the blood supply to a portion of the heart muscle is impaired, leading to necrosis of the heart muscle.

Following myocardial infarction, patients typically have poor quality sleep, which is characterized by an increased number of awakenings, reduced REM sleep and reduced sleep efficiency. Daytime sleep episodes are also more common in such patients. SLEEP-RELATED BREATHING DISORDERS have been implicated as a cause of myocardial infarction during sleep due to the associated HYPOXEMIA. Cardiac ARRHYTHMIAS are known to be more common in patients with sleep-related breathing disorders. (See also DEATHS DURING SLEEP, OBSTRUCTIVE SLEEP APNEA SYNDROME.)

myoclonus   Term that refers to brief muscle contractions detectable by electromyographic recording. The term is used to denote muscle activity that lasts less than one second in duration. However, in sleep-related NOC-TURNAL MYOCLONUS or PERIODIC LIMB MOVEMENT DISORDER, the muscle activity exceeds one second in duration and has a recurring pattern of characteristic frequency (20 to 40 seconds). (See also PERIODIC LEG MOVEMENTS.)

N

nadir The lowest point of a biological rhythm. The nadir may be applied to a CIRCADIAN RHYTHM, such as body TEMPERATURE, which has its nadir during the major sleep episode, typically two to three hours before awakening. (See also CHRONOBIOLOGY.)

naps Brief sleep episodes taken outside of the major sleep episode. Naps vary in duration, from five minutes to four or more hours. The time that naps are most likely to occur is in the mid-afternoon, when there is a reduced degree of alertness because of the biphasic circadian pattern of alertness. Some cultures will take a SIESTA in the mid-afternoon; consequently, nighttime sleep is reduced in duration.

Frequent daytime naps are seen in sleep disorders, particularly those associated with EXCESSIVE SLEEPINESS. The naps that occur in NARCOLEPSY are typically short in duration—often five minutes of sleep will be refreshing—and are characterized by the presence of REM SLEEP. Naps taken by persons with disorders that cause fragmentation and disruption of nighttime sleep, such as the OBSTRUCTIVE SLEEP APNEA SYNDROME, are commonly of longer duration, lasting 30 minutes or more, and are largely composed of non-REM sleep. The refreshing quality of naps varies from individual to individual, but typically naps in narcoleptics are found to be very refreshing, whereas the naps in patients with obstructive sleep apnea syndrome are often perceived as inducing even greater sleepiness and sometimes are associated with headaches upon awakening.

Persons who go into deep, SLOW WAVE SLEEP in naps are often difficult to awaken until their time of spontaneous awakening. If aroused prior to that time, they often feel very lethargic, confused and unrefreshed.

Naps are to be discouraged in individuals who have a primary complaint of INSOMNIA, particularly PSYCHOPHYSIOLOGICAL INSOMNIA or insomnia related to psychiatric disorders. Any daytime sleep will take away sleep from the nighttime sleep episode, thereby leading to greater nighttime sleep disturbance.

Naps commonly occur in children from infancy and gradually reduce in number and in duration as the child develops. Young children who have disturbed nighttime sleep often benefit from a daytime nap, and the elimination of the nap may contribute to sleep difficulties at night. However, in some children excessive sleeping during the daytime contributes to nighttime sleep disturbances. Napping in children has been shown largely to be culturally determined, particularly in older children. For example, in a study of children in Zurich, 21% at age five had daytime naps compared with 5% of five-year-olds surveyed in Stockholm.

As multiple daily naps are indicative of a sleep disturbance, one should consider disorders of excessive sleepiness as being the cause. Naps that are taken at times when maximal alertness is to be expected, for example about two hours after awakening and about four hours before the time of usual sleep onset at night, are particularly important in considering whether napping behavior is reflective of an underlying sleep disorder. Mid-afternoon naps are of less significance.

narcolepsy   A disorder of excessive sleep that is associated with CATA-PLEXY and other REM sleep phenomena, such as SLEEP PARALYSIS and HYPN-AGOGIC HALLUCINATIONS. This disorder was first described by JEAN GELINEAU in 1880. Since that time it has been recognized as a common cause of excessive sleepiness. The sleepiness is characterized by brief episodes of lapses into sleep that occur throughout the day, usually lasting less than an hour. Sometimes only five or 10 minutes of sleep is sufficient to refresh the patient with narcolepsy.

The daytime episodes of sleep are often accompanied by DREAMS and a sensation of inability to move the body (sleep paralysis) upon awakening, which are typically associated with RAPID EYE MOVEMENT (REM) SLEEP. The sleepiness in narcolepsy usually becomes manifest when the individual is in a quiet situation, such as relaxing, reading or watching television, as well as in situations with minimal participation, such as while attending meetings, movies, theater or concerts. Sleep is also liable to be induced when the patient with narcolepsy travels in a moving vehicle, such as an automobile, train, bus or airplane. Due to the induction of sleepiness while driving, motor vehicle accidents are more common in individuals who have narcolepsy.

Sometimes the episodes of sleep that occur during the daytime occur quite suddenly and the individual is unable to prevent them, in which case they are often termed "sleep attacks." When the sleepiness is severe, it can occur while the individual is talking, eating, walking or actively conversing.

In addition to the excessive sleepiness, the characteristic and unique feature of narcolepsy is the presence of cataplexy, the onset of muscular weakness that occurs with emotional stimuli. A sudden, intense emotional response, such as laughter, anger, surprise, elation or pride, can induce a loss of muscle tone manifested by a weakness in the legs, with an occasional fall to the ground. If the precipitating stimulus continues, the sufferer may have a continuing state of paralysis that affects all skeletal muscles, and the individual will be completely paralyzed, in a state sometimes called "status cataplecticus." During episodes of cataplexy, consciousness, memory and the ability to breathe and move the eyes are retained. In milder forms of cataplexy, the weakness may occur in one or more groups of muscles, so that the jaw may droop or the head may sag or the wrist may go limp. Sometimes the weakness is not evident to observers, but is perceived as an unusual sensation by the sufferer. The symptoms of cataplexy can be dramatically eliminated by the use of tricyclic ANTIDEPRESSANTS, including protriptyline, clomipramine and imipra-mine. Other medications that have been shown to be helpful in the treatment of cataplexy are gamma-hydroxybutyrate and L-tyrosine. (See STIMULANT MEDICATIONS.) Episodes of cataplexy may be rare or infrequent, or may occur on a daily basis, causing severe incapacity.

In addition to excessive sleepiness and cataplexy, patients with narcolepsy often have other features indicative of an abnormality of REM sleep, such as sleep paralysis and hypnagogic hallucinations. Sleep paralysis is an inability to move upon awakening from sleep and is often perceived as a frightening sensation of being unable to breathe. Episodes usually last only a few seconds following which the individual comes to full wakefulness and is able to move. These episodes are thought to be partial manifestations of REM sleep that occur in the transition from REM sleep to wakefulness.

In addition, when REM sleep occurs at the onset of sleep, vivid, dream-like images are often perceived. Termed hypnagogic hallucinations, these images may be frightening. The sufferer may imagine that someone is in the bedroom or the house is on fire, yet have difficulty in being able to respond to these images. These images occur in the transition from wakefulness to sleep, usually during nocturnal sleep, but they also occur during sleep episodes in the daytime. Less frequently the episodes will occur upon awakening from a sleep episode, at which time the episodes are termed hypnopompic hallucinations.

An additional feature of narcolepsy is AUTOMATIC BEHAVIOR, which is characterized by a seemingly normal behavior that occurs when an individual is tired or sleepy. These episodes of behavior are not recalled afterward. An example: When driving a car and arriving at a destination the individual may not recall the trip. Sometimes rather unusual behavior can occur during such states, so that a narcoleptic patient may erroneously put clothing in a refrigerator or stove and afterward not recall having done so. These episodes of inappropriate behavior are less common than normal behavior for which the individual is amnesiac.

See Chapter 5: Excessive Daytime Sleepiness and Narcolepsy.

narcolepsy-cataplexy syndrome   See NARCOLEPSY.

narcotics   The word *narcotic* is derived from the Greek word *narkosis,* meaning a benumbing. Narcosis is a nonspecific and reversible form of depression of the central nervous system, marked by stupor that is produced by drugs. The term *narcotics* primarily refers to the opioid derivatives of opium. The opioids include MORPHINE, pentazocine, oxycodone, heroin and CODEINE. The narcotic derivatives have been used in sleep medicine for the treatment of RESTLESS LEGS SYNDROME, particularly the medication oxycodone. Codeine has been shown to be helpful in improving sleepiness in some patients with NARCOLEPSY; however, because of its potential for addiction it is rarely used.

The narcotic derivatives mainly affect the central nervous system and can induce analgesia, sleepiness, mood changes, respiratory depression, constipation, nausea and vomiting. These medications affect specific receptors in the central nervous system that can be blocked by agents such as naloxone. (See also MORPHEUS.)

nasal congestion   Normally breathing occurs through the nose during sleep, unless there is upper airway obstruction—when mouth breathing is necessary. Nasal congestion produces impaired nasal breathing during sleep, whether the congestion is due to acute nasal stuffiness or allergic rhinitis. It can also exacerbate preexisting OBSTRUCTIVE SLEEP APNEA SYNDROME or can induce apneas in a person who otherwise does not have apnea during sleep. Nasal infection and congestion need to be treated in any patient with obstructive sleep apnea syndrome to avoid a worsening apnea.

Nasal congestion can be treated surgically by submucous resection, the removal of polyps or treatment with mucosal medications. Medications used to treat allergic rhinitis include antihistamines, topical steroids and related medications.

Patients with the obstructive sleep apnea syndrome who are treated by CPAP (CONTINUOUS POSITIVE AIRWAY PRESSURE) may have an exacerbation or a new onset of allergic rhinitis. Initial treatment by nasal decongestants often will settle the nasal congestion; however, medications such as the antihistamines, anticholinergics or steroids may be required to allow the patients to continue the CPAP. (See also NASAL SURGERY.)

nasal positive pressure ventilation (NPPV)   A new treatment modality that can be useful for patients who have SLEEP-RELATED BREATHING DISORDERS that are not responsive to CONTINUOUS POSITIVE AIRWAY PRESSURE devices (CPAP). Nasal positive pressure ventilation (NPPV) consists of the application of intermittent positive pressure ventilation through a nasal mask. Because of the increased ventilatory pressure, compared with continuous positive airway pressure devices, the lungs can be inflated in patients who otherwise have difficulty inspiring. This method is particularly useful for the treatment of CENTRAL SLEEP APNEA SYNDROME, especially in those with NEUROMUSCULAR DISEASES that prevent adequate VENTILATION during sleep, as well as for patients with KYPHOSCOLIOSIS.

nasal surgery   Occasionally performed to relieve SNORING or the OBSTRUCTIVE SLEEP APNEA SYNDROME. Surgery to reduce the bulk of the nasal mucosa, submucuous resection, produces initial improvement in the severity of obstructive sleep apnea. However, it is unusual for the syndrome to be completely relieved by this procedure. As a result, submucous resection has infrequently been performed for the obstructive sleep apnea syndrome. It can be useful in combination with other surgical treatments, such as the UVULOPALATOPHARYNGOPLASTY (UPP) operation.

Submucuous resection in combination with UPP is only useful for those patients with a major degree of NASAL CONGESTION. Some patients who are prescribed the nasal CPAP (CONTINUOUS POSITIVE AIRWAY PRESSURE) system find that the nasal congestion prevents the routine use of CPAP. Surgical management of mucous congestion can improve airflow, thereby allowing the patient to tolerate CPAP more easily.

Submucous resection is required for sleep apnea due to severe deviation of the nasal septum. A major improvement in nasal breathing can result from the surgery. Mild septal deviation does not require corrective surgery because little beneficial effect on the sleep apnea is likely to be seen.

Nasal obstruction may occur at the nares, particularly in patients who have previous submucous resection with a subsequent nose droop. Choanal obstruction at the posterior nasopharynx may also be treated and is more likely to occur in patients who have cranial facial abnormalities contributing to the obstructive sleep apnea syndrome. (See also AIRWAY OBSTRUCTION, PHARYNX, SURGERY AND SLEEP DISORDERS.)

National Narcolepsy Registry   A registry of patient information and DNA samples established by the NATIONAL SLEEP FOUNDATION to further genetic research of NARCOLEPSY. The registry is housed at the Sleep-Wake Disorders Center at Montefiore Medical Center in New York. The director is Michael Thorpy, M.D. The blood samples are stored and the DNA extracted at the Human Genetics Program of the Department of Molecular Genetics at Albert Einstein College of Medicine under the chairmanship of Raju Kucherlapati, Ph.D.

As of February 1998 more than 800 patients had volunteered for the registry. Emphasis is primarily on obtaining at least 100 sibling pairs and multiplex with narcolepsy, but all affected individuals and their families are encouraged to participate.

For additional information, contact the National Narcolepsy Registry, c/o The National Sleep Foundation, 1552 K St. NW, #500, Washington, D.C. 20005. E-mail: natsleep@erols.com; Web: www. sleepfoundation.org.

National Sleep Foundation   (NSF)   A nonprofit organization dedicated to improving the quality of life for the millions of Americans who suffer from sleep disorders and to the prevention of catastrophic accidents related to sleep deprivation or sleep disorders. The NSF was founded in 1990 with a grant from the American Sleep Disorders Association (now called the American Academy of Sleep Medicine). For further information, contact the National Sleep Foundation, 1522 K Street NW, #500,

Washington, D.C. 20005. E-mail: natsleep @erols.com; Web: www.sleep-foundation.org.

neuroleptics   Medications that have beneficial effects upon mood and thought and are used primarily to treat severe PSYCHIATRIC DISORDERS. This group of drugs, also known as the antipsychotic medications, has side effects that are characterized by abnormal neurological function. The neuroleptic medications include the phenothiazines and medications such as haloperidol. These medications can have pronounced sedative effects and are often used for patients with psychiatric disorders to control the underlying psychiatric state and also to improve sedation at night. The haloperidol and thioridazine are also commonly used for patients with DEMENTIA in order to produce nocturnal sedation. (See also MOOD DISORDERS, NOCTURNAL CONFUSION.)

neuromuscular diseases   Term applied to those disorders that are due to an abnormality of the muscle or its nerve supply. Typically these disorders will lead to muscle weakness and feelings of fatigue. Many neuromuscular disorders affect the muscles of VENTILATION, and SLEEP-RELATED BREATHING DISORDERS occur. (See also ALVEOLAR HYPOVENTILATION, CENTRAL SLEEP APNEA SYNDROME, PULMONARY HYPERTENSION.)

nicotine   Stimulant that can interfere with the quality of sleep. It may produce a SLEEP ONSET INSOMNIA if taken immediately prior to the sleep episode, or it may prevent sleep from recurring if a cigarette is smoked during the night. People who have disorders of EXCESSIVE SLEEPINESS, such as OBSTRUCTIVE SLEEP APNEA SYNDROME, are liable to fall asleep while smoking in bed. A fire may result and can be a major cause of accidental death during sleep.

Nicotine is contained in cigarette tobacco. The content of nicotine in tobacco varies between 1% and 2% and the average cigarette delivers approximately 1 milligram of nicotine (range 0.05 to 2.0 milligrams). Nicotine is also present in chewing tobacco and can be obtained in a gum form (Nicorette). Nicorette has 2 milligrams of nicotine contained in small pieces of gum and is often used by smokers in an attempt to prevent or decrease some of the withdrawal effects when trying to stop smoking.

Nicotine produces an alerting pattern in the ELECTROENCEPHALOGRAM. In addition, it can produce hand tremor, decreased skeletal muscle tone and reduction in deep tendon reflexes.

Tolerance develops to some of the effects of nicotine with chronic use. Withdrawal syndromes may occur in individuals who are chronic smokers and are characterized by daytime DROWSINESS, headaches, increased appetite and sleep disturbances.

Help for quitting the cigarette habit is available from a variety of programs or organizations, such as Smokenders, the American Lung Association, ASH (Action on Smoking and Health), based in Washington, D.C., the American Cancer Society's FreshStart Program, and local or state affiliates of GASP (Group Against Smoking Pollution). A popular book about the history of the cigarette in America and the development of the cigarette habit is Robert Sobel's *They Satisfy* (Garden City, New York: Anchor Books/Doubleday, 1978). (See also INSOMNIA, SMOKING.)

night blindness   A disorder of persons who have difficulty seeing at night but whose vision is relatively normal during the daytime or when in bright light. Night blindness is an early symptom of deficiency of vitamin A, a vitamin that is important in maintaining the integrity of the retina. With vitamin A deficiency, the retina degenerates and vision decreases. In addition, there usually are changes of the conjunctiva, which becomes dry, and there may be accumulations of foam-like lesions on the surface of the conjunctiva. These lesions, called Bitot's spots, can deteriorate and cause ulceration, with breakdown of the cornea, resulting in complete blindness.

Vitamin A deficiency occurs in developing countries, and blindness in children is not uncommon. Night blindness usually responds well to the daily administration of 30,000 IU of vitamin A for one week.

night fears   Fears common in children, particularly around the time of nursery school. The fears usually represent insecurity about some aspect of growing up, whether it is beginning school or being left with a baby-sitter, which leads to the development of fears at bedtime. Anxiety may not be apparent during the daytime; however, when the child goes to bed and is alone in the dark, mental images may begin and turn into fantasies. Commonly, a child may say there is a monster under the bed or hiding behind the curtains. In such situations, the parent should reassure the child that there is nothing to be afraid of; however, exhaustive searches in the bedroom are unnecessary and will not aid in relaxing the child. The best way to manage these concerns is for the parents to demonstrate love and concern for the child, and look for the daytime anxieties that are the cause of the nighttime fears.

Fear of the dark is also common in older children and the fear can be exacerbated by some event during the daytime, such as watching a scary movie. The parents should not insist that the child sleep in the dark but should accommodate the child by leaving a door partly open or using a night-light in the bedroom or hall. The sounds of other family members moving around the house can reassure the child that he or she is protected by the parents, which will help to reduce some of the fears of the dark.

NIGHTMARES commonly occur in children, and bad DREAMS are associated with the REM state of sleep. Nightmares may be a reflection of daytime concerns. Because nightmares are so common, reassurance at the time is all that is required to settle the child. The child may come into the parent's bedroom and wish to remain for the night, particularly if the dream was especially frightening, but this is to be discouraged (see FAMILY BED).

Sometimes night fears are a technique used to stall going to bed at night, and parents should be aware if their children are using these fears to manipulate their bedtime hours. It is important for the parents to establish limits, and if parents suspect this is the cause of the night fears, then appropriate management may be necessary or a form of LIMIT-SETTING SLEEP DISORDER may develop.

A child with recurrent or frequent fears or nightmares may require intervention with psychological counseling, but this is unnecessary for the majority of healthy children. (See also CONFUSIONAL AROUSALS, REM SLEEP, SLEEP TERRORS, SLEEP ONSET ASSOCIATION DISORDER.)

nightmare   A frightening dream that usually produces an awakening from the dreaming stage of sleep. It often consists of having been chased or of personal injury. The nightmare sufferer will sit upright in bed in an intensely scared state. Dream recall is immediate, and the person is fully awake, often with a petrified look, breathing rapidly and with a rapid heart rate. Sometimes the nightmares may not cause awakenings, and the frightening content of the dream will be recalled upon awakening the next morning.

Nightmares are very common in childhood, particularly between the ages of three and six years; however, it is not uncommon for nightmares to be reported from the age of two years. Nightmares appear to be a common phenomenon, occurring in 10% to 50% of children between the ages of three and five years; treatment is usually unnecessary. The child should be reassured and usually can return to sleep without great difficulty.

The tendency for nightmares appears to decrease with increasing age; however, episodes commonly occur after the age of 60 years. When episodes occur in adulthood they may be associated with underlying PSY-CHIATRIC DISORDERS, particularly borderline personality disorders, schizophrenia or schizoid personality disorder. However, 50% of adults with nightmares have no psychiatric diagnosis. Emotional stress is clearly associated with an increased frequency of nightmares, as well as traumatic event stress. The use of medications, especially L-DOPA and the beta adrenergic blockers, used for the treatment of hypertension or cardiac disease, are often precipitants of nightmares.

Treatment for nightmares is not necessary in childhood, whereas adults can benefit from attempts to reduce emotional stress or withdrawal of precipitating medications. In some instances, suppression of episodes can occur with medications such as the tricyclic ANTIDEPRESSANTS. However, their abrupt withdrawal may lead to an increase in the nightmare frequency. (See also REM SLEEP, STRESS.)

night owl   See EVENING PERSON.

night person   See EVENING PERSON.

night shift   Work during the nocturnal hours, typically from 11 P.M. through to 7 A.M. (Work from 3 P.M. till 11 P.M. is usually called an EVENING SHIFT.) Night shift workers typically have disturbed chronobiological rhythms because of the altered sleeping pattern. A night worker will usually attempt to sleep upon returning home from the night work but often has a short sleep period of four hours (from about 8 A.M. to 12 noon). A nap in the late afternoon or evening is usually required before going to work.

Typically, night shift workers will revert to a normal time of sleeping, from 11 P.M. to 7 A.M., on the days off work. However, because of the fluctuating time for sleep, the sleep pattern is usually disrupted on the days off, and brief sleep episodes can occur at other times of the day. Most shift workers find it very difficult to maintain full alertness during the night shift-work, particularly if the work is monotonous and boring. However, if the shift worker has a circadian drop of body temperature that occurs during the shift work hours, it may be extremely difficult to maintain full alertness, particularly between 4 A.M. and 7 A.M. Studies of night shift work have failed to show complete adaptation to the shift work, even after 10 years of shift-work experience. (See also CHRONOBIOLOGY, SHIFT-WORK SLEEP DISORDER.)

night sweats   See SLEEP HYPERHIDROSIS.

night terrors   See SLEEP TERRORS.

nitrazepam   See BENZODIAZEPINES.

noctiphobia   Term synonymous with nyctophobia; refers to an irrational fear of night and darkness that may be a manifestation of ANXIETY DISORDERS. Some children may experience noctiphobia during their early childhood, but they outgrow it. (See also ANXIETY, NIGHTMARE.)

nocturia   Term referring to frequent urination at night, compared with the daytime; synonymous with nycturia. Patients with nocturia will have a full bladder, causing them to arise several times from sleep to go to the bathroom. Urinary frequency may be due to a variety of urological problems, including infections, local tumors, such as bladder or prostate tumors, bladder prolapse or other disorders affecting sphincter control. Patients with sleep disturbance typically will have an increase in the number of episodes of nocturia at times of the sleep disturbance. Some patients with insomnia may arise five or six times at night to go to the bathroom, and each time will typically void only a small amount of urine.

There is a strong association between the development of OBSTRUCTIVE SLEEP APNEA SYNDROME and the need for nocturia. Relief of the obstructive sleep apnea syndrome relieves the nocturia, as does the treatment of insomnia in patients who have nocturia related to insomnia. If urinating occurs during sleep, then the term SLEEP ENURESIS is used.

Many other medical disorders can produce nocturia, such as diabetes and bladder disorders, as well as medications, particularly diuretics.

nocturnal   Pertaining to night, night-related. It does not necessarily imply a sleep-related phenomenon. Although many nocturnal disorders are sleep-related, some occur during the night hours, when the person is either awake or asleep, such as nocturnal epilepsy. The term is used to differentiate night from day, and is the opposite of the word *diurnal.*

nocturnal cardiac ischemia   Ischemia (lack of oxygen that causes damage to the tissue) of the myocardium (heart muscle) that occurs during the major sleep episode. Cardiac ischemia may be symptomatic, in which case it is often termed nocturnal angina, or the ischemia may be asymptomatic. It may be detected by electrocardiographic monitoring during sleep, either by Holter monitoring (a 24-hour electrocardiograph) or during nocturnal polysomnographic monitoring. When symptomatic, cardiac ischemia produces a chest pain that is described as a tightness within the chest, often like a vise. The pain may be felt in the jaw, left arm or the back. The pain may be mild, in which case the person may not believe it is of cardiac origin, or it may be severe, requiring acute medical attention.

Patients who have nocturnal cardiac ischemia will also usually have daytime ischemic episodes. However, nocturnal cardiac ischemia may be independent of any prior or current daytime ischemic features, and it may be related solely to underlying pathological disorders that occur during sleep, such as the OBSTRUCTIVE SLEEP APNEA SYNDROME. Episodes of nocturnal cardiac ischemia are more common in the later half of the night, particularly during REM SLEEP. Severe cardiac ARRHYTHMIAS and even sudden DEATH DURING SLEEP may result.

Cardiac ischemia is usually a feature of coronary artery disease—either intrinsic disease, such as atherosclerosis or coronary artery spasms, or valvular disease, such as aortic stenosis.

Patients at most risk for coronary artery disease are overweight males. Other risk factors include HYPERTENSION, cigarette smoking, a family history of cardiac disease and an elevated cholesterol level.

Electrocardiographic monitoring during sleep may demonstrate cardiac ischemia, which is evidenced by ST wave changes of 1 millimeter or greater, either elevation or depression. Polysomnographic monitoring may demonstrate either the cardiac ischemia or predisposing disorders, such as SLEEP-RELATED BREATHING DISORDERS.

Patients demonstrating cardiac ischemia require further cardiac investigations, which may include cardiac exercise testing with echocardiography or coronary angiography.

Nocturnal cardiac ischemia needs to be differentiated from other causes of chest pain that occur during sleep, such as left ventricular failure producing PAROXYSMAL NOCTURNAL DYSPNEA, gastroesophageal reflux or peptic ulcer disease.

Treatment of nocturnal cardiac ischemia rests on treatment of the underlying cardiac disease. Anti-anginal agents, such as long acting nitroglycerine, may need to be given before bedtime. Other medications and surgical management of coronary artery disease need to be considered. If underlying sleep-related disorders induce cardiac ischemia, such as the CENTRAL SLEEP APNEA SYNDROME, OBSTRUCTIVE SLEEP APNEA SYNDROME or CENTRAL ALVEOLAR HYPOVENTILATION SYNDROME, then treatment of these disorders is necessary.

nocturnal confusion   A typical occurrence in patients who have DEMENTIA. Patients will arise from sleep at night in a confused state, not knowing where they are, and start to behave as if it is daytime rather than nighttime. The activity of such patients may pose some major problems for caretakers and often can lead to institutionalization of the patient. The nocturnal confusion can be worsened by some HYPNOTICS or acute underlying medical illnesses. Attention to good SLEEP HYGIENE and the judicious use of sedative medications may be helpful.

nocturnal dyspnea   Respiratory difficulty that occurs during sleep at night. This commonly occurs in association with lung or cardiac disease. Nocturnal dyspnea (also known as paroxysmal nocturnal dyspnea) is typically seen in patients who have leftsided heart failure that causes fluid to accumulate in the lungs, thereby producing discomfort and difficulty in breathing and leading to an awakening with a sensation of respiratory distress. It may also be due to other disorders that produce difficulty in breathing at night, for example, CAHS (CENTRAL ALVEOLAR HYPOVENTILATION SYNDROME), CHRONIC OBSTRUCTIVE PULMONARY DISEASE or OBSTRUCTIVE SLEEP APNEA SYNDROME.

Marked OBESITY can cause compression of the lower lung fields, thereby leading to impaired VENTILATION during sleep and a sensation of dyspnea. Most often, individuals with nocturnal dyspnea will use several pillows in order to sleep in a semi-reclining position, which assists in improving ventilation during sleep. Sometimes nocturnal dyspnea may be so severe that a person needs to sleep upright in a chair for the entire night.

Treatment of many sleep-related respiratory disorders will relieve nocturnal dyspnea and allow improved quality of nocturnal sleep.

nocturnal eating (drinking) syndrome   Disorder characterized by one or more awakenings that occur during the night with a desire for food or drink. Sleep cannot be reinitiated until the intake has been completed, after which sleep occurs easily. This sleep disorder usually occurs in children, although it can occur in adults. Typically, an infant would require nursing at the breast, or bottle feeding, after which the baby will return to sleep. The older child may request something to eat or drink and is unable to sleep until the requested food or drink has been taken. This disorder is also seen in adults who occasionally will awaken with a strong desire to eat. Again, sleep cannot be initiated until the desired food or drink has been ingested.

An infant's ability to sleep through the night without the need for food or drink is usually attained by the age of six months. Frequent awakenings may lead to the production of a disturbed sleep-wake pattern, with the need for sustenance at frequent intervals.

The need for food or drink in infants generally persists until the child is weaned completely, typically by age three to four months. However, if bottle feeding or drinks are allowed to be given throughout the night until an older age, then the sleep disturbance may occur.

Caregiver factors are very important in the development of this sleep disorder. In infants and children, the caregiver needs to recognize appropriate hunger signals; repeated demands without true need should not be complied with.

The increased weight gain may be a source of concern, anxiety and depression.

Approximately 5% of the population from six months to three years of age may exhibit the nocturnal eating (drinking) syndrome and the prevalence in adults is unknown.

Adults who ingest more than 50% of their caloric intake during the sleeping hours are regarded as having the nocturnal eating (drinking) syndrome. This condition is frequently associated with increasing weight gain and concern over frequent nocturnal awakenings.

Treatment of this disorder involves weaning the young child from the breast or bottle, the recognition of any true need for sustenance during sleep, the elimination of compliance with the false demands of children, behavior modification with sleep consolidation, and eliminating the need in adults to awake and eat or drink. There have been reports that there may be benefits from reducing carbohydrate intake, and increasing protein intake, before sleep. In the adult, hypoglycemia can occur during sleep and, if indicated, a glucose tolerance test may be necessary to explore this possibility. (Hypoglycemia is a disorder that is associated with intermittent low blood sugar levels. Treatment may require an adult to eat small portions of food at frequent intervals to stabilize the blood sugar level.)

nocturnal emission   Ejaculation of sperm that occurs during sleep in relationship to a dream that is sexually motivated. (A common term for this phenomenon is *wet dream*.) According to the Kinsey study of American males, approximately 85% of the male population will experience one or more "wet dreams" during their lifetime. The highest incidence of nocturnal emissions occurs during the late teens and diminishes with age. Nocturnal emissions occur in association with the SLEEP-RELATED PENILE ERECTIONS that occur during REM SLEEP.

nocturnal enuresis   See SLEEP ENURESIS.

nocturnal leg cramps   A painful feeling associated with muscle tightness or tension in the calves of the legs, but occasionally in the feet. The tightening of the muscle lasts a few seconds and usually stops spontaneously, but the discomfort may persist for up to about 30 minutes. When the nocturnal cramps occur during sleep, they will cause an awakening. Episodes may also occur during the daytime; however, patients with daytime cramps rarely have episodes during sleep. Some patients have a predisposition for having only sleep-related cramps.

Nocturnal cramps have also been called by the term *charley horse*, derived from the old term for a horse that was lame due to the stiffness of its muscles.

The cause of the muscle cramps is poorly understood, but metabolic disturbances, such as diabetes or calcium abnormalities, can contribute. The cramps also appear to be more common during pregnancy.

The peak age of onset of nocturnal cramps appears to be in adulthood, but they can occur in children. However, this type of cramping has never been reported in infants or very young children.

This discomfort can be relieved by stretching the involved muscle, by movement and massage of the muscle, or by local heat to the affected area. Quinine is an effective medication.

The disorder needs to be distinguished from other forms of muscle disorder that can occur during sleep, such as PERIODIC LIMB MOVEMENT DISORDER, sleep-related seizures, NOCTURNAL PAROXYSMAL DYSTONIA and sleep-related tonic spasms, which all have differing clinical features and history.

nocturnal myoclonus   Term applied by Charles Symonds in 1953 for repetitive leg jerks that occur during sleep. As the movements are of longer duration than typical myoclonic jerks, the term PERIODIC LEG MOVEMENTS is preferred. When the movements reach sufficient frequency to disrupt sleep, the resulting disorder is called the PERIODIC LIMB MOVEMENT DISORDER. (See also RESTLESS LEGS SYNDROME.)

nocturnal paroxysmal dystonia (NPD)   A neurological disorder that produces abnormal movement activity during sleep, particularly non-REM sleep. This disorder produces dystonic or dyskinetic movements that are characterized by a twisting or writhing type of movement. Nocturnal paroxysmal dystonia appears to be of central nervous system origin (caused by mechanisms inside the brain) and seems to have a long course lasting many years without spontaneous resolution.

Episodes of nocturnal paroxysmal dystonia have occurred in infancy or can occur for the first time as late as the fifth decade. It appears to have an equal prevalence in men and women, and episodes do not subside spontaneously but have been known to occur for at least 20 years.

Polysomnographic investigation has demonstrated that the episodes occur during stage two sleep and rarely can occur in stages three and four sleep; they do not occur during REM sleep. Immediately prior to the onset of the abnormal motor movement activity the ELECTROENCEPHALOGRAM shows evidence of an arousal or a brief awakening. Other forms of investigation, including brain imaging, have failed to reveal any specific central nervous system pathology to account for the disorder. Patients with generalized tonic-clonic seizures may have abnormal epileptiform activity seen on routine daytime electroencephalograms.

The abnormal movement needs to be differentiated from other forms of sleep-related movement disorders, such as the REM SLEEP BEHAVIOR DISORDER, which occurs predominantly during REM sleep and can be easily discerned by polysomnography. Other forms of parasomnia activity, including SLEEP TERRORS and SLEEPWALKING, are easily differentiated by their characteristic features. There may be difficulty in differentiating from SLEEP-RELATED EPILEPSY, particularly that of frontal lobe origin. Electroencephalographic patterns consistent with epilepsy are rarely seen in paroxysmal dystonia and suggest that nocturnal paroxysmal dystonia is not an epileptic phenomenon. Polysomnographic documentation of episodes has failed to show any preceding or following epileptic features.

Nocturnal paroxysmal dystonia is responsive to the anticonvulsive medication carbamazepine (Tegretol).

nocturnal penile tumescence (NPT) test   A test of the ability to attain an adequate erection during sleep. This test involves monitoring the erectile ability during an all-night polysomnogram (see POLYSOMNOGRAPHY).

nocturnal sleep episode   The typical nighttime or major sleep episode that is determined by the daily rhythm of sleep and wakefulness.

noise   A common cause of sleep disturbance. Environmental noise, due to traffic, aircraft or neighbors, can cause a person to have difficulty in initiating or maintaining sleep and can contribute to an EARLY MORNING AROUSAL. It is one of many environmental effects that can produce an environmental sleep disorder. In addition to its more obvious effect of causing awakenings and insomnia, noise can also disturb the quality of sleep by inducing brief arousals, which do not lead to full awakenings. This disturbance may lead to EXCESSIVE SLEEPINESS that can be documented by a MULTIPLE SLEEP LATENCY TEST.

Environmental noise can be eliminated from the bedroom by ensuring tight seals around windows and doors and the use of heavy curtains.

Earplugs or the use of a white noise machine can be helpful for some patients. (Overuse or improper use of ear plugs, however, can lead to a buildup of wax, which might necessitate removal by a physician.) Alternatively, HYPNOTICS, which prevent the arousals and the awakenings, can be useful, particularly in the short term.

The subjective assessment of noise can vary among individuals. Some good sleepers may be totally oblivious to loud sounds during the night and sleep is undisturbed. However, others find even the quietest sounds especially disturbing. It is well-recognized that the mother of the newborn infant is able to sleep yet responds to the softest whimper of her baby, which may not be heard by her sleeping spouse. Patients who, for other reasons, have impaired sleep quality at night characterized by a complaint of insomnia are usually especially sensitive to environmental sounds.

SNORING, which can reach very loud levels, as high as 80 or 90 decibels, is a common cause of disturbance to a sleeping spouse. Although many bed partners are able to sleep beside a snorer without being bothered, loud snoring is usually very disruptive. Often there will be complaints not only from the bed partner but also from other people sleeping in the house, either children or relatives. Snoring may be of concern even to strangers, particularly when the snorer sleeps in a hotel or motel room. Loud snoring is commonly associated with the OBSTRUCTIVE SLEEP APNEA SYNDROME. Snoring not associated with the syndrome is often termed PRIMARY SNORING.

non-REM-stage sleep   Sleep is composed of two main sleep stages: non-REM and REM sleep. Non-REM is further divided into stages one, two, three and four sleep. (See also SLEEP STAGES.)

nonrestorative sleep   Sleep regarded as nonrefreshing or insufficient to produce full daytime alertness. Many disorders that produce sleep interruption, such as the OBSTRUCTIVE SLEEP APNEA SYNDROME and PERIODIC LIMB MOVEMENT DISORDER, can produce unrestful sleep. But in SLEEP STATE MISPERCEPTION sleep may be normal and full, yet the patient may awaken with the complaint of not feeling fully refreshed.

non-24-hour sleep-wake syndrome   Characterized by a regular pattern of one-to-two-hour delays in the sleep onset and wake times; also known as the hypernyctohemeral syndrome. (*Hyper,* over, above; *nychthemeron,* a full period of a night and a day.) This rare disorder is one of the CIRCADIAN RHYTHM SLEEP DISORDERS. The non-24-hour sleep-wake syndrome is a sleep pattern that is similar to that seen in human subjects who live in a time isolation facility, free of ENVIRONMENTAL TIME CUES. Such subjects have a sleep-wake 25-hour pattern induced by the time period of the ENDOGENOUS CIRCADIAN PACEMAKER. Such patients complain of difficulty in falling asleep at night, or difficulty in awakening in the morning. Typically, this pattern is most disruptive when the major sleep episode occurs during the daytime and is least disruptive when the sleep episode occurs during the nocturnal periods. Attempts to control the sleep pattern by the use of HYPNOTICS are usually unsuccessful.

Because the sleep pattern severely interferes with daytime activities, individuals with this pattern are either self-employed or have flexible work patterns.

Some individuals with this sleep pattern have psychopathology characterized by being schizoidal or having an avoidant personality disorder. The syndrome is also present in blind adults and has been described as occurring congenitally in blind infants.

Polysomnographic studies have rarely been reported but would be expected to show normal sleep duration and quality that occurs with a progressive daily delay in sleep onset time.

The differential diagnosis of non-24-hour sleep-wake pattern includes DELAYED SLEEP PHASE SYNDROME, which is characterized by a stable sleep onset and awake time. The IRREGULAR SLEEP-WAKE PATTERN has a variable sleep onset time, with occasional sleep episode advances.

There are few reports of treatment attempts in patients with the non-24-hour sleep-wake syndrome, but recent evidence about LIGHT THERAPY being able to advance or delay sleep-onset time holds promise of enabling maintenance of a stable sleep-wake pattern. (See also FREE RUNNING, TEMPORAL ISOLATION.)

NPD   See NOCTURNAL PAROXYSMAL DYSTONIA.

NREM-REM sleep cycle   This term denotes a recurrent cycle of non-REM alternating with REM sleep that occurs throughout the major sleep episode. This term is synonymous with the terms sleep cycle and sleep-wake cycle. Any non-REM sleep stage may alternate with REM sleep to form the NREM portion of the NREM-REM sleep cycle. In a typical adult sleep period of 6.5 to 8.5 hours, there are five non-REM-REM sleep cycles. The duration of the cycle increases from about 60 minutes in infancy to 90 minutes in young adulthood. (See also NON-REM-STAGE SLEEP, REM SLEEP.)

NREM sleep   See NON-REM-STAGE SLEEP and SLEEP STAGES.

NREM sleep period   Usually applies to the NREM sleep portion of the NREM-REM SLEEP CYCLE. The non-REM period usually consists mainly of stages two, three and four sleep. (See also NON-REM-STAGE SLEEP.)

O

obesity   Defined as a body weight that is greater than the ideal body weight. The Metropolitan Life Insurance Co. weight tables are a commonly used source of determining ideal weight; these tables determine weight according to the patient's age, weight, sex and height. Morbid obesity is regarded as 100 pounds of weight over the ideal body weight as expressed on the Life tables.

Obesity is a common feature of OBSTRUCTIVE SLEEP APNEA SYNDROME and is most graphically portrayed in the story of Joe the Fat Boy in *The Pickwick Papers* by Charles Dickens. The PICKWICKIAN SYNDROME, which applies to persons with obesity, sleepiness and evidence of right-sided heart failure, was reported in the medical literature in 1954; since that time the relationship between obesity and sleepiness has been increasingly recognized.

Up to 80% of patients with obstructive sleep apnea syndrome are overweight, and the syndrome itself is exacerbated by obesity. Reduction of body weight sometimes reduces the severity of obstructive sleep apnea syndrome, although this is not a universal finding. Many patients find that there is a critical weight at which symptoms of obstructive sleep apnea become evident, and there may be little improvement in the symptoms until that weight is reached. For some people, reduction of body weight by as little as five or 10 pounds causes a major degree of improvement in symptoms, whereas in other patients even 100 pounds of weight loss may not produce any useful improvement.

In general, because there is a possibility that the obstructive sleep apnea syndrome can be improved, all patients are recommended to obtain an ideal body weight. For some morbidly obese patients, weight reduction by surgical means has been shown to produce a profound weight loss with a major degree of clinical improvement in obstructive sleep apnea syndrome.

The theory that effective treatment of obstructive sleep apnea syndrome would increase activity, and thereby lead to improved weight reduction, has not been demonstrated in research studies. Even following a TRACHEOSTOMY, which is usually performed in the most severe cases of the syndrome (the majority of whom are obese), five and 10 years after the surgery a significant loss of weight is not seen. Some patients, despite optimum treatment of their sleep apnea syndrome, will put on more weight.

Obesity appears to affect obstructive sleep apnea in three ways: it may contribute to the narrowing of the upper airway by increasing the bulk of tissues in the pharyngeal and neck region; the increased bulk of tissues may cause the tongue to prolapse back, thereby contributing to the blockage (occlusion) of the upper airway during sleep. Second, the excessive weight on the chest wall may contribute to impaired VENTILATION during sleep; this appears to be a more significant factor in females with large, pendulous breasts. Third, the large abdominal size affects diaphragm function.

For most patients with obstructive sleep apnea syndrome, obesity impairs diaphragmatic function during sleep, thereby impairing the function of the lungs (perfusion of the basal lung fields). The resulting right-to-left shunt allows unoxygenated blood to pass through the heart, which in turn causes arterial oxygen desaturation. Many extremely obese patients find they are unable to breathe adequately when lying on their backs because of this effect and therefore sleep in a semi-reclining or even in a sitting position.

In addition to surgical management of the obesity, which is typically reserved for patients over 300 pounds in weight, dietary programs, such as liquid diets, can be very effective in producing a rapid weight reduction. However, the long-term effects of the liquid diet programs have not been demonstrated, and initial results tend to suggest an early recurrence of the lost weight. Some patients find the more well-known dietary programs to be very effective, such as Weight Watchers or Overeaters Anonymous. Dietary suppressant medications, such as the amphetamine derivatives, are not only ineffective but are also potentially dangerous, as their cardiac stimulant properties may lead to serious cardiac ARRHYTHMIAS.

Although weight reduction is important for all overweight patients with obstructive sleep apnea syndrome, it cannot be relied upon as a primary form of treatment except in the mildest cases. As a primary treatment strategy weight reduction is poorly achieved by patients, and during the weight reduction attempts the patient's life may be at risk because of the effects of obstructive sleep apnea syndrome. Therefore, any recommendations for weight reduction must be pursued concurrently with effective treatment of the obstructive sleep apnea syndrome, which is most commonly carried out by either a CONTINUOUS POSITIVE AIRWAY PRESSURE device or upper airway surgery. (See also DIET AND SLEEP, SURGERY AND SLEEP DISORDERS.)

obesity hypoventilation syndrome   Applied to the condition of obese individuals who suffer severe hypoventilation during sleep and wakefulness. The hypoventilation causes a lowering of the oxygen level and an elevation of carbon dioxide, usually above 60 millimeters of mercury. The term describes any number of disorders characterized by hypoventilation during sleep, including OBSTRUCTIVE SLEEP APNEA SYNDROME, CENTRAL SLEEP APNEA SYNDROME and CENTRAL ALVEOLAR HYPOVENTILATION SYNDROME.

obstructive sleep apnea syndrome   A disorder characterized by repetitive episodes of UPPER AIRWAY OBSTRUCTION that occur during sleep and are usually associated with a reduction in the blood oxygen saturation. It is synonymous with upper airway sleep apnea. The clinical features of this disorder were clearly described by Charles Dickens in his novel *The Pickwick*

Papers. It was only in the 1960s that its pathophysiological basis could be understood.

Several hundred apneic episodes can occur during a night of sleep, thereby leading to severe sleep disruption and fragmentation, with the development of EXCESSIVE SLEEPINESS during the daytime. The apneic episodes are most severe during the REM stage of sleep, in part due to the associated loss of muscle tone, but also because of the change in metabolic control of VENTILATION.

The disorder is associated with loud SNORING, which is indicative of intermittent upper airway obstruction that at times can be complete and cause a cessation of airflow and obstructive apnea. The loud snoring is disturbing to bed partners or others, which often leads to the presentation of the patient to a SLEEP DISORDERS CENTER.

A typical feature of obstructive sleep apnea syndrome is excessive sleepiness. Sleepiness occurs whenever the patient is in a relaxed situation, varies from mild to severe and can lead to automobile ACCIDENTS. Typically patients with the obstructive sleep apnea syndrome fall asleep while reading, watching TV or even while attending business or social meetings. The patient may purposefully take a daytime nap, but the NAPS are usually not sufficiently refreshing. Awakenings are associated with a dull, groggy feeling and sometimes a headache.

Obstructive sleep apnea syndrome is also associated with very restless sleep, particularly in children who have varied positions in bed, often sleeping on their hands and knees. Occasionally the restlessness can result in a fall out of bed, but more typically movements of the arms and legs greatly disturb the sleep of a bed partner.

Primary or secondary enuresis can occur during sleep, particularly in children. (See SLEEP ENURESIS.) Gastroesophageal reflux may also be produced by obstructive sleep apnea syndrome.

Obstructive sleep apnea syndrome can be investigated by means of all-night POLYSOMNOGRAPHY, with appropriate measurement of breathing, oxygen saturation and heart rate. All-night polysomnography confirms the diagnosis and also allows determination of its severity. Apneic episodes of more than 60 seconds in duration, oxygen desaturation that falls below 70% and an APNEA-HYPOPNEA INDEX of greater than 50 episodes per hour of sleep are features that indicate severe obstructive sleep apnea syndrome.

Electrocardiographic changes typically occur in association with apneas and oxygen desaturation. A slowing of the heart rate during the apneic pause followed by reflex tachycardia (ARRHYTHMIA characterized by speeding of the heart rate) during the few breaths of hyperventilation commonly occurs and is termed the brady-tachycardia (arrhythmia characterized by slowing and speeding of the heart rate) syndrome. This electrocardiographic pattern, when it occurs solely during sleep, is diagnostic of obstructive sleep apnea syndrome. Occasionally, sinus pauses lasting 10 or more seconds, episodes of atrial tachycardia or ventricular arrhythmias can occur.

Other investigations include documentation of the degree of severity of daytime sleepiness by means of the MULTIPLE SLEEP LATENCY TEST (MSLT). Mean sleep latencies of less than five minutes are commonly seen in patients with severe sleep apnea syndrome. Studies of the upper airway, including FIBEROPTIC ENDOSCOPY, can determine both the site of upper airway obstruction and the potential for success of operative procedures such as UVULOPALATOPHARYNGOPLASTY or TONSILLECTOMY AND ADENOIDECTOMY.

In addition, cephalometric radiographs of the upper airway will help demonstrate skeletal abnormalities and also the soft tissue changes of the upper airway.

Consequences of the obstructive sleep apnea syndrome include social difficulties related to the snoring and excessive daytime sleepiness; increased risk of motor vehicle accidents because of the sleepiness; cardio-vascular consequences, which can include a MYOCARDIAL INFARCTION during sleep or sudden death during sleep; severe oxygen desaturation during sleep, which can be associated with development of pulmonary hyperten-sion and right-sided heart failure.

Treatments of obstructive sleep apnea syndrome include behavioral as well as medical or surgical measures. Weight reduction is an essential rec-ommendation for any overweight patient (see OBESITY) with obstructive sleep apnea syndrome. SMOKING may cause irritation and swelling of the upper airway, thereby exacerbating the upper airway obstruction as well as impairing pulmonary function, leading to deterioration of blood-gas exchange.

ALCOHOL exacerbates obstructive sleep apnea syndrome by causing cen-tral nervous system depression resulting in the increasing severity of apneic events.

The most effective medical treatment for obstructive sleep apnea syn-drome is by use of a nasal CONTINUOUS POSITIVE AIRWAY PRESSURE (CPAP) device.

Surgical management of obstructive sleep apnea syndrome includes adeno-tonsillectomy—uvulopalatopharyngoplasty surgery in which the soft tissue at the level of the soft palate is removed. Other surgical proce-dures involve enlarging the air space at the back of the tongue by jaw sur-gery; this may be indicated in some patients who have severe obstructive sleep apnea syndrome. TRACHEOSTOMY is also an effective treatment for severe obstructive sleep apnea syndrome, particularly for those who are unable to respond to nasal CPAP therapy.

RESPIRATORY STIMULANTS can be partially effective in treating the obstruc-tive sleep apnea syndrome. Medroxy-progesterone and protriptyline are most commonly used but have the potential for complications and may not be entirely effective.

Excessive daytime sleepiness due to obstructive sleep apnea syndrome needs to be distinguished from other disorders of excessive sleepiness.

NARCOLEPSY and PERIODIC LIMB MOVEMENT DISORDER can produce excessive sleepiness and can occur concurrently with the obstructive sleep apnea syndrome. Other breathing disorders, such as CENTRAL SLEEP APNEA SYNDROME or CENTRAL ALVEOLAR HYPOVENTILATION SYNDROME, can be differentiated from obstructive sleep apnea syndrome by polysomnography. Patients who present with the primary complaint of INSOMNIA need to be differentiated from patients with other insomnia disorders, such as PSYCHOPHYSIOLOGICAL INSOMNIA or insomnia associated with psychiatric disorders.

Effective treatment of obstructive sleep apnea syndrome can lead to a dramatic resolution of the clinical symptoms and features. Respiration during sleep will return to normal without apneic episodes or oxygen desaturation. Electrocardiographic changes can be improved.

Case History

A 45-year-old tour guide noticed the gradual onset of excessive sleepiness over a five-year period. He was also a very loud snorer and the snoring, as well as the excessive sleepiness, were major concerns. The snoring bothered his wife, who had to sleep in another room because the snoring would disturb her sleep. As he was a tour guide, and often slept in hotels, he was unable to share a room with others because of the loudness of his snoring. During a trip to eastern Europe, the hotel maid had awoken him in the middle of the night because of complaints about his snoring from people in other rooms. He recalled that 25 years earlier, during a ski trip, he had to be separated from the rest of the group because of his snoring.

His daytime sleepiness would occur whenever he was in a quiet situation. He would fall asleep when sitting and watching TV in the evening or while reading. He was a smoker and, as a result of dropping cigarettes beside his favorite chair, had burnt holes in the carpet. He had fallen asleep while driving on at least two occasions and frequently would find himself veering to the side of the road because of sleepiness while driving. His wife was particularly concerned about his driving and therefore did most of it herself when they were together in the car.

He was a very restless sleeper and this contributed to his wife seeking refuge in another bed in another room. He also had a dry mouth upon awakening and occasionally would have severe morning headaches that would last for one to two hours. He was 5 feet 10 inches tall and weighed 210 pounds, which was the heaviest that he had ever been. Five years previously he had weighed 185 pounds and had tried to lose weight but found it very difficult to do so.

A physical examination showed an elevated blood pressure with diastolic level of 95. He had a very compromised posterior oropharynx, which appeared to be the site of his upper airway obstruction. He had bilateral conjunctivitis that was probably due to the chronic and constant sleep disturbance.

He underwent polysomnographic evaluation and had 222 obstructive sleep apneas, the longest being 66 seconds, and he had 161 episodes of shallow breathing (HYPOPNEAS). The oxygen saturation value fell from a baseline level of 93% while awake, to a low of 77% during the most severe apneas. He underwent a daytime multiple sleep latency test, which confirmed severe sleepiness with a mean sleep latency of 5.3 minutes. However, he did not have any REM sleep during the naps.

He underwent a repeat night of polysomnographic monitoring while using a nasal continuous positive airway pressure (CPAP) device. During the recording he had only 10 obstructive sleep apneas during the adjustment phase. When the CPAP system was adjusted to a pressure of 10 centimeters of water, he was entirely free of apnea episodes. His oxygen level did not fall below 90% at that pressure. The study demonstrated a great improvement in the quality of sleep, with a REM sleep rebound as well as a great increase in the amount of slow wave sleep. Upon awakening in the morning he felt much more alert and was energetic for the rest of the day.

He was prescribed a CPAP system to use on a regular basis at night and with this treatment his sleepiness was eliminated. He was able to drive without getting sleepy and stay up and watch his favorite TV programs without falling asleep. In addition to the improvement in his breathing at night and his sleepiness, the CPAP system also eliminated his snoring and restlessness, and his wife was able to return to sleeping in the same bed.

Ondine's Curse   From Act III of *Ondine* by Jean Giraudoux; means the inability to breathe during sleep.

> Ondine: Hans, you too will forget.
> Hans: Live! It's easy to say. If at least I could work up a little interest in living, but I'm too tired to make the effort. Since you left me, Ondine, all the things my body once did by itself it does now only by special order . . . It's an exhausting piece of management I've undertaken. I have to supervise five senses, two hundred bones, a thousand muscles. A single moment of inattention and I forget to breathe. He died, they will say, because it was a nuisance to breathe . . .

It was first described by John Severinghouse and Robert Mitchell in 1962 in three patients who had long episodes of cessation of breathing that occurred particularly while asleep. They needed assisted ventilation during sleep, but the patients were able to breathe voluntarily during the day. The term CENTRAL SLEEP APNEA SYNDROME is now most commonly used to refer to similar forms of sleep-induced apnea.

A number of neurological disorders have been associated with Ondine's Curse, such as brain stem lesions affecting the respiratory centers or spinal cord lesions. Patients with Ondine's Curse require assisted VENTILATION at night, usually by means of a positive pressure ventilator.

oneiric   Derived from the Greek *oneirus,* which means a dream; an event or activity pertaining to dreaming. Oneirism refers to an abnormal dream-like state of consciousness and is occasionally used to describe the unusual behavior that occurs in REM SLEEP in disorders such as REM SLEEP BEHAVIOR DISORDER and FATAL FAMILIAL INSOMNIA.

ontogeny of sleep   There are major changes in sleep from infancy to old age. See Chapter 9: Sleep Across the Life Cycle.

oral appliances   Appliances that are indicated for use in patients with primary snoring or mild OBSTRUCTIVE SLEEP APNEA SYNDROME (OSAS) who do not respond to or are not candidates for treatment with behavioral measures such as weight loss or sleep-position change. Patients with moderate to severe OSAS should have an initial trial of nasal CONTINUOUS POSITIVE AIRWAY PRESSURE (CPAP) because greater effectiveness has been shown with this intervention than with the use of oral appliances.

Oral appliances are indicated for patients with moderate to severe OSAS who are intolerant of or refuse treatment with nasal CPAP. Oral appliances are also indicated for patients who refuse treatment or are not candidates for TONSILLECTOMY AND ADENOIDECTOMY, craniofacial operations or TRACHEOSTOMY.

At least 37 different oral appliances have been developed to maintain airway patency during sleep. They can be categorized into two groups: devices that hold the mandible anteriorly in relation to the maxilla, and devices that hold the tongue in an anterior position. Commercially available oral appliances include the following: Herbst Appliance, Mandibular Repositioner, Nocturnal Airway Patency Appliance, Snore Guard, TONGUE RETAINING DEVICE, Klearway, PM Positioner and Therasnore.

orexin   See HYPOCRETIN.

orthopnea   Term used for shortness of breath that occurs in the recumbent position, not necessarily associated with nocturnal sleep. (See also NOCTURNAL DYSPNEA, OBESITY.)

owl and lark questionnaire   Survey developed in 1977 by James Horne and Olov Ostberg to determine morning or evening activity preference. This questionnaire determines the time of day that individuals are most active, least active or sleeping. Individuals who are alert until late evening, and do not arise early in the morning, are termed owls, whereas those who are early to bed and awaken early in the morning are termed larks. There is a range of preference for morning or evening tendency, and the most extreme forms of evening tendency are seen in patients who have the DELAYED SLEEP PHASE SYNDROME. Conversely, the most extreme form of a tendency to being a morning person is seen in someone who has the ADVANCED SLEEP PHASE SYNDROME. (See also CIRCADIAN RHYTHM SLEEP DISORDERS.)

oximetry The measurement of oxygen levels that reflects the oxygen presence in the blood. Two forms of oximetry are commonly used, the predominant form being an infrared oximeter that measures the oxygen saturation of the capillaries by infrared light waves. Typically, an infrared oximeter has a probe that attaches to a patient's ear and the infrared light shines through the tissues and gives an estimation of the oxygen saturation. Such oximeters are most accurate for oxygen saturation levels greater than 50%. They are routinely used during POLYSOMNOGRAPHY to determine oxygen saturation values in patients who have respiratory disturbance, such as patients with OBSTRUCTIVE SLEEP APNEA SYNDROME or CENTRAL SLEEP APNEA SYNDROME.

In infants, a transcutaneous partial pressure of oxygen oximeter is used that gives a more stable assessment of the blood oxygen level. These oximeters are less liable to damage the sensitive skin of infants compared with the probe of the infrared oximeters, which can get quite hot. The infrared oximeter can give a pulse to pulse determination of oxygen saturation according to each heartbeat, whereas the transcutaneous oximeter can give only a trend of oxygen change, which requires several minutes for equilibration.

oxygen Oxygen is an effective treatment for some SLEEP-RELATED BREATHING DISORDERS associated with HYPOXEMIA. CHRONIC OBSTRUCTIVE PULMONARY DISEASE, OBSTRUCTIVE SLEEP APNEA SYNDROME, CENTRAL SLEEP APNEA SYNDROME and CAHS (CENTRAL ALVEOLAR HYPOVENTILATION SYNDROME) are disorders where the nocturnal use of oxygen may be indicated.

Studies of patients with chronic obstructive pulmonary disease have demonstrated that 15 hours of oxygen therapy at 3 liters per minute administered by nasal prongs is associated with improved survival. However, similar levels of oxygen given to patients with the obstructive sleep apnea syndrome have produced prolonged apneic episodes during sleep with elevations of carbon dioxide. Low-flow oxygen at approximately 0.5 or 1 liter per minute, however, can be useful for some patients with sleep apnea. But the reports are variable, and in some studies oxygen has not been beneficial; therefore it should initially be administered under polysomnographic control.

Some patients with obstructive sleep apnea treated by CONTINUOUS POSITIVE AIRWAY PRESSURE (CPAP) may still have sleep-related hypoventilation that is not caused by UPPER AIRWAY OBSTRUCTION. The administration of oxygen through the CPAP mask may be an effective way of dealing with this residual hypoxemia. (See also HYPOXIA.)

P

pacemaker   In sleep medicine, this term is often used to denote a group of neurons responsible for maintaining a biological rhythm. Most often it is used for the circadian pacemaker, a term used to refer to the SUPRACHI-ASMATIC NUCLEUS, which determines the rhythms of sleep and wakefulness, or rest and activity in animals. Many pacemakers are present in the body for the timing of different rhythms, such as cardiac rhythm or the control of the MENSTRUAL CYCLE. Some pacemakers are believed to be a subtle network of cells, such as the system that may be responsible for the circadian rhythm of body TEMPERATURE.

The term *pacemaker* is used in cardiology for an artificial device that maintains cardiac rhythm. A cardiac pacemaker may be required for certain sleep disorders, such as REM SLEEP-RELATED SINUS ARREST, which may induce a fatal episode of sinus arrest. Sometimes patients with bradycardia occurring during sleep, due to the OBSTRUCTIVE SLEEP APNEA SYNDROME, have a pacemaker inserted as a temporary measure. Treatment of the obstructive sleep apnea syndrome will reverse the bradycardia and episodes of sinus arrest associated with the syndrome. However, when investigative facilities for obstructive apnea are unavailable or where treatment cannot be immediately initiated, a temporary pacemaker may be necessary. A permanent pacemaker usually is not required for cardiac ARRHYTHMIAS due to obstructive sleep apnea syndrome. (See also CIRCADIAN RHYTHMS, CIRCADIAN TIMING SYSTEM, NREM-REM SLEEP CYCLE.)

pain   Pain is commonly thought to be a major cause of sleep disturbance; however, research studies have shown that most patients with chronic pain do not have complaints regarding sleep. Acute pain is associated with sleep disturbance, but psychological and environmental factors, such as hospitalization, probably add to the sleep disturbance for this group. In a study of patients with chronic pain compared with a group of patients with insomnia of psychiatric cause, the insomnia patients had more sleep disturbance than the patients with chronic pain.

Several disorders have sleep complaints that may have a basis in pain. Patients with rheumatoid arthritis have frequent awakenings and disturbed sleep; however, sleep is usually not greatly dis-turbed unless there is an acute exacerbation of the arthritis. Patients with FIBROSITIS SYNDROME complain of NONRESTORATIVE SLEEP, which is predominantly a complaint upon awakening. Polysomno- graphic studies show the presence of alpha activity throughout the sleep recording of these patients.

Tricyclic ANTIDEPRESSANTS can be useful for treating pain and also for the sleep disruption and alpha sleep seen in patients with fibrositis syndrome.

HYPNOTICS can be useful in improving the quality of sleep of the patient in acute pain, such as is seen postoperatively.

panic disorder   A psychiatric condition characterized by discrete episodes of intense fear that occur unexpectedly and without any specific precipitation. Panic disorder can occur during sleep and is associated with a sudden awakening with intense fear. A number of somatic symptoms occur with panic disorder, including shortness of breath, dizziness, palpitations, trembling, sweating, choking, chest discomfort, numbness and a fear of dying. Panic attacks can be associated with the symptoms of agoraphobia, in which there is a fear of being in certain places or situations. For example, an individual may have the feeling of needing to escape when outside of the home alone, in wide open spaces, in a crowd or traveling in a vehicle. Most panic attacks occur during the daytime and only rarely do panic attacks occur during sleep.

A panic episode that occurs during sleep is characterized by a sudden awakening during NON-REM-STAGE SLEEP, particularly stage two sleep (see SLEEP STAGES), with a feeling of intense fear of dying. Other somatic symptoms may be present.

The panic disorders are most commonly seen in young adults. There may be a prior history of childhood separation anxiety, and the disorder tends to run in families; it is more common in females.

The cause of panic disorder is unknown; however, infusions of lactate can precipitate episodes in susceptible individuals.

Panic disorder needs to be differentiated from anxiety disorder, in which anxiety is generalized and less focused on a specific situation or place. Panic disorder also has to be distinguished from SLEEP TERRORS, which typically occur from stage three/four sleep and are heralded by a loud scream. Patients with sleep terror episodes are confused or disoriented compared with patients with panic disorders, who are more typically aware of their surroundings. Agoraphobia is also not a feature of patients who have sleep terror episodes. The SLEEP CHOKING SYNDROME has some features that are similar to panic disorder; however, the focus of the anxiety is on the symptom of choking that occurs during sleep, and agoraphobia is not present, nor are daytime panic attacks.

In addition to discrete episodes of panic occurring during sleep, patients with panic disorders may have other features of difficulty in initiating and maintaining sleep, and they demonstrate a prolonged sleep latency and frequent awakenings with reduced total sleep time on polysomnographic investigation. The sleep disturbance appears to parallel the course of the underlying panic disorder.

Treatment of panic disorder is mainly pharmacological. Alprazolam (see BENZODIAZEPINES) has been demonstrated to be effective in suppressing episodes. Tricyclic ANTIDEPRESSANTS and beta-blockers have also been reported as being effective.

paradoxical sleep   See RAPID EYE MOVEMENT SLEEP.

paradoxical techniques   Procedures commonly used for the treatment of INSOMNIA. These techniques involve instituting wakeful activity, such as reading, writing or watching television, whenever the patient is unable to sleep. The premise is that by trying to remain awake sleep will occur naturally. (Very often sleep disturbance may be due to the strong attempts made to fall asleep.) The patient undergoing a paradoxical technique of trying to remain awake, by diverting the attention away from sleep, allows sleep to occur more rapidly. (See also AUTOGENIC TRAINING, BEHAVIORAL TREATMENT OF INSOMNIA, BIOFEEDBACK, COGNITIVE FOCUSING, SLEEP RESTRICTION THERAPY, STIMULUS CONTROL THERAPY, SYSTEMIC DESENSITIZATION.)

parasomnia   Term used for the disorders of arousal, partial arousal and sleep stage transition. A parasomnia represents an episodic disorder in sleep, such as SLEEPWALKING, rather than a disorder of sleep or wakefulness per se. The parasomnias may be induced or exacerbated by sleep but do not produce a primary complaint of INSOMNIA or EXCESSIVE SLEEPINESS. According to the INTERNATIONAL CLASSIFICATION OF SLEEP DISORDERS, the parasomnias are divided into four groups: the first, the disorders of arousal, comprises sleepwalking, SLEEP TERRORS and CONFUSIONAL AROUSALS; the second, the sleep-wake transition disorders, comprises SLEEP STARTS, SLEEP TALKING, NOCTURNAL LEG CRAMPS and RHYTHMIC MOVEMENT DISORDERS; the third, a group usually associated with REM sleep, consists of NIGHTMARES, SLEEP PARALYSIS, IMPAIRED SLEEP-RELATED PENILE ERECTIONS, SLEEP-RELATED PAINFUL ERECTIONS, REM SLEEP-RELATED SINUS ARREST and REM SLEEP BEHAVIOR DISORDER; and the fourth group of other parasomnias includes SLEEP BRUXISM, PRIMARY SNORING, SLEEP ENURESIS, SLEEP-RELATED ABNORMAL SWALLOWING SYNDROME, NOCTURNAL PAROXYSMAL DYSTONIA, SUDDEN UNEXPLAINED NOCTURNAL DEATH SYNDROME and BENIGN NEONATAL SLEEP MYOCLONUS.

The parasomnias comprise those disorders that are regarded as primary or major sleep disorders and do not comprise the occurrence of medical or psychiatric events during sleep that otherwise might not cause a complaint of insomnia or excessive sleepiness. Such disorders, for example, the tremor of Parkinson's disease, are not included in the section entitled "parasomnias."

Parkinsonism   Group of neurological disorders characterized by muscular rigidity, slowness of movements and tremulousness. The term is derived from the most well-known neurological disorder that produces these symptoms, Parkinson's disease. Associated with the neurological disorders are sleep complaints, typically INSOMNIA. Patients often have difficulty in maintaining both a regular sleep pattern and a full period of wakefulness during the daytime. In addition, there may be specific complaints related to the lack of body movement that occurs during sleep, such as the inability to arise to go to the bathroom or the inability to turn over in bed. Muscular disorders, such as leg cramping or jerking of the limbs, can also occur during sleep. Vivid dreams and NIGHTMARES, and REM sleep behaviors, may occur in patients with Parkinsonism.

paroxysmal nocturnal dyspnea   Term referring to recurrent episodes of shortness of breath that occur when an individual lies in the recumbent position, typically during nocturnal sleep. This condition occurs in individuals with heart failure in whom the ventricular dysfunction causes an increase in the pulmonary venous pressure, thereby allowing fluid to pass from the blood vessels into the alveoli of the lung, impairing respiratory gas exchange. Upon assuming the sitting or standing position, the fluid is cleared from the lungs, and the shortness of breath diminishes. Individuals who suffer from paroxysmal nocturnal dyspnea require several pillows in order to be able to assume a semi-reclining position during sleep. In such a position, the accumulation of fluid in the lungs is reduced and sleep may occur with fewer disturbances. The term ORTHOPNEA is also used for shortness of breath that occurs in the recumbent position but is not necessarily associated with nocturnal sleep. (See also NOCTURNAL CARDIAC ISCHEMIA.)

paroxysmal nocturnal dystonia   See NOCTURNAL PAROXYSMAL DYSTONIA.

pemoline   See STIMULANT MEDICATIONS.

penile erections during sleep   See ERECTIONS DURING SLEEP.

peptic ulcer disease   This disease can awaken individuals at night because of a pain or discomfort present in the abdomen. Spontaneous pain occurs during sleep that is typically a dull, steady ache, usually within one to four hours after sleep onset. The pain can produce arousals and awakenings during sleep that lead to a complaint of INSOMNIA.

   Peptic ulcer disease can be associated with SLEEP-RELATED GASTROESOPHAGEAL REFLUX with acid indigestion, HEARTBURN, and a sour, acid taste in the mouth. The pain of peptic ulcer disease often radiates to the chest or back. There is typically a hunger-like sensation, often with nausea, and there may be a cramping discomfort. The pain becomes intense and constant if perforation of the ulcer occurs.

   Treatment of peptic ulcer disease is by reduction of gastric acid secretion and by such medications as rantidine (Zantac) or cimetidine (Tagamet). (See also ESOPHAGEAL PH MONITORING.)

periodic breathing   A breathing pattern that consists of shallow episodes alternating with an increased depth of breathing. This can be seen at any age and commonly is seen in infants with breathing disorders (see INFANT SLEEP DISORDERS). It is also a typical pattern of the SLEEP-RELATED BREATHING

DISORDERS, such as the OBSTRUCTIVE SLEEP APNEA SYNDROME or CENTRAL SLEEP APNEA SYNDROME. The periodicity of the breathing may induce a slight reduction in central respiratory drive that allows the upper airway to collapse, thereby exacerbating or inducing an obstructive apneic event.

Periodic breathing is seen in normal, healthy individuals at high altitudes due to the low level of inspired oxygen. This pattern of breathing is usually relieved by the administration of oxygen or by treatment with medications such as acetazolamide.

periodic hypersomnia   See RECURRENT HYPERSOMNIA.

periodic leg movements   This term is synonymous with periodic limb movements, nocturnal myoclonus and periodic movements of sleep. It refers to periodic leg movements that occur with a stereotyped pattern of 0.5 to 5 seconds duration in one or both legs. The movement is typically a rapid partial flexion of the foot at the ankle, extension of the big toe and partial flexion of the knee and hip.

periodic limb movement disorder   A disorder of recurrent episodes of leg movements that occur during sleep that can be associated with a complaint of either INSOMNIA or EXCESSIVE SLEEPINESS. Episodes of leg movements may be infrequent during sleep or may occur up to several thousand times during a typical sleep episode.

The leg movements are of short duration, lasting 0.5 to 5 seconds, and recur repetitively at intervals of approximately 20 to 40 seconds. The movements can occur in either leg or both simultaneously or asynchronously. The episodes typically occur in non-REM sleep and are usually absent during REM sleep. Often they cluster throughout the night so that there may be a run of 50 movements followed by uninterrupted sleep before a second or even a third cluster of movements.

Patients with periodic limb movement disorder present with the complaint of being unrested upon awakening in the morning. There may be tiredness and fatigue during the day and there may be frequent awakenings during the major sleep episode. Typically this disorder has been present for many years, often having been present since childhood. If the frequency of the episodes is sufficient to cause severe disruption of the nocturnal sleep episode then daytime sleepiness may result. Usually this sleepiness is somewhat vague and nonspecific at the onset but may become more severe with the increasing duration of the disorder.

People with the RESTLESS LEGS SYNDROME will typically have periodic limb movement disorder during sleep. The episodes of limb movements can be exacerbated by metabolic disorders, such as chronic uremia or hepatic disease. Medications, such as the tricyclic ANTIDEPRESSANTS, can aggravate this disorder and the withdrawal of central nervous system depressants, such as the HYPNOTICS, BENZODIAZEPINES and BARBITURATES, can also exacerbate it.

222 periodic movements of sleep

Typically the patient is unaware of the leg movements, because they occur only during sleep; polysomnographic documentation may be required to establish the presence of the disorder. The leg movements are often associated with upper limb movements and hence the term periodic limb movement disorder is preferred over such terms as periodic leg movements in sleep.

Treatment may be by means of medications that suppress the arousals related to the movements or the use of the newer dopaminergic agents such as pramipexole.

periodic movements of sleep   See PERIODIC LEG MOVEMENTS.

persistent psychophysiological insomnia   This term was first presented in the *Diagnostic Classification of Sleep Disorders* that was published in the journal SLEEP in 1979. The simpler term, PSYCHOPHYSIOLOGICAL INSOMNIA, is the preferred term for the persistent type of psychophysiological insomnia. (See also ADJUSTMENT SLEEP DISORDER.)

pharynx   Derived from the Greek for "the throat"; refers to the musculo-membranous passage among the mouth, posterior nares and the larynx and the esophagus. The pharynx is often divided into the portion above the level of the soft palate, which is called the nasopharynx, a lower portion between the soft palate and the epiglottis, called the oropharynx, and the hypopharynx, which lies below the tip of the epiglottis and opens into the larynx and esophagus. It has been suggested that the portion of the pharynx that lies behind the soft palate be called the velopharynx.

The pharynx is the prime site of obstruction in patients who have the OBSTRUCTIVE SLEEP APNEA SYNDROME. Evaluation of the pharynx may involve FIBEROPTIC ENDOSCOPY of the upper airway or cephalometric radiographs.

Most patients with obstructive sleep apnea syndrome have obstruction at the level of the soft palate caused by an elongated soft palate and narrowing of the air passage at that level. Patients with obstruction of the pharynx at the soft palate level may be suitable for the UVULOPALATOPHARYNGOPLASTY procedure for the relief of SNORING and the obstructive sleep apnea syndrome. Commonly the obstruction in the airway is at the oropharyngeal or hypopharyngeal level, in which case procedures to bring the tongue forward, such as hyoid myotomy or mandibular advancement surgery, may be helpful. Mechanical devices, including the TONGUE RETAINING DEVICE, or other dental appliances, such as the Equalizer, can be useful in maintaining a patent posterior pharyngeal airway in some patients. A more effective means is by the use of a CONTINUOUS POSITIVE AIRWAY PRESSURE DEVICE, which applies a positive air pressure to the posterior pharynx, thereby preventing the collapse of the pharyngeal tissue.

phase advance   A chronobiological term applied to an advancement of a rhythm in relationship to another variable, most commonly clock time. (See also PHASE DELAY, PHASE SHIFT.)

phase delay   The delay of a rhythm in relation to another variable, usually clock time. (See also PHASE SHIFT.)

phase shift   A displacement of a rhythm in relationship to some other variable, usually clock time.

phasic event   A brain muscle or autonomic event of an episodic or fluctuating nature that occurs during a sleep episode. Such a phasic event is seen during REM sleep and can comprise muscle twitches or the rapid eye movements. Usually, phasic events have a duration that is measured in terms of milliseconds, and they last one to two seconds at the most.

pH monitoring   Technique used to evaluate the acidity of esophageal contents in order to determine if gastroesophageal reflux has occurred.

   PH monitoring is usually performed over a 24-hour period or over the sleep episode to determine whether gastroesophageal reflux occurs in association with sleep or daytime activities. Esophageal reflux can be the cause of esophageal disorders, such as esophagitis, or sleep-related disorders, such as respiratory distress during sleep. (See also SLEEP-RELATED LARYNGOSPASM, SLEEP-RELATED GASTROESOPHAGEAL REFLUX, OBSTRUCTIVE SLEEP APNEA SYNDROME.)

phylogeny   The evolution or development of a plant or animal. The phylogeny of sleep is based on studies of the evolutionary physiology of vertebrate sleep, which have revealed three distinct phylogenetic stages. The first type of sleep, which is found in fish and amphibians, is termed "primary sleep" and comprises different sleep-like forms of rest. This type of sleep appears to be a non-differentiated form compared to the sleep patterns found in higher vertebrates. An "intermediate sleep" form is found in reptiles and is characterized by activated and nonactivated stages, which divide sleep into two distinct phases. Nonactivated sleep has a more pronounced, synchronized, electrical cerebral activity, with features that are indicative of SLOW WAVE SLEEP.

   The third type of sleep, a "paradoxical phase of sleep" seen in birds, is characterized by desynchronization of the electroencephalogram and a reduction in muscle tone. Suggestive of REM SLEEP, this type of sleep is differentiated from the slow activity that is more pronounced in mammals.

   On the evolutionary scale, slow wave sleep appears to have arisen about 200 million years ago, and paradoxical sleep approximately 50 million years later.

This evolution of sleep correlates with the degree of development of overall cerebral electrical activity and the level of development of the higher regions of the brain. The evolution of the thalamo-cortical system is of particular importance in the development of sleep. This system first began in amphibians, became more specialized in reptiles, and is most clearly developed in mammals. The development of mammalian sleep is clearly related to the development of the thalamo-cortical pathways. The development of REM sleep appears to arise from the early forms of activated sleep.

Pickwickian syndrome   Term applied to individuals who are overweight, with ALVEOLAR HYPOVENTILATION, an elevated carbon dioxide level and abnormally low oxygen level in the blood, and, most commonly, to patients who have severe OBSTRUCTIVE SLEEP APNEA SYNDROME, who are sleepy during the daytime, are loud snorers, obese and have impairment of daytime blood gases. The term was derived from the description of Joe the fat boy in *The Posthumous Papers of the Pickwick Club*, published on March 31, 1836. Charles Dickens modeled his description of the sleepy boy upon someone who very clearly had all the typical features of obstructive sleep apnea syndrome.

Although the term *Pickwickian syndrome* had been used prior to the 1950s, it was brought to more general attention in a paper published in 1956 by Burwell et al. The term may apply to disorders of impaired respiration during sleep other than obstructive sleep apnea, and it frequently is used to describe people who have right-sided heart failure in association with the other typical features.

It is preferable to use more specific terms than Pickwickian syndrome to describe patients who have sleep disorders characterized by OBESITY, hypersomnolence, snoring and alveolar hypoventilation, such as the obstructive sleep apnea syndrome or CENTRAL ALVEOLAR HYPOVENTILATION SYNDROME.

pineal gland   A small, pea-sized protuberance situated at the back of the brain above the brain stem. Rene Descartes in the 17th century regarded the pineal as the seat of the soul. The pineal gland is markedly influenced by light because its primary hormone, MELATONIN, is released at night and is suppressed during the day. The circadian pattern of melatonin levels peaks between 1 A.M. and 5 A.M. and is maximal around the time of puberty. Melatonin is an important hormone in the regulation of circadian rhythms. It also appears to be important in the control of reproduction and in normal sexual development.

The pineal gland is innervated (nerve fibers go to the gland) by sympathetic fibers that arise in the superior cervical ganglion of the neck. Light impulses from the retina pass through the SUPRACHIASMATIC NUCLEUS of the hypothalamus. Pathways extend from the suprachiasmatic nucleus to the spinal cord and innervate the superior cervical ganglion and from there pass to the pineal gland. (See also CIRCADIAN RHYTHMS.)

placebo   A sham or false treatment that most commonly is in the form of a tablet with no effective ingredient, used for either the psychological effects or for control purposes in research studies. The term is derived from the Latin, meaning "I will please." (See also MEDICATIONS.)

polysomnogram   The continuous and simultaneous recording of physiological variables during sleep; includes the ELECTROENCEPHALOGRAM (EEG), the ELECTRO-OCULOGRAM (EOG) and the ELECTROMYOGRAM (EMG). In addition, the electrocardiogram (ECG) (a graph of the electrical activity of the heart) records respiratory airflow, respiratory movements, blood oxygen saturation and lower limb movement activity. Other commonly taken measures include intraesophageal pressure, intraesophageal pH changes, end-tidal carbon dioxide values and penile tumescence.

The polysomnogram is the recording upon which sleep disorder specialists rely in order to obtain objective documentation of a patient's physiological status during sleep. It typically consists of a paper tracing, approximately 1,000 pages long. However, it may be recorded on magnetic tape or on a computer disc.

The polysomnogram is scored in a standard manner according to epochs of 20 or 30 seconds in duration, and sleep is scored by the Alan Rechtschaffen and Anthony Kales method. (See also POLYSOMNOGRAPHY, SLEEP DISORDER CENTERS.)

polysomnography   Studies of sleep require the measurement of several physiological variables, including activity of the brain, the eyes and the muscles. Sleep is typically recorded on an electroencephalograph machine, which has the ability of measuring not only the ELECTROENCEPHALOGRAM (EEG) but also the electromyographic (EMG) (see ELECTROMYOGRAM) activity and electrooculography (EOG) (see ELECTRO-OCULOGRAM). The EEG records the brain activity, the EMG records the muscle activity and the EOG monitors eye movements.

The electroencephalogram electrodes are placed on the scalp in the routine manner; however, only a few electrodes are required. For reporting sleep, an electrode is centrally placed on the head (in the C3 or C4 position), and this electrode is referred to an electrically neutral lead usually placed on the mastoid bone behind the ear (at either A1 or A2 position). This produces a unipolar recording, which measures the difference in the electrical activity between the C3 position and the A1 electrode. The electrodes are usually attached to the head by means of collodion, a temporary glue, in order to prevent their dislodgment during a whole night's recording. (Electrodes may be attached to the face with surgical tape, but collodion is used to attach electrodes to the scalp.)

The electromyogram is usually recorded from chin-muscle activity. Two electrodes are placed just beneath the tip of the chin and the difference between recorded potentials is measured, giving a bipolar recording.

With the electro-oculogram, the electrodes are attached to the outer canthus of each eye to record eye movements. Usually two eye channels are measured, so when the eyes move conjugately, the tracings appear as mirror images of each other. The electro-oculogram electrodes are referred to a reference electrode. Because the retina is negatively charged with respect to the surface of the eye, movements of the eye induce a potential difference, which is recorded by the electrodes.

In addition to measuring sleep activity, polysomnography often involves the measurement of other physiological variables during sleep, such as respiratory movements, airflow, electrocardiogram, blood-oxygen saturation, carbon dioxide levels, urometry, skeletal muscle activity, pH monitoring and penile tumescence (erections of the penis) to help in analyzing the cause of impotence.

The electrical signals of a polygraph go in just one direction—from the patient to the polygraph—so there is little possibility of the patient receiving an electrical shock. The tracings for each sensor are recorded on a continuous roll of moving paper, which becomes the record of a night's sleep, and that record is known as a POLYSOMNOGRAM. Typically, a patient will be asked to come to the sleep laboratory an hour or two before the patient's usual bedtime. The electrodes are attached at the appropriate place to enable recording of each desired measure. An entire night of sleep will be recorded on the polygraph, creating almost a thousand pages of chart paper monitoring of EEG waves, eye movements, muscle activity and the other physiological variables.

For clinical or research studies, the different parameters can be measured according to different arrays called a montage, depending upon the clinician's preference and the particular variables under investigation. A standard recording for a patient with the disorder of OBSTRUCTIVE SLEEP APNEA SYNDROME might be as follows: two electroencephalogram measures, one at the C3 position and one at the O2 position, as well as electro-oculogram and chin electromyogram recordings. Leg movement activity can be recorded by means of electromyographic measures of the right and left anterior tibialis muscles in order to help confirm body movements associated with arousals that may occur because of apnea episodes. In order to determine airflow, thermistors that determine temperature changes of inspired and expired air may be placed at both left and right nasal passages and another at the mouth. A small microphone may be utilized in order to determine sounds of SNORING. Respiratory movements are detected by means of bellows pneumographs placed around the abdomen and chest or, alternatively, mercury strain gauges can be placed on the chest and abdomen. An electrocardiogram is recorded by chest leads. An infrared, transcutaneous sensor may be used for recording oxygen saturation values, and end-tidal carbon dioxide levels may be recorded by means of a small tube placed in one of the nostrils attached to a capnograph.

Patients undergoing polysomnography for suspected seizure disorders may have additional electroencephalogram channels recorded, whereas a patient undergoing studies for SLEEP-RELATED PENILE ERECTIONS would have sleep measured along with measurements of penile tumescence during sleep.

Although patients typically undergo polysomnography over their habitual sleep period for a minimum of eight hours of recording, in many clinical situations it may be necessary for the patient to undergo more than one night of recording in order to obtain adequate information. (See also SLEEP DISORDER CENTERS.)

pons   Region of the brain stem that lies between the medulla and the midbrain; important in the maintenance of sleep and wakefulness because it contains the locus ceruleus, raphe nuclei and reticular nuclei. Although the pons is clearly defined by the external anatomical landmarks, the nuclei extend across boundaries. Various and incompatible terms have been used to describe the reticular regions of nuclei.

The raphe nuclei, which are likely to be important in the regulation of phasic events of REM sleep, contain serotonin. Although the raphe nuclei of the pons were thought to be important in the maintenance of slow wave sleep, the region around the nuclei appears to be more important.

The pons is also the site of the pontogeniculooccipital (PGO) waves (see PGO SPIKES), which are large phasic potentials generated from the pons immediately prior to the onset of REM sleep. (See also SLEEP ATONIA.)

post-traumatic hypersomnia   A disorder of EXCESSIVE SLEEPINESS that occurs within 18 months of a traumatic event involving the central nervous system. This disorder may consist of a changed sleep pattern, such as a long sleep duration at night, as well as frequent sleep episodes during the day on a background of excessive sleepiness.

Polysomnographic studies of this disorder have shown a slightly prolonged nocturnal sleep period or relatively normal nocturnal sleep with excessive sleepiness, evident on MULTIPLE SLEEP LATENCY TESTING. The daytime sleep episodes are generally of non-REM sleep. It is possible that some patients with this disorder have microsleep episodes that impair daytime functioning and may be detectable only by 24-hour polysomnographic monitoring.

Diagnosis of this disorder is made in part upon the temporal association with the head trauma. Other disorders of excessive sleepiness contribute to motor vehicle accidents, which may lead to head trauma. Patients suspected of having post-traumatic hypersomnia should have other disorders of sleepiness ruled out by appropriate polysomnographic investigation.

Treatment of post-traumatic hypersomnia is largely symptomatic and rests on the use of daytime STIMULANT MEDICATIONS, such as methylphenidate or pemoline, to alleviate the sleepiness.

pramipexole A clinically effective nonergot dopamine agonist used in the treatment of RESTLESS LEGS SYNDROME (RLS).

The limited studies available suggest that it is effective in treating restless legs syndrome and suppresses periodic limb movements. Doses are from 0.125 milligram to 4.5 milligrams. Side effects that have been encountered include nausea, constipation, and insomnia. Sleepiness and visual hallucinations occur more commonly than with placebo. The brand name for pramipexole is Mirapex. (See also L-DOPA, PERIODIC LEG MOVEMENTS.)

pregnancy-related sleep disorder Sleep disorder characterized by either EXCESSIVE SLEEPINESS or INSOMNIA occurring during the course of pregnancy. Typically the disorder is a biphasic one, with the onset of sleepiness during the first trimester and insomnia in the third trimester. In some women, parasomnia activity, such as NIGHTMARES and SLEEP TERRORS, can occur in association with the pregnancy.

Complaints of tiredness, fatigue and sleepiness are common during the first trimester, sometimes even before the pregnancy has been diagnosed. The TOTAL SLEEP TIME can be increased and a pregnant woman will frequently have the need to take a nap.

Normal pregnancy is associated with changes in the quality of nighttime sleep and an alteration in daytime alertness. Typically in the first trimester there is an increased sleepiness with a heightened desire to take a daytime nap. For some women who experience ANXIETY related to the pregnancy, insomnia may occur, related to the emotional components of the pregnancy and not due to any pregnancy-related physical condition. CAFFEINE or NICOTINE withdrawal may add to the sleep disruption.

During the second trimester, the tendency for daytime napping disappears; however, the quality of the nocturnal sleep episode starts to deteriorate. SLEEP LATENCY, the number of awakenings and the SLEEP EFFICIENCY tend to increase at this time.

Some of the sleep disturbances in the later months of the pregnancy may be related to the increase in the physical complaints at this time, such as an uncomfortable sleep position due to back discomfort, increased urinary frequency and fetal movements.

Because of increased abdominal pressure, it might be expected that sleep-related breathing abnormalities would increase. However, respiratory disturbance has not been described in pregnancy, and this may be due to the increased progesterone levels at this time that act as a respiratory stimulant. TIDAL VOLUME is increased by PROGESTERONE.

Polysomnographic studies have demonstrated a gradual reduction of deeper stages three/four sleep during the pregnancy (see SLEEP STAGES), with its absence in the later stage of pregnancy in some women. The sleepiness may be clinically evident and documented by MULTIPLE SLEEP LATENCY TESTING. The polysomnographic features of the nocturnal sleep disturbance are typically those of an increased sleep latency, frequent awakenings, increased stage one sleep and reduced sleep efficiency.

There is some evidence to suggest that postpartum psychoses may be related to the sleep state changes that occur in late pregnancy. Following delivery, REM sleep decreases markedly and normalizes over the subsequent two weeks, and there is a gradual recovery of stage four sleep after delivery.

Following delivery, the disturbed quality of sleep generally resolves itself unless other factors intervene, such as postpartum depression, in which case insomnia or hypersomnia due to MOOD DISORDERS may occur. There may now be sleep-related problems because of the frequent awakening of the newborn, but those problems are environmentally caused rather than a physical complaint associated with the post-pregnancy period. The new mother can minimize the effects of sleep deprivation that often occur because she interrupts her sleep to respond to the newborn, by taking turns with her spouse to respond to the newborn if the cries are not food-related, or, if she is bottle-feeding, by keeping the baby nearby so it is easier to go back to sleep after attending to the newborn, or by taking naps during the day at the same time that the newborn naps so that she does not try to get through the next night of interrupted sleep completely exhausted.

The onset of fatigue, tiredness and excessive sleepiness (of relatively short duration) in a woman of childbearing age should suggest the possibility of pregnancy-related sleep disorder. Other disorders contributing to sleep disruption, such as NARCOLEPSY or PERIODIC LIMB MOVEMENT DISORDER, should be considered in the differential diagnosis.

Treatment of pregnancy-related sleep disorder is purely supportive mainly by SLEEP HYGIENE measures. Pregnant women should not take hypnotic medications. However, if the sleep disturbance is associated with the development of severe anxiety or DEPRESSION, and the maternal or fetal well-being is at risk, sedative hypnotics may be indicated in the third trimester, but only under the guidance of an obstetrician. (See also INFANT SLEEP DISORDERS, INSUFFICIENT SLEEP SYNDROME, SLEEP-RELATED BREATHING DISORDERS.)

pregnancy and sleep   See PREGNANCY-RELATED SLEEP DISORDER.

premature infant   Infant born after the 27th week of pregnancy and before full term, who weighs between 1,000 grams (2.2 pounds) and 2,500 grams (5.5 pounds). Premature infants are more likely to have SLEEP-RELATED BREATHING DISORDERS characterized by APNEA. This disorder, apnea of prematurity, often spontaneously resolves as the infant ages. Premature infants have a greater risk of suffering from SUDDEN INFANT DEATH SYNDROME than full-term infants. (See also INFANT SLEEP, INFANT SLEEP APNEA, INFANT SLEEP DISORDERS.)

premature morning awakening   See EARLY MORNING AROUSAL.

primary snoring   A disorder characterized by loud sounds that come from the back of the mouth during breathing in sleep and in the absence of impaired breathing. This disorder is differentiated from the OBSTRUCTIVE SLEEP APNEA SYNDROME, in which loud snoring is associated with impaired VENTILATION during sleep, sleep disruption and abnormal cardiovascular features. Usually, primary snoring is noted by a disturbed bed partner. The snorer is typically unaware of the loud snoring; however, there may be a brief gasp or choking sensation at the termination of a loud snore.

The snoring is usually rhythmical, with a continuous sound made during inspiration and expiration that can be worsened by body position, such as sleeping on the back. Sometimes this form of snoring is eliminated when the snorer lies on the side. (See also SNORING.)

progesterone   A female sex hormone, used in sleep medicine in the form of medroxyprogesterone (see RESPIRATORY STIMULANTS), for stimulation of respiration to treat some SLEEP-RELATED BREATHING DISORDERS.

progressive relaxation   The sequential relaxation of muscle groups to assist in sleep onset for those with INSOMNIA. This method of relaxation was first proposed by Edmund Jacobson and is occasionally referred to as JACOBSONIAN RELAXATION or SLEEP EXERCISES. (See also DISORDERS OF INITIATING AND MAINTAINING SLEEP, PSYCHOPHYSIOLOGICAL INSOMNIA.)

prolactin   A hormone released from the pituitary gland that accompanies GROWTH HORMONE release. This hormone is under the close control of the neurotransmitter DOPAMINE, which inhibits prolactin secretion. Prolactin is secreted during sleep and has a CIRCADIAN RHYTHM that is tied to the sleep-wake cycle but is not related to specific sleep stage activity.

Prolactin is secreted in higher amounts during pregnancy and lactation and also appears to be important in the maintenance of the reproductive system in both males and females.

Medications that affect dopamine levels will influence the secretion of prolactin. Phenothiazines (antipsychotic drugs) that inhibit dopamine action can produce elevated levels of prolactin whereas bromocriptine, a dopamine agonist (a drug that acts in the same manner as dopamine), will suppress the release of prolactin. (See also CORTISOL.)

proposed sleep disorders   A category of the INTERNATIONAL CLASSIFICATION OF SLEEP DISORDERS that lists various disorders for which there is insufficient information available to substantiate the presence of a particular disorder. This category also contains newly described disorders not yet substantiated by replicated data in the medical literature—for example, the SLEEP CHOKING SYNDROME. In addition, disorders representing one end of the spectrum of normality are included here—for example, SHORT SLEEPER and LONG SLEEPER.

protriptyline   See ANTIDEPRESSANTS.

Provera   See RESPIRATORY STIMULANTS.

Provigil   See MODAFINIL.

Prozac   See ANTIDEPRESSANTS.

pseudoinsomnia   See SLEEP STATE MISPERCEPTION.

psychiatric disorders   A psychiatric diagnosis is the most frequent diagnosis given to patients with the complaint of INSOMNIA who are seeking help at SLEEP DISORDER CENTERS; almost all patients with DEPRESSION have some sleep complaint. (Insomnia due to acute situational stress is more common in the general population.)

The MOOD DISORDERS, typically disorders due to mania, hypermania or depression, are common causes of the complaint of insomnia, especially EARLY MORNING AROUSAL. Patients with bipolar disorder, such as manic-depressive disorder, will often show periods of short sleep duration during the manic episodes, alternating with episodes of EXCESSIVE SLEEPINESS during the depressive phase. Typically, patients with depression do not have true hypersomnia, that is, the total sleep time during a 24-hour period is not increased above normal levels. However, an excessive amount of time spent in bed is a common feature of depressed patients.

ANXIETY DISORDERS cause sleep disruption, characterized by prolonged sleep latency with frequent awakenings and poor sleep efficiency. These features are most commonly seen in patients who have general anxiety disorders; however, poor sleep quality is also seen in patients who have PANIC DISORDERS. More typically, panic disorder causes an acute event during sleep, with an awakening and feelings of fear and intense anxiety. These abrupt and infrequent episodes during sleep at night are usually accompanied by similar panic attacks during wakefulness. Patients with panic disorders may also suffer from agoraphobia, which is characterized by a fear of being in certain situations where escape may be difficult, such as in a crowded environment or a moving vehicle. The features of agoraphobia and daytime panic episodes are important in order to differentiate panic disorder from awakenings with panic due to other disorders, such as SLEEP TERRORS, which may have a similar presentation.

Patients with the PSYCHOSES, such as schizophrenia or schizoaffective disorder, may have very severe sleep disturbance. This disturbance is characterized by sleep onset difficulties, with small amounts of nocturnal sleep that can alternate with prolonged episodes of sleep. This pattern of sleep may lead to a complete sleep reversal, with no sleep at night and the major sleep episode during the day. Patients with a psychosis can have REM sleep disorders characterized by a reduced REM sleep latency and increased REM density, which is similar to that seen in patients with depression. However, these polysomnographic features are not invariably present, as they are in the depressive disorders.

ALCOHOLISM is associated with severe sleep disturbance due to the acute ingestion of alcohol; it is initially associated with an increase in SLOW WAVE SLEEP, but is followed by a withdrawal effect of sleep disruption, which is seen as the alcohol is metabolized. The chronic alcoholic who abstains from drinking alcohol will have severe sleep disruption. This may be characterized by disrupted REM sleep, hallucinations and NIGHTMARES, as well as disturbed sleep related to autonomic hyperactivity as a result of the alcohol withdrawal. Drinking alcohol during the day will cause impaired daytime functioning because of increased lethargy and sleepiness; that effect is often exacerbated if there was too little sleep the night before.

Other psychiatric disorders, such as substance abuse, adjustment disorder, dissociative and somatoform disorder, can also be associated with either difficulty in initiating and maintaining sleep or excessive sleepiness.

psychophysiological insomnia   A form of INSOMNIA that develops because of learned associations that negatively impact on sleep. Typically, individuals with psychophysiological insomnia tend to react to stress with an increased level of agitation and tension that is often evident by physiological arousal with increased muscle tension and vasoconstriction. With psychophysiological insomnia, there is an overconcern about the inability to fall asleep, which makes it harder to fall asleep. This apprehension may exist throughout the daytime when thinking about the likelihood of little sleep that night.

Sometimes individuals with psychophysiological insomnia can fall asleep at times when it is unexpected, such as relaxing in a chair in the early evening. This reflects their ability to fall asleep when unconcerned about sleep, but when in situations of wanting to fall asleep, the harder the person tries, the less likely it is that sleep will occur. Conditioning factors that contribute to this insomnia include lying in bed awake. The usual sleep environment becomes negatively associated with good sleep. Therefore many individuals with this type of insomnia find that when sleeping in bedrooms other than their own, sleep can occur relatively easily.

Psychophysiological insomnia may be precipitated by a stressful event and may develop subsequent to an ADJUSTMENT SLEEP DISORDER so that after the precipitating event has resolved, the negatively learned associations with sleep continue, and the insomnia becomes chronic. This type of insomnia often becomes fixed over a period of time as intermittent life stress may exacerbate or produce recurrence of psychophysiological insomnia.

Although elements of anxiety and depression are present, particularly in relation to the sleep period, there is little evidence of overt psychopathology. Patients with this form of insomnia do not meet standard psychiatric criteria for the diagnosis of a general anxiety disorder or depression.

Psychophysiological insomnia is uncommon in childhood or adolescence. It will usually present for the first time in the twenties or thirties. More typically, individuals will seek help in middle age. It appears to be more common in females, and there may be a familial tendency.

Polysomnographic monitoring of sleep usually demonstrates a prolonged sleep latency, multiple awakenings, early morning awakening and a reduced sleep efficiency. There may be an increase in the lighter stage one sleep and reduction in a deeper slow wave sleep. Increased muscle tension during sleep can be demonstrated by muscle activity monitoring. Not infrequently, individuals with psychophysiological insomnia will show a reversed "first night effect" in which they sleep much better in the lab on the first night because of the change in their habitual environment; however, the learned negative associations with sleep return by the second night, which demonstrates the reduced quality of sleep.

Psychophysiological insomnia needs to be differentiated from a number of other insomnia disorders. INADEQUATE SLEEP HYGIENE can produce a chronic form of insomnia due to alterations in the timing of sleep, excessive CAFFEINE intake, altered meal times or the ingestion of dietary factors that can adversely affect sleep (see DIET AND SLEEP). An environmental sleep disorder can develop because of such factors as light, noise, abnormal temperature or an uncomfortable or adverse sleeping environment. If anxiety or depression are major factors and warrant a psychiatric diagnosis of either anxiety or mood disorder, the appropriate psychiatric treatment is indicated. If the sleep disturbance is the result of an acute stressful situation, and lasts less than three weeks, then a diagnosis of adjustment sleep disorder is made.

Treatment of psychophysiological insomnia involves redeveloping positive associations with the sleeping environment. Attention to good sleep hygiene is essential, and behavioral management is the most appropriate form of treatment. Relaxation therapy, such as JACOBSONIAN RELAXATION, specific behavioral treatments that may involve STIMULUS CONTROL THERAPY OR SLEEP RESTRICTION THERAPY can be helpful. A short or intermittent course of HYPNOTICS may be useful; however, chronic and long-term use of hypnotics is to be discouraged.

psychoses   PSYCHIATRIC DISORDERS characterized by the presence of delusions, hallucinations, inappropriate effect, incoherence and catatonic behavior, which lead to impaired social and work functioning. Sleep disturbance, either INSOMNIA or EXCESSIVE SLEEPINESS, is a common feature of these disorders.

Psychoses can be produced by organic neurological disorders, as well as by DEMENTIA, ALCOHOLISM, drug effects, schizophrenia, AFFECTIVE DISORDERS, paranoid states and autism.

The sleep disturbances associated with psychoses are typically sleep disruption, with a severe difficulty in initiating sleep. There may be an inadequate amount of sleep because of hyperactivity associated with the psychotic disorder, which leads to a partial or complete reversal of the sleep-wake cycle. Daytime sleepiness may result due to the disturbed sleep at night or the disrupted sleep-wake pattern.

Polysomnographic studies of patients with psychoses have shown varied sleep patterns; some patients will even show normal sleep. Typically there is an increased SLEEP LATENCY, decreased total sleep time, reduced SLEEP EFFICIENCY with frequent awakenings, and reduced SLOW WAVE SLEEP. There may be features of disturbed REM sleep, such as shortened REM latency, increased REM density and varied percentages of REM sleep.

Treatment of the psychoses is by pharmacological means and typically involves the use of phenothiazine medications. The drug therapy may produce sedation, insomnia or withdrawal syndromes. Institutionalization may be required for patients with psychoses who have a severe impairment of their ability to adequately function in society.

pulmonary hypertension   An increased pressure in the pulmonary arteries that leads to hypertrophy and dilation of the right side of the heart. The most potent stimulus for pulmonary constriction leading to pulmonary hypertension is alveolar HYPOXIA. Hypoxia may be produced by SLEEP-RELATED BREATHING DISORDERS that impair ventilation of the lungs. Pulmonary hypertension can be a consequence of severe OBSTRUCTIVE SLEEP APNEA SYNDROME or CENTRAL ALVEOLAR HYPOVENTILATION SYNDROME.

pupillometry   The measurement of pupil diameter and activity. Large, stable pupils are associated with alertness, and small, unstable pupils are associated with decreased alertness and sleepiness. Variations and fluctuations in pupil size can be measured by a pupillometer. The pupillometry test is mainly used as a research procedure to determine sleepiness and has little diagnostic usefulness.

Q–R

quiet sleep   Term used to describe NON-REM-STAGE SLEEP that is seen in infants and animals when the specific sleep phases from one through four are unable to be clearly determined. Quiet sleep usually refers to an encephalographic pattern of sleep in the absence of eye movement recordings or muscle tone recording. The term "non-REM" is preferred when specific SLEEP STAGES are able to be determined. Quiet sleep is distinguished from ACTIVE SLEEP, in which there is an increase in body movement and faster electroencephalographic patterns.

rapid eye movements   The presence of rapid eye movements during sleep was first discovered by Eugene Aserinsky and NATHANIEL KLEITMAN in 1953. This historic discovery of REM sleep led to the recognition that sleep was not a homogeneous state but consisted of two major divisions, REM sleep and non-REM sleep.

Rapid eye movements are seen during wakefulness but are also characteristic of the rapid eye movement stage of sleep (REM sleep). The EEG pattern and muscle tone distinguish the presence of REM sleep from wakefulness, although the pattern of the rapid eye movements usually differs and is characteristic in REM sleep. The movements often occur in discrete bursts in REM sleep. In addition, the presence of the sawtooth EEG pattern in association with the rapid eye movements assists in the determination of REM sleep. The eye movements are conjugate (move together) and can occur in a vertical, horizontal or diagonal direction. The rapid eye movements can be seen under the closed eyelids.

With the discovery of the association of dreaming and rapid eye movement sleep it was initially thought that the rapid eye movements reflected visual scanning of the content of dreams. Subsequent research suggested this was not the case; the rapid eye movements bore no relation to the dream content. (See also REM PARASOMNIAS, REM SLEEP, REM SLEEP LATENCY, REM SLEEP ONSET, REM SLEEP PERCENT, REM SLEEP PERIOD.)

rapid eye movement sleep (REM sleep)   One of the five stages of sleep that are scored according to the method of Alan Rechtschaffen and Anthony Kales. REM sleep is defined by the appearance of a relatively low voltage, mixed frequency EEG activity and episodic, rapid eye movements that occur simultaneously. The EEG pattern resembles stage one sleep (see SLEEP STAGES), with the exception that there are fewer vertex sharp transients and, sometimes, distinctive "saw tooth" waves. The muscle activity is usually at its lowest degree of tone as the skeletal muscles become paralyzed in this sleep stage (see REM ATONIA).

The loss of muscle tone is due to a hyperpolarizing inhibitory activation of the alpha motor neuron. The REM phasic activity is due to excitatory input on the motor-neurone, which is superimposed on a background of inhibitory input. All striated muscle is affected by the phasic jerks and twitches that occur during REM sleep. Rapid eye movements, contractions of the middle ear musculature and the irregular contractions of the respiratory muscles are all components of this phasic muscle activity.

REM sleep typically comprises about 20% to 25% of normal adult sleep. However, the percentage in childhood is greater, with up to 50% of sleep being REM sleep in infancy.

Usually there are five NREM-REM SLEEP CYCLES in a full night of sleep, with REM sleep occurring in episodes of increasing duration from 10 to 30 minutes.

REM sleep is also associated with other physiological changes, such as an increased oxygen consumption of the brain compared with that during non-REM sleep, variability of blood pressure and heart rhythm, variable respiratory rate and altered blood gas control. Body TEMPERATURE control also differs during REM sleep compared with non-REM sleep.

Certain pathological events are more likely to occur during REM sleep, such as obstructive sleep apneas (see OBSTRUCTIVE SLEEP APNEA SYNDROME) and blood oxygen desaturation. Some disorders occur solely during REM sleep, such as the REM SLEEP BEHAVIOR DISORDER, NIGHTMARES and SLEEP-RELATED PAINFUL ERECTIONS. The presence of penile erections during REM sleep is an important finding in the differentiation of IMPOTENCE due to organic versus psychogenic causes. Normal erections during REM sleep in a patient complaining of impotence generally reflect a psychogenic cause of the impotence.

rebound insomnia   INSOMNIA that occurs upon acute withdrawal of hypnotic medication. This form of insomnia more commonly occurs in persons who are on high dosages of HYPNOTICS, particularly short-acting hypnotics. It is less likely to occur in persons who take hypnotic agents for a brief period of time.

Rebound insomnia is characterized by increased sleep disruption with a greater number of awakenings and sleep stage changes that occur upon cessation of the medication. It can be reduced by a gradual decrease in dosage prior to withdrawal. All patients withdrawing from hypnotic medication should be reassured that some sleep disruption is likely for the first few days following cessation of drug treatment. But as long as good SLEEP HYGIENE is instituted, and other causes of insomnia are not present, sleep should return to normal within a few days. (See also BARBITURATES, BENZODIAZEPINES, HYPNOTIC-DEPENDENT SLEEP DISORDER.)

reciprocal interaction model of sleep   First proposed by J. Allan Hobson, Robert McCarley and Peter W. Wyzinski in 1975 to explain the cellular interactions in the regulation of REM sleep. They suggested that there are two sets of cells, the REM-off cells and REM-on cells, that are located in the pontine region of the brain stem. The REM-on cells cause the initiation of REM sleep, and the REM-off cells cause the termination of REM sleep. The REM-on cells are situated near the REM-on cells in a similar region of the brain stem and include the serotonergic cells of the RAPHE NUCLEI. Since the original proposal, the model has been modified to include both explanations of non-REM sleep and waking. (See also SEROTONIN.)

recurrent hypersomnia   A group of disorders characterized by recurrent episodes of EXCESSIVE SLEEPINESS that occur weeks or months apart. These disorders may be associated with other symptoms, such as gluttony or hypersexuality. The combination of recurrent hypersomnia, gluttony and hypersexuality is also known as the KLEINE-LEVIN SYNDROME, which was first described by Willi Kleine in 1925 and Max Levin in 1929. However, a form of recurrent hypersomnia can exist without features of gluttony or hypersexuality; it is then called recurrent hypersomnia monosymptomatic type.

Recurrent hypersomnia more commonly occurs in adolescents or young adults. Typically an episode of excessive sleepiness will occur over a one-to-two-week period followed by weeks or months of normal daytime alertness. There often are personality disturbances, such as withdrawal, irritability and lethargy. Persons with this disorder may eat excessively and start to eat any food in sight. The hypersexuality is characterized by excessive discussion or display of sexual behavior along with public masturbation.

Episodes occur very infrequently and, on average, occur twice a year. Some patients may go many years without an episode or may have as many as one episode each month.

During the period of hypersomnolence, there can be great impairment of social and occupational functioning. The behavior changes can be so intense that the patient requires hospitalization.

Polysomnographic investigation has tended to show excessive sleepiness with high sleep efficiencies and reduced awake time during sleep. A loss of the deeper stage three and four sleep has been demonstrated; however, MULTIPLE SLEEP LATENCY TESTING during the daytime has shown the presence of sleep onset REM periods on one or more naps.

The disorder is believed to be in part due to a hypothalamic dysfunction. There have been some reports of abnormal hormone secretory patterns during sleep. GROWTH HORMONE and PROLACTIN secretion may be abnormal.

A recurrent form of hypersomnia, MENSTRUAL-ASSOCIATED SLEEP DISORDER, also occurs in relationship to the MENSTRUAL CYCLE and is characterized by insomnia and hypersomnia.

Recurrent hypersomnia needs to be differentiated from hypersomnias due to central nervous system tumors and other causes of excessive sleepi-

ness, such as IDIOPATHIC HYPERSOMNIA, NARCOLEPSY and INSUFFICIENT SLEEP SYN-
DROME. Excessive sleepiness due to PSYCHIATRIC DISORDERS, such as major
DEPRESSION or bipolar depression, may present similarly, with the exception
of the gluttony and hypersexuality.

Treatment of recurrent hypersomnia is largely supportive. Lithium carbonate has been reported to stabilize the behavior in some patients but not
in others. The effect of STIMULANT MEDICATIONS in improving alertness is
usually only very temporary. (See also DISORDERS OF EXCESSIVE SOMNOLENCE,
MOOD DISORDERS.)

relaxation exercises   A variety of techniques to enhance muscle relaxation in order to reduce muscle tension and help sleep onset. Various
forms of relaxation exercises are utilized; however, one of the most commonly used is the JACOBSONIAN RELAXATION method. BIOFEEDBACK exercises
can also enhance relaxation. (See also SLEEP EXERCISES.)

REM atonia   The atonia (loss of muscle tone) of REM sleep causes the
skeletal muscles to become flaccid so that the arms and legs are paralyzed.
REM sleep cannot be scored if the ELECTROMYOGRAM (EMG) muscle activity
is increased. Only a few muscles have the ability to move during REM
sleep, such as the eye muscles, the auditory muscles, and the diaphragm
for respiration. Occasional phasic (short burst) muscle activity is seen during the atonia of REM sleep.

Some disorders, such as the REM SLEEP BEHAVIOR DISORDER, are associated
with a variable degree of muscle activity that episodically occurs during
REM sleep and leads to the behavior that is characteristic of the disorder.
The polygraphic features of REM sleep behavior disorder indicate a disrupted and dissociated form of REM sleep. The REM behavior disorder is
not too dissimilar to an experimental condition seen in cats with neurological lesions placed in the pontine region of the brain stem. Cats with
such lesions have the absence of the REM atonia and are able to move
around during REM sleep. It has been proposed that there are two systems
in the nervous system that control muscle tone and movement during
REM sleep: a locomotor system and a system that determines atonia. Usually the locomotor system is inhibited by REM sleep simultaneously with
activation of the system producing the muscle atonia during REM sleep.
(See also RAPID EYE MOVEMENT SLEEP.)

REM parasomnias   Abnormalities that occur during sleep that are not
associated with excessive sleepiness or insomnia but are usually associated
with REM sleep; a subdivision of the parasomnias and the INTERNATIONAL
CLASSIFICATION OF SLEEP DISORDERS. The parasomnias in this section include
NIGHTMARES, SLEEP PARALYSIS, IMPAIRED SLEEP-RELATED PENILE ERECTIONS, SLEEP-
RELATED PAINFUL ERECTIONS, REM SLEEP-RELATED SINUS ARREST, and REM SLEEP
BEHAVIOR DISORDER.

REM rebound   An increase in the amount, duration and density of REM sleep that occurs following the curtailment of a variety of techniques that have suppressed REM sleep. For example, REM rebound can occur following medication suppression of REM sleep by such drugs as the tricyclic ANTIDEPRESSANTS or MONOAMINE OXIDASE INHIBITORS, commonly used for the treatment of DEPRESSION.

Another means of producing REM sleep deprivation is by mechanically arousing an individual whenever REM sleep is detected during a polysomnographic recording. This procedure not only reduces REM sleep but also causes frequent arousals during the major sleep episode. Following this method of REM sleep deprivation there is a rebound of REM sleep.

Some disorders, such as OBSTRUCTIVE SLEEP APNEA SYNDROME, can markedly interfere with the ability of the subject to maintain REM sleep; its relief by either TRACHEOSTOMY or CONTINUOUS POSITIVE AIRWAY PRESSURE devices can lead to an initial REM rebound. REM sleep episodes lasting several hours can sometimes be seen in these situations.

A REM rebound is often accompanied by an increase in awareness of having had long and complex DREAMS. Occasionally NIGHTMARE activity may be exacerbated by the REM rebound. ALCOHOL is also a REM suppressant drug and its withdrawal, particularly in the chronic alcoholic, can lead to a REM rebound, with an increase in nightmares.

REM sleep   See RAPID EYE MOVEMENT SLEEP.

REM sleep behavior disorder   Disorder characterized by the acting out of dream content during the dreaming stage (REM SLEEP) of sleep. Typically, affected persons will have a predominance of violent activity that occurs during sleep and involves punching, kicking, running or other movements of the limbs. These movements may injure a bed partner, which precipitates the disorder being brought to medical attention. The episodes usually occur about 90 minutes after the onset of sleep when the person goes into REM sleep; however, it can occur throughout the major sleep episode. Very often episodes may be precipitated by withdrawal from ALCOHOL or other HYPNOTICS. The disorder has also been described as occurring in association with NARCOLEPSY. There may be partial manifestations of the disorder, evidenced by episodes of SLEEP TALKING or limb movements that may antedate the development of the more physically active behavior.

The most common age of presentation is after age 60; however, episodes have been reported to occur in childhood and in individuals of any age with neurological disorders such as cerebral vascular disease, degeneration or tumors of the brain stem, and DEMENTIA. It has also been described in association with multiple sclerosis. Recent evidence indicates that REM sleep behavior disorder can be a precursor to the development of Parkinson's disease.

The majority of persons with REM sleep behavior disorder appear to be male, and there is some evidence to suggest a familial pattern.

An identical disorder has been described in animals who have suffered lesions in the brain stem. Cats with lesions affecting the locomotor inhibitory region of the brain stem often will have motor activity during REM sleep.

Polysomnographic monitoring of persons with this disorder has shown an intermittent absence of muscle tone. Concurrent rapid eye movements indicative of REM sleep alternate with high muscle activity lasting a few seconds prior to the immediate resumption of REM sleep. There may be an increase in the density of the rapid eye movements and also in the total amount of SLOW WAVE SLEEP.

REM sleep behavior disorder must be differentiated from SLEEP-RELATED EPILEPSY or other disorders of arousal, such as SLEEPWALKING or SLEEP TER-RORS. Nightmares may be somewhat similar but are characterized by less motor activity and lack of the typical polysomnographic features of REM sleep behavior disorder.

Treatment of REM sleep behavior disorder involves securing the bed-room—such as removing sharp objects from nightstands—so the individual does not suffer injury. Clonazepam (see BENZODIAZEPINES) in a dose of 0.5 to 1 milligram, given before sleep at night, has been shown to be very effective in suppressing the behavior. Occasionally tricyclic antidepressants have been shown to be effective as well.

Case History

A 58-year-old real estate executive had episodes of excessive body activity in association with dreams at night. On occasion, he would hit the nightstand or his wife while moving about excessively during sleep. These episodes had occurred over the previous five years. He did have a history of sleepwalking as a child; however, this went away in adolescence and had never reoccurred. The current activity during sleep was characterized by a lot of violent activity, particularly boxing or fighting an individual, and was very different from his childhood sleepwalking episodes. At times, his wife, who was lying quietly beside him, would become the focus of his dream activity and occasionally would get in the way of some of his more violent movements. On one occasion, his activity caused him to fall out of bed and he cut his head on the nightstand. All of the activity was associated with dream content, and he appeared to be actually trying to act out dreams during sleep. He was on no medication at this time, and had sought help from several physicians. His baseline blood work and brain scan were normal. There was no evidence of any underlying neurological disorder. He underwent an all-night POLYSOMNOGRAM, which demonstrated much restlessness during REM sleep with an abnormal amount of muscle activity; REM sleep was very fragmented.

A diagnosis of REM sleep behavior disorder was made on the clinical history and the polysomnographic data. He was prescribed clonazepam (0.5 milligram) to take before sleep at night. With this medication, the activity abruptly subsided and he had a quiet night's sleep. The patient noticed considerable improvement over the subsequent two months; however, some activity reoccurred and the dosage was increased to 1 milligram, whereupon the episodes subsided and remained absent over the subsequent months.

REM sleep deprivation   REM SLEEP deprivation can be produced by mechanically preventing REM sleep from occurring, or by the use of REM suppressant medications. A patient may be mechanically aroused whenever a polygraph shows that he is entering REM sleep; however, this tends to produce frequent arousals and therefore the effects of REM deprivation may be masked by the effects of the frequent arousals or awakenings. A variety of medications, including antidepressant medications such as tricyclic ANTIDEPRESSANTS or MONOAMINE OXIDASE INHIBITORS, as well as BENZODIAZEPINES, STIMULANTS and ALCOHOL, can usually inhibit REM sleep.

The initial effects of REM sleep deprivation are an increase in brain activity; aggressive and sexual behavior may be increased. Psychological difficulties have been reported as the result of REM deprivation; however, recent evidence tends to suggest that this is an unlikely effect.

Positive effects of REM deprivation can include improvement of DEPRESSION, and several studies have shown this to be clinically useful.

The most pronounced effect of REM sleep deprivation is REM REBOUND, with a dramatic increase in the amount and duration of REM sleep episodes. (See also DREAMS.)

REM sleep and dreaming   In 1953, Eugene Aserinsky and NATHANIEL KLEITMAN at the University of Chicago made a major scientific development in the study of dreams when they recognized physiological changes during dreaming and rapid eye movements (REM). Over the next few years, joined by WILLIAM C. DEMENT, the researchers compared dream recall during REM versus NREM SLEEP PERIODS. By 1957, the results of these experiments were published: Subjects awakened 191 times during REM periods had dream recall 80% of the time, or in 152 of the awakenings. By contrast, subjects were awoken 160 times during NREM periods, with only 6.9% or 11 dream recalls. (See also REM SLEEP.)

REM sleep latency   The interval from sleep onset to the first appearance of REM sleep during a sleep episode. In normal, healthy adults, REM sleep usually occurs approximately 90 minutes after the onset of non-REM sleep. A short REM latency is seen in patients who have DEPRESSION and may be a biological marker of depression. Treatment of depression in such patients often leads to a normalization of the REM latency. REM latencies of less than 65 minutes are regarded as being shorter than normal. A short REM latency may also be seen in patients who acutely withdraw from a REM suppressant medication, such as tricyclic ANTIDEPRESSANTS, ALCOHOL or MONOAMINE OXIDASE INHIBITORS.

In NARCOLEPSY, the REM sleep latency is usually reduced. Patients may sometimes go directly into REM sleep. However, this is not always present. The presence of REM sleep during a daytime MULTIPLE SLEEP LATENCY TEST has more diagnostic usefulness. The occurrence of REM sleep within 10 minutes of initiating a daytime nap is regarded as supportive evidence of narcolepsy. Two or more sleep onset REM periods during a multiple sleep latency test that is performed following a night of normal sleep is diagnostic of narcolepsy.

Infants (see INFANT SLEEP) have a much greater percentage of REM sleep (in contrast to adults) and will frequently initiate their short sleep episodes by an immediate occurrence of REM sleep; therefore, a short REM sleep latency is commonly seen.

REM sleep-locked   This term has been used for the close association between CHRONIC PAROXYSMAL HEMICRANIA (a type of headache) and REM SLEEP. Episodes of chronic paroxysmal hemicrania during sleep always occur in association with REM sleep. (See also SLEEP-RELATED HEADACHES.)

REM sleep onset   The occurrence of REM sleep at sleep onset; occasionally used instead of the longer SLEEP ONSET REM PERIOD, which is the preferred term.

REM sleep percent   The proportion of total sleep time that is filled by REM sleep. For adults, a typical night of sleep is comprised of 20% to 25% REM sleep; in an infant, REM sleep equals 50% of the total sleep time. The percentage of REM sleep falls slightly from young adulthood to old age. (See also RAPID EYE MOVEMENT SLEEP.)

REM sleep period   Occasionally used for an episode of REM SLEEP that occurs during the major sleep episode. The term is discouraged from use because the word "period" implies a cyclical event; therefore, REM sleep period may be confused with the NREM-REM SLEEP CYCLE.

REM sleep-related sinus arrest   A disorder of cardiac rhythm that produces episodes of sinus arrest during REM SLEEP in otherwise healthy individuals. This disorder has been described in young adults and appears to be associated with symptoms that include acute discomfort, sudden palpitations, light-headedness, feeling of faintness and blurred vision. Some individuals with this disorder have reported episodes of syncope (fainting) that have occurred during the nocturnal hours.

The diagnosis is based entirely upon the presence of episodes of sinus arrest of at least 2.5 seconds in duration, which suddenly occur during REM sleep. Episodes as long as 9 seconds have been reported. Additional investigations, including coronary angiography and electrical conduction studies, are normal.

The episodes of ARRHYTHMIA are not associated with sleep-related respiratory disturbance or oxygen desaturation. They occur in clusters and do not induce arousals or awakenings.

This disorder must be differentiated from the cardiac irregularity characterized by brady-tachycardia that is typically seen in the OBSTRUCTIVE SLEEP APNEA SYNDROME.

If the episodes are frequent in occurrence and long in duration, consideration should be given to implantation of a ventricular inhibited pacemaker in order to prevent episodes of cardiac arrest.

RERA   See RESPIRATORY EFFORT–RELATED AROUSAL.

respiratory disturbance index (RDI)   Also known as APNEA-HYPOPNEA INDEX. RDI is a measure of the number of apneas, both central and obstructive, plus the number of hypopneas, expressed per hour of sleep. A respiratory disturbance index of greater than five is regarded as an abnormal frequency of respiratory events during sleep. This index is commonly used as a measure of the severity of the sleep apnea syndromes. Many authors regard the term RDI as preferable to the apnea-hypopnea index because it is more descriptive for those not familiar with the term HYPOPNEA. (See also APNEA, CENTRAL SLEEP APNEA SYNDROME, OBSTRUCTIVE SLEEP APNEA SYNDROME.)

respiratory effort   Applies to respiratory muscle activity; typically measured during sleep to determine the degree of respiratory impairment. Patients who have cessation of respiratory movements during sleep, as is seen during an apneic episode, will have no respiratory effort, whereas patients with the OBSTRUCTIVE SLEEP APNEA SYNDROME may have an increased degree of respiratory effort, particularly immediately prior to the termination of the obstructive event. Respiratory effort does not imply that there is a transfer of air between the atmosphere and the lung because complete airway obstruction may occur despite the presence of respiratory effort.

Respiratory effort can be measured by means of a mercury-filled strain gauge, a bellows pneumograph or inductive plethysmography. (See also APNEA, CENTRAL SLEEP APNEA SYNDROME.)

respiratory effort–related arousal (RERA)   An arousal associated with increasing negative esophageal pressure which is terminated by a sudden change in pressure to a less negative level with an arousal. The event lasts 10 seconds or longer.

244 respiratory stimulants

Five or more RERAs per hour are regarded as abnormal and in association with other symptoms are sufficient to produce a diagnosis of OBSTRUCTIVE SLEEP APNEA SYNDROME. (See also CENTRAL SLEEP APNEA SYNDROME.)

respiratory stimulants   Drugs used in SLEEP DISORDERS MEDICINE for the stimulation of VENTILATION in SLEEP-RELATED BREATHING DISORDERS such as CENTRAL SLEEP APNEA SYNDROME or OBSTRUCTIVE SLEEP APNEA SYNDROME. (See also CHEYNE-STOKES RESPIRATION, INFANT SLEEP DISORDERS.)

restless legs syndrome   A disorder associated with discomfort experienced in both legs as well as the uncontrollable urge to keep moving the legs. This discomfort is described as a crawling, tickling, itching sensation in the legs and is usually found in the calf, feet and sometimes in the thigh. It is rarely experienced as a pain. This syndrome was first described by K.A. Ekbom in 1945, and it is recognized as a cause of difficulty in falling asleep at night. The legs are moved around in bed to find a comfortable position, and often the patient has to get out of bed to walk around. Rubbing the calves and exercising the muscles often produces a temporary relief.

The discomfort is typically present at sleep onset, although it often can occur during wakeful episodes during the night. Sometimes the sensation is also experienced during the daytime when lying down or sitting.

The discomfort may be very intense and has been said to have driven sufferers, on rare occasion, to commit suicide.

Since restless legs syndrome is typically associated with PERIODIC LEG MOVEMENTS, treatment may be required for both conditions. Polysomnographic evaluation of restless legs syndrome demonstrates movement of the legs that occurs at sleep onset and a prolonged SLEEP LATENCY. There may be further episodes of leg movements occurring during wakeful episodes throughout the night. Intermittent periodic leg movements can be seen in sleep throughout the polysomnographic recording.

Restless legs syndrome needs to be differentiated from other disorders that produce abnormal movements during sleep. SLEEP STARTS are whole body jerks that occur only at sleep onset. The restless movements that occur during REM SLEEP BEHAVIOR DISORDER typically occur during REM sleep at night and are associated with more violent movements, reflecting the acting out of DREAMS. NOCTURNAL PAROXYSMAL DYSTONIA is a disorder associated with abnormal posturing of the limbs; it typically occurs during non-REM sleep and not at sleep onset.

Although the cause of this disorder is unknown, relief of the discomfort is available by using a variety of medications including the anticonvulsants as well as the HYPNOTICS. Carbamazepine (see ANTIDEPRESSANTS) may be helpful in some patients; however, many patients do not respond to this medication. The most effective BENZODIAZEPINE is clonazepam, which is also effective against the periodic leg movements that can occur in association with restless legs syndrome. However, other benzodiazepines, such as tri-zolam, and narcotic derivatives, such as oxycodone, have also been shown to be useful in some patients.

L-DOPA has been shown to be effective in reducing the number of episodes of both restless legs syndrome and periodic leg movement during sleep. Other dopaminergic agents such as PRAMIPEXOLE have also proved to be very effective and now have become the medications of choice.

restlessness   Term applied to increased body movements occurring during sleep. Restlessness (a restless sleep) is often an indication of an underlying sleep disorder, and therefore investigation by appropriate polysomnographic studies may be indicated. Although occasional awakenings are not uncommon in normal, healthy sleepers, in general sleep should be relatively quiet for most individuals.

Restlessness predominantly occurs during disorders that produce INSOMNIA, such as PSYCHOPHYSIOLOGICAL INSOMNIA, or insomnia due to psychiatric disorders. However, it can also occur in other disorders that disrupt sleep, such as the OBSTRUCTIVE SLEEP APNEA SYNDROME, the REM SLEEP BEHAVIOR DISORDER and the RESTLESS LEGS SYNDROME.

Individuals who complain of insomnia will often describe how they stay motionless during sleep with the hope it will enhance sleep onset and reduce the amount of times they awaken during sleep. However, lying in bed awake often makes the individual aware of discomfort related to body position. Restlessness occurs because of the need to keep changing position. Some disorders may be directly associated with discomfort of body position, such as PREGNANCY-RELATED SLEEP DISORDER or the restless legs syndrome. However, in the majority of individuals who suffer from insomnia due to psychophysiological or psychiatric causes, the discomfort experienced is a result of being in a single position for a prolonged period of time while awake. Very often the discomfort is exacerbated by the increased muscular tension and ANXIETY that accompany insomnia. The generalized restlessness that accompanies insomnia often leads to the individual getting out of bed and going to another room or walking about for a period of time before returning to bed. Although the SLEEP SURFACE is sometimes responsible for the discomfort, in most cases it is not the primary cause unless there was a recent change in the sleep surface.

Patients with the obstructive sleep apnea syndrome can be particularly restless. The termination of the apneic events is associated with an increase in body movements, and not uncommonly there are reports of an arm being raised from the bed or the legs changing position. The movements may become excessive and lead the individual to fall out of bed. Not uncommonly, children will adopt a hands/knees position in order to improve their breathing at night.

In the elderly population, in addition to the increased number of causes of insomnia, the REM sleep behavior disorder is associated with increased motor activity during sleep. In this disorder, the individual will tend to act out DREAMS and so there may be quite violent arm and leg movements. Restlessness may be the primary complaint of a spouse.

The restless legs syndrome is characterized by a discomfort experienced in the legs in which the legs have to be moved to relieve the discomfort. Typically, patients will get out of bed in order to walk around thereby easing the pain. Once sleep onset has occurred, generally the legs are still; however, brief interruptions or awakenings of sleep will often be associated with an increase in the leg movements.

Although a number of parasomnias, such as SLEEPWALKING, can be associated with abnormal movement activity, restlessness is usually not a common feature, in part due to the episodic nature of the movements. SLEEP-RELATED EPILEPSY generally produces infrequent episodes during sleep, and therefore a complaint of restless sleep is uncommon.

Restoril   See BENZODIAZEPINES.

reversal of sleep   A 12-hour shift in the onset of the major sleep episode. Reversal of sleep has been performed experimentally to determine the effect on circadian rhythmicity. Sleep itself is less efficient when acutely moved, and there is usually a decrease in deep stages three/four sleep and REM sleep (see SLEEP STAGES). Total sleep time is shorter than before the shift, and the REM SLEEP LATENCY is reduced.

Following an acute reversal of the sleep pattern there are changes in underlying circadian rhythms in that some will shift with the change in the sleep pattern, but others will remain fixed at the previous phase. For example, the pattern of cortisol secretion and body temperature adjusts very slowly over a period of one to two weeks to the new time of sleep. Some body rhythms, such as urine volume and electrolyte excretions, shift to the new pattern of sleep within a few days, as does growth hormone secretion.

Reversal of sleep is also applied to individuals who are on a stable pattern of sleeping during the day and awakening at night. In such individuals, the pattern of circadian rhythmicity has adjusted to the new time of sleep and therefore there is no dissociation between circadian rhythms. This pattern is sometimes seen in individuals who have a severe form of the DELAYED SLEEP PHASE SYNDROME. An acute reversal of the sleep pattern also occurs in shift workers and individuals who cross many time zones. (See also CIRCADIAN RHYTHMS, SHIFT-WORK SLEEP DISORDER, TIME ZONE CHANGE (JET LAG) SYNDROME.)

reversed first night effect   Typically, sleep is of better quality on the first night of polysomnographic recording in the laboratory, and of much reduced quality during the second night. This pattern can be seen in patients with IDIOPATHIC INSOMNIA or PSYCHOPHYSIOLOGICAL INSOMNIA. (See also FIRST NIGHT EFFECT.)

rhythmic movement disorder   A disorder characterized by repetitive abnormal movements during sleep such as HEADBANGING, BODYROCKING or leg rolling. These movements usually occur during the lighter stages of sleep or immediately prior to sleep onset; however, rarely they can occur during deep sleep stages or RAPID EYE MOVEMENT (REM) SLEEP. Usually treatment is limited to securing the environment so that banging into solid objects does not harm the individual. For example, a child in a crib may need to have padding affixed to crib bars to prevent injury. Medication treatment is usually not effective although the BENZODIAZEPINES have been helpful in some patients. See also HEAD ROLLING.

rhythms   This term applies to a cyclical process and in sleep medicine mainly applies to the sleep-wake rhythm. Rhythms that occur within a 24-hour cycle are called CIRCADIAN RHYTHMS. Rhythms less than 24 hours are called ultradian (see ULTRADIAN RHYTHM), and those greater than 24 hours are called infradian.

The most frequently studied rhythms in human physiology are the circadian rhythms, of which the sleep-wake cycle, body TEMPERATURE and cortisol pattern are examples.

The term "biological rhythm" applies to the rhythmicity of biological variables; however, this is not to be confused with BIORHYTHM, a term that is not used in CHRONOBIOLOGY. Biorhythms are patterns of human behavior that are determined by astrological signs and have no scientific validity.

Ritalin   See STIMULANT MEDICATIONS.

S

SAD   See SEASONAL AFFECTIVE DISORDER.

sandman   A personification of sleep or sleepiness that refers to someone who goes around sprinkling sand in the eyes as a way of inducing sleep. The term developed from the gritty sensation that often occurs in the eyes upon awakening in the morning. The term *dustman* was first reported in P. Egan's *Tom and Jerry* in 1821: "till the dustman made his appearance and gave the hint to Tom and Jerry that it was time to visit their beds." The term referred to getting sleepy and the sensation of dust being in the eyes. Over the years, *dustman* became associated with garbage and refuse, and therefore the term was changed from *dustman* to *sandman*. The term *sandman* is still commonly used in children's fairy tales.

Sanorex   See STIMULANT MEDICATIONS.

sawtooth waves   A form of THETA ACTIVITY that occurs during REM SLEEP and is characterized by a notched appearance on the wave form. This notched appearance looks like the teeth of a saw, hence the term *sawtooth waves*. These episodes of EEG activity occur in bursts that last up to 10 seconds and are a characteristic of REM sleep.

schizophrenia   Group of psychiatric disorders (see PSYCHOSES) characterized by disturbances of thought process, with delusions and hallucinations. Specifically there is a low level of intellectual and social functioning that typically occurs before middle age. Sleep disturbances are common in schizophrenic patients and are characterized by INSOMNIA or alterations in the sleep-wake cycle.

During acute schizophrenia, there may be a reduction in the TOTAL SLEEP TIME, and an alteration in the timing of REM SLEEP, with a short REM SLEEP LATENCY, similar to that seen in DEPRESSION. The amount of SLOW WAVE SLEEP may be reduced, but the amount of REM sleep is usually normal.

The sleep symptoms often parallel the course of the underlying schizophrenia, which usually requires psychiatric management.

SCN   See SUPRACHIASMATIC NUCLEUS.

seasonal affective disorder (SAD)   A disorder that most often occurs in the mid-to-late fall as the nights grow longer. The increased tendency for DEPRESSION is believed to be in part related to the reduced light exposure at that particular time of year. A clinical diagnosis of SAD is made if, for at least two consecutive winters, someone experiences being depressed, sleeping too much, overeating, craving carbohydrates, a diminished sex drive and working less productively. Such individuals are relatively depression-free during the rest of the year, when there is more light. Exposure to light of more than 2,000 lux (a unit of illumination) for two or more hours in the morning from 6 A.M. to 8 A.M. can improve mood and decrease the seasonal affective disorder. But there may be a mid-afternoon reduction in mood associated with the circadian variation in daytime alertness. A shorter exposure of light at that time may improve the symptoms and reduce the need for a mid-afternoon nap.

Although SAD is uncommon—an estimated half a million people are affected in the United States—a related seasonal condition has been found in 25% of the general population whereby clinically depression is absent but there are mood swings related to the winter and diminished light. In the northern United States, light deprivation and related mood swings seem to begin in October, achieve their most severe form in January and go into remission by the end of February. Bright light systems are commercially available. (See also CIRCADIAN RHYTHMS, LIGHT THERAPY, MOOD DISORDERS.)

sedative-hypnotic medications   See HYPNOTICS.

sedative medications   See HYPNOTICS.

seizures   Term commonly used to denote a clinical manifestation of an epileptic discharge. (The term *epilepsy* applies to a disorder of abnormal brain electrical activity, whereas the term *seizure* applies to the clinical manifestation.) Patients may have epilepsy but may not have seizures if their disorder is under good control with anticonvulsant medications. Rarely some forms of epilepsy do not have seizure manifestations, such as ELECTRICAL STATUS EPILEPTICUS OF SLEEP.

Seizures often occur during sleep and are typically characterized by abnormal motor activity, sometimes producing SLEEPWALKING episodes or enuresis (bed-wetting, see SLEEP ENURESIS). Epilepsy is a major cause in children of secondary enuresis. Rarely SLEEP TERROR episodes may be due to epilepsy. Some abnormal movement disorders, such as NOCTURNAL PAROXYSMAL DYSTONIA, can occur during sleep and have features similar to those of seizures. These disorders can be differentiated from seizures by appropriate encephalographic monitoring during sleep.

Seizure disorders can affect an individual of any age; however, some seizures are more commonly seen in childhood. Infantile spasms associated with hypsarrhythmia (abnormal EEG pattern) or the tonic seizures of Lennox-Gastaut syndrome (atonic seizures) are seen in young children. Petit mal epilepsy and generalized tonic-clonic (grand mal) seizure disorder are common in prepubertal and postpubertal children.

In adults, including the elderly, partial complex seizures (temporal lobe or psychomotor) are more commonly seen. Generalized seizures can also occur as a result of central nervous system lesions, such as a stroke. A stroke typically produces a focal motor seizure that may become generalized, with whole body tonic-clonic movements similar to that seen in grand mal epilepsy.

Most seizure disorders can be adequately controlled by anticonvulsant medications such as phenytion, phenobarbital, or carbamazepine (see ANTI-DEPRESSANTS). (See also BARBITURATES, BENIGN EPILEPSY WITH ROLANDIC SPIKES.)

selective serotonin reuptake inhibitors (SSRIs)   See ANTIDEPRESSANTS.

serotonin   A neurotransmitter that is found in cells of the central nervous system, particularly within the brain stem. Serotonin is a naturally-occurring agent in the blood that has the effect of producing vasoconstriction. It is believed to be involved in the regulation of sleep because inhibition of the synthesis of serotonin in animals has led to very profound INSOMNIA. Michel Jouvet in 1969 first proposed that serotonin is involved in the maintenance of sleep, particularly SLOW WAVE SLEEP. The RAPHE NUCLEI of the brain stem are the primary site of the serotonin-containing neurons that are involved in sleep regulation.

Precursors of serotonin, such as tryptophan, have been shown to induce drowsiness in animals; however, the effects in man are unclear. Research studies on L-tryptophan (see HYPNOTICS) have suggested a beneficial effect on reducing SLEEP LATENCY and improving the depth of sleep. L-tryptophan is a commonly used OVER-THE-COUNTER MEDICATION in patients who have sleep disturbance; however, it has a relatively weak hypnotic effect. L-tryptophan has recently been withdrawn from the market in the United States because of an association with potentially fatal eosinophilia-myalgia syndrome.

Several ANTIDEPRESSANTS that inhibit the re-uptake of serotonin—the so-called serotonin blockers—tend to decrease REM SLEEP. Serotonin reuptake blockers, such as fluvoxamine, zimeldine, femoxitine and fluoxetine, have been reported to be effective in suppressing the CATAPLEXY of NARCOLEPSY. The tricyclic antidepressants that inhibit the uptake of serotonin have pronounced effects in decreasing REM sleep. It has been proposed that the antidepressant effect of these medications is due to this suppression effect on REM sleep.

serotonin reuptake inhibitors   See ANTIDEPRESSANTS.

SESE   See ELECTRICAL STATUS EPILEPTICUS OF SLEEP.

settling   Popular term that is often used to describe an infant who sleeps through the night and does not awaken for feedings during the night. Settling typically occurs within the first three months of life. (See also INFANT SLEEP, INFANT SLEEP DISORDERS.)

shift-work sleep disorder   Disorder that affects workers who work the night shift and who typically have a disturbed sleep-wake pattern. Since most nighttime shift work is performed between 11 P.M. and 7 A.M., sleep is typically delayed until after the shift. SLEEP ONSET would begin anywhere between 6 A.M. and 12 noon. In addition, on days off the shift worker may attempt to return to a more normal sleep-wake pattern, with sleep occurring during the night hours when he would usually be working. As a consequence of the delayed sleep pattern when working the NIGHT SHIFT and the alteration and timing in sleep on days off, complaints of INSOMNIA or EXCESSIVE SLEEPINESS are common. See Chapter 8: Circadian Rhythm Sleep Disorders.

short sleeper   An individual who consistently sleeps less than someone of the same age. Typically, the total sleep time is less than 75% of the lowest normal sleep time for someone of that age. Although exact limits for the total sleep times of a particular individual are unknown, a sleep episode of less than five hours in any 24-hour day, before the age of 60 years, is regarded as an unusually short sleep episode. (After the age of 60, the nocturnal sleep period is usually reduced in duration, but daytime sleep episodes are more common, so the normal total sleep within any 24-hour period is still typically greater than five hours in duration.)

Sleep lengths in short sleepers may vary from two hours to five hours in duration; however, most short sleepers sleep for only three to five hours, without any tendency for daytime sleepiness. Monitoring of sleep-wake patterns by means of an activity monitor may be useful in documenting the sleep length of short sleepers over a period of weeks or months.

Short sleepers, because of a complaint of INSOMNIA at night, often have the expectation that they should sleep for eight hours. Excessive time spent in bed awake is considered an inability to fall asleep and, hence, induces a complaint of insomnia. Although the pattern of short sleep has its onset in early adolescence, when the more typical adult sleep pattern is being established, it is not usually regarded as a problem until adulthood, when a full eight-hour sleep period is desired. An adolescent short sleeper very often has fewer complaints about the sleep period and usually enjoys the luxury of being able to stay up late at night.

Studies have indicated that most short sleepers are males and the prevalence of this disorder is rare. There is some evidence to suggest it is more common in families.

A psychological profile of short sleepers by Ernest Hartmann, Frederick Baekeland and George Zwilling indicated that they generally are not psychiatrically disturbed but tend to be high achievers who are efficient and who have a tendency to hypomania, an increase in activity, with an elevated, expansive mood.

A survey by Daniel Kripke, R. Simons, L. Garfinkel and E. Hammond that involved over one million individuals indicated that people with a nocturnal sleep period of less than five hours had a shorter life expectancy than those with more usual sleep durations.

Objective documentation of the sleep patterns of short sleepers is relatively sparse. It is difficult to confirm the habitual tendency to short sleeping because of the difficulty in monitoring someone for 24 hours a day for many consecutive days. Studies that have been performed have tended to show normal amounts of stages three and four sleep, with reduced lighter sleep stages and REM sleep. There is no evidence for any sleep disorder causing disrupted nighttime sleep or for a tendency to daytime sleepiness.

Short sleepers need to be differentiated from individuals who have psychopathology that may cause a short-term reduction in total sleep time, such as is seen during the manic phase of manic-depressive disease.

Short sleepers also have to be differentiated from those who have short sleep but then make up for it by an excessively long sleep episode, such as on the weekends. Those individuals are classified as having insufficient sleep and may be chronically sleep deprived.

No treatment is indicated or necessary for a short sleeper other than the reassurance that the sleep length is normal for that individual and that an appropriate time spent in bed will allay concerns regarding insomnia. Many short sleepers, particularly in middle or old age, are concerned about being awake at night when others are sleeping; it should be suggested that they find activities to occupy them during their period of wakefulness. (See also ACTIVITY MONITOR, INSUFFICIENT SLEEP SYNDROME, MOOD DISORDERS.)

short-term insomnia   Defined as lasting up to three weeks, usually in association with a situational stress—such as an acute loss, work or marital stress—or due to a serious medical illness. SLEEP HYGIENE and nondrug procedures are primarily recommended for the treatment of this type of sleep disturbance. However, sleep-promoting medications, such as the BENZODIAZEPINES, could be considered. This form of insomnia is equivalent to ADJUSTMENT SLEEP DISORDER; however, other causes of insomnia, such as jet lag or shift work, when seen within three weeks of their onset, could also be regarded as short-term insomnia. (See also HYPNOTICS.)

SIDS   See SUDDEN INFANT DEATH SYNDROME.

siesta   A voluntary nap usually taken in the mid-afternoon by certain cultural and ethnic groups, such as the Latin Americans and the Spanish. Many societies adopt the midafternoon siesta to avoid the hottest part of the day, particularly in tropical environments. A siesta usually lasts two hours and is taken at a point in the biphasic circadian ALERTNESS cycle when there is an increased amount of sleepiness, typically between 2 P.M. and 4 P.M. Prolonged siestas are taken at the expense of nighttime sleep so that total sleep time within any 24-hour period is still one-third of the day, or about eight hours. Longer siestas of four hours may be accompanied by a short nocturnal sleep episode of a similar duration. Most persons in cultures where siestas are typical tend to stay up later at night because the NAP necessitates shorter nocturnal sleep.

Many cultures that take a siesta will purposely have a large midday meal, which is an additional stimulus to taking a midafternoon nap. Consequently, the evening meal is often taken at a later hour, approximately 9 to 10 P.M.

It is believed by many that the sleep pattern seen in prepubertal children of eight or nine hours of nocturnal sleep along with a daytime of maximal alertness is preferable. Therefore in many societies the tendency for a daytime nap or siesta is discouraged. The avoidance of a midafternoon nap is especially important for persons who suffer from sleep disorders such as INSOMNIA, as it may lead to a further breakdown and disruption of nighttime sleep. (See also CIRCADIAN RHYTHMS, NAPS.)

Siffre, Michel   A speleologist (cave expert) who began an experiment on July 16, 1962, of living in an underground cavern in the Alps between France and Italy. The underground cavern contained an ice glacier at a depth of 375 feet below the surface. Siffre stayed in a tent on the underground ice shelf for 59 days and recorded his sleep-wake pattern while isolated from ENVIRONMENTAL TIME CUES. The sleep-wake pattern showed a rhythm of 24 hours and 30 minutes over the course of the experiment. This study was one of the first demonstrations of man's FREE RUNNING pattern of sleep and wakefulness in an environment isolated from time cues. (See TEMPORAL ISOLATION.)

sigma rhythm   Previously-used term for SLEEP SPINDLES. Sigma rhythm is derived from the shape of the Greek "sigma" character.

situational insomnia   See ADJUSTMENT SLEEP DISORDER.

sleep   A behavioral state characterized by rest, immobility and reduced perception of environmental stimuli in which cognition and consciousness are suspended. Sleep occurs when the brain waves slow, and the erratic activity of many parts of the brain starts to coalesce into a coordinated synchronized background rhythm. The heart rate slows, the muscles relax, and the wakeful brain mentation calms to the point that a satisfying sense of contentment occurs as we mentally drift away from our environment into peaceful unconsciousness. See also BEDTIME, DREAM CONTENT,

DREAMS, DREAMS AND CREATIVITY, SLEEP DEPRIVATION, SLEEP DURATION, SLEEP NEED, SLEEP ONSET, SLEEP STAGES.

Sleep   A leading scholarly journal originally published bimonthly by Raven Press, Ltd., but now published by the American Academy of Sleep Medicine. A peer-reviewed journal, *Sleep* contains scholarly articles on all aspects of sleep (clinical, experimental, biochemical, etc.), reporting sleep research findings as well as announcements, book reviews and a bibliography of recent literature in sleep research. *Sleep* is listed in *Index Medicus, Current Contents* and *PASCAL/CNRS.*

sleep apnea   Cessation of breathing that occurs during sleep. APNEA in association with complete cessation of respiratory movements is termed "central sleep apnea" whereas apnea that occurs in association with upper airway obstruction is called "obstructive sleep apnea." A mixed form of apnea may occur if there is an initial central apnea that is continuous with an obstructive apnea. Sleep apnea is differentiated from episodes of partial obstruction, which are termed HYPOPNEAS, in which there is an incomplete reduction of airflow (but a reduction of 50% or more) associated with a reduction in blood oxygen saturation.

Some people have frequent episodes of sleep apnea and may develop a sleep apnea syndrome. CENTRAL SLEEP APNEA SYNDROME or OBSTRUCTIVE SLEEP APNEA SYNDROME are the two apnea syndromes seen in infancy, childhood or adulthood. A physiological form of central sleep apnea may occur in premature infants and is called APNEA OF PREMATURITY. (See also INFANT SLEEP APNEA, SLEEP-RELATED BREATHING DISORDERS.)

sleep atonia   Term denoting the decrease of muscle activity during sleep. As sleep gets deeper, from the early stages of NON-REM STAGE SLEEP through to SLOW WAVE SLEEP, muscles reduce in activity and tone. The most pronounced reduction of muscle tone is during REM SLEEP, when the alpha motor neurons of the spinal cord are inhibited by the medullary region of Magoun and Rhines. The medullary inhibitory region is stimulated by the caudal region of the locus ceruleus.

Bilateral-lateral pontine lesions in cats can cause destruction of the region around the locus ceruleus, thereby preventing stimulation of the medullary inhibitory region, leading to a retention of muscle tone during REM sleep. Cats with such lesions will tend to "act out" DREAMS. A similar situation has recently been discovered in humans in whom muscle activity persists during REM sleep and the patient also "acts out" dreams. This disorder, which has been called the REM SLEEP BEHAVIOR DISORDER, is most commonly seen in persons over the age of 60 years, although it has been described in younger individuals, usually in association with neurological lesions of varied types. The majority of cases of REM sleep behavior disorder have no known neurological cause. (See also PONS.)

sleep bruxism   Stereotyped movement disorder that involves clenching or grinding the teeth during sleep. Some individuals have bruxism when awake during the day; others have bruxism predominantly while asleep. When bruxism occurs during sleep, it commonly produces an unpleasant grinding sound that may be disturbing to a bed partner; it can also interfere with the sufferer's quality of sleep by causing brief arousals. When the grinding occurs over many years, the cusps of the teeth can be worn down, and this may be detected during a routine dental examination. The constant grinding during sleep often leads to discomfort in the muscles of the jaw and there may also be gum damage. Bruxism is a cause of an atypical headache and may also produce a temporomandibular joint discomfort.

Bruxism typically occurs in healthy adults or children, but it is more common in children who have a central nervous system disorder such as cerebral palsy. Exacerbation of the bruxism may occur with psychological stress.

Although the majority of the population will at some time grind their teeth, if only infrequently, up to 5% of the population have more persistent teeth grinding. The onset of teeth grinding among healthy infants occurs at a mean age of 10 months, affecting male and female children equally.

Studies of bruxism during sleep have shown that it can occur during all stages but is most common during stage two sleep (see SLEEP STAGES). Rarely will it occur predominantly in REM sleep.

Bruxism may be helped by the use of a dental appliance, the mouth guard, which is worn during sleep. Attention to underlying psychological stress by using appropriate psychological or psychiatric treatment may also be helpful. For many individuals, the disorder does not require a specific treatment. Particularly in children, it appears to be a transient phenomenon.

sleep choking syndrome   Disorder characterized by choking episodes that occur during sleep and do not have an apparent organic or psychiatric cause. The patient awakens with a sudden and intense feeling of being unable to breathe associated with a choking sensation. The episodes occur typically in the early part of the night. Once awake, there is a sensation of fear, ANXIETY and the feeling of impending death. Within a few seconds, the anxiety abates as the awareness develops that breathing is unimpaired. This disorder commonly occurs either nightly or almost every night.

The sleep choking syndrome is not associated with any objective evidence of difficulty in breathing. There is no stridor, hoarseness or change in color noted in these patients. Bed partners are usually not aware of the episodes until reported to them the next morning.

The episodes most commonly occur in females in early to middle adulthood.

sleep cure   See SLEEP THERAPY.

sleep cycle   See NREM-REM SLEEP CYCLE.

sleep deprivation   One of the most intriguing questions in sleep research is, "Why do we need to sleep?" As this is a difficult question to answer, experimenters have studied the opposite phenomenon of what happens if you do not sleep. Sleep deprivation has been studied extensively to determine the effect of sleep loss, as well as the loss of specific components of sleep, such as REM SLEEP.

Although it is clear that most people who are deprived of sleep become sleepy, no one had ever tried staying awake for a prolonged period of time until 1959, when PETER TRIPP, a New York disc jockey, stayed awake for some 200 hours as a fund-raising publicity stunt. Toward the end of Tripp's 200-hour vigil, psychotic features became evident, with hallucinations. As a result of this unscientific experiment of sleep deprivation, it was erroneously believed that the loss of sleep would be accompanied by severe mental deterioration.

The first opportunity to scientifically study somebody who had been deprived of sleep occurred in 1964 when RANDY GARDNER, a San Diego resident, remained awake for 260 hours. During the later part of his stint of wakefulness, he was observed by the sleep researcher WILLIAM C. DEMENT, and subsequently studied by Dr. Laverne Johnson in the sleep laboratory at the San Diego Naval Hospital. Toward the end of the attempt at keeping awake, it was clear that Gardner was in a state of partial sleep and wakefulness that could not be separated. One of the intriguing questions that arose was whether he would have a prolonged sleep episode following the wakefulness. After the 11 days, Gardner slept for 14 hours and 40 minutes and appeared entirely refreshed upon awakening. He subsequently remained awake for 24 hours before having a second sleep episode of normal duration of approximately eight hours. Gardner did not have any psychiatric disturbance related to the sleep deprivation; subsequent sleep episodes demonstrated that the accumulated lost sleep was not made up by the body, as a short sleep episode appeared to be fully refreshing.

Subsequent research studies have given conflicting results, with some brief psychiatric disturbances following sleep deprivation of up to 10 days. However, prolonged and complete sleep deprivation is usually not possible because of the intrusion of brief sleep episodes, even though the subject is active and conversant.

There are major changes in mood and performance, with fatigue, irritability, impaired perception and orientation, and inattentiveness due to sleep deprivation. These features begin after about 36 hours of sleep deprivation and are most notable during the time that would usually be the time of the habitual sleep period. Even during the first night of sleep deprivation, subjects have great difficulty in maintaining full alertness at the time that correlates with the low point in body TEMPERATURE, typically between 4 A.M. and 6 A.M. This particular time is most crucial in studies of sleep deprivation because a few minutes of inattention will allow a non-active subject to fall asleep.

Activity and mood following one night of sleep deprivation do not show a linear decrease from the time of the last sleep episode but rather there is a cyclical fluctuation in the relation to the circadian pattern of alertness and sleepiness. The mid-afternoon following a night of sleep deprivation is a time of increased sleepiness and decreased alertness, which is related to the physiological, biphasic pattern of alertness. However, there is increasing alertness in activity a few hours later although the level of activity may be much reduced.

There are some neurological features of sleep deprivation, such as weakness of the muscles and tremulousness of the limbs, as well as incoordination and unsteadiness.

Short episodes of sleep deprivation have been beneficial in some situations. It is often used as an activating procedure for the diagnostic monitoring of patients with suspected seizure disorders. Total sleep deprivation has also been demonstrated to improve mood in patients suffering from DEPRESSION. See Chapter 1: Sleep: An Overview.

sleep diary   See SLEEP LOG.

sleep disorder centers   Facilities designed for the diagnosis, evaluation and treatment of patients with sleep disorders. A comprehensive sleep disorder center has the expertise and facilities for diagnosing and evaluating disorders that occur during sleep as well as disorders of EXCESSIVE SLEEPINESS during the day. The disorders that are able to be evaluated cover all medical specialties and age groups from infancy to old age. The first sleep disorder center in the United States was developed in the early 1970s at the Stanford University Medical Center. By the end of 1988, 110 sleep disorder centers had been accredited in the United States. Similar centers are being developed in many other countries, including Japan, England and Germany.

A typical sleep disorder center comprises a specialist in SLEEP DISORDERS MEDICINE, usually a physician, and consultants from a variety of different medical specialties, including otolaryngology, pulmonary medicine, cardiology, neurology and psychiatry. Patients typically undergo a full clinical evaluation that may involve seeing a psychologist and, if necessary, patients will undergo polysomnographic testing.

A sleep disorder center will have at least one recording room for POLYSOMNOGRAPHY, and typically will have two or three rooms. These rooms consist of a hotel-like bedroom with specialized monitoring equipment housed in an adjacent control room. Patients will undergo all-night polysom-nographic monitoring as needed, which may be followed by an assessment of excessive daytime sleepiness by MULTIPLE SLEEP LATENCY TESTING. Some patients require several nights of polysomnographic monitoring to determine an accurate diagnosis, or to provide for treatment under polysomnographic monitoring. Bathroom and kitchen facilities are usually available for the patient's comfort.

The development of quality standards for sleep disorder centers throughout the United States is provided through the American Academy of Sleep Medicine. Sleep disorder centers are accredited if they meet the standards and guidelines of the American Academy of Sleep Medicine. (See also ACCREDITATION STANDARDS FOR SLEEP DISORDER CENTERS, FIRST NIGHT EFFECT, REVERSED FIRST NIGHT EFFECT.)

sleep disorder centers, accreditation standards for   See ACCREDITATION STANDARDS FOR SLEEP DISORDER CENTERS.

sleep-disordered breathing   Term applied to a variety of breathing disorders that can occur during sleep, such as the OBSTRUCTIVE SLEEP APNEA SYNDROME, CENTRAL SLEEP APNEA SYNDROME or CENTRAL ALVEOLAR HYPOVENTILATION SYNDROME. Chronic respiratory diseases including nocturnal asthma can also produce sleep-related breathing abnormalities, characterized by reduction in blood oxygen saturation during sleep as well as disrupted sleep. Sleep-disordered breathing may consist of a pattern of hyperventilation or hypoventilation with or without apneic episodes. The term *sleep-disordered breathing* has also been applied to the APNEAS and HYPOPNEAS that occur during sleep and is often expressed as the RESPIRATORY DISTURBANCE INDEX. (See also CHRONIC OBSTRUCTIVE PULMONARY DISEASE, SLEEP-RELATED ASTHMA, SLEEP-RELATED BREATHING DISORDERS.)

sleep disorders medicine   A clinical specialty concerned with the diagnosis and treatment of disorders of sleep and wakefulness. In the last 25 years, there has been a rapid development of this subspecialty area due to the recognition of the importance of sleep in health and disease. It is estimated that approximately 100 million people in all age groups in the United States have a disturbance of sleep and wakefulness, which can manifest itself in many different ways. SUDDEN INFANT DEATH SYNDROME affects some 7,000 normal infants every year. Approximately 250,000 people have a disorder of EXCESSIVE SLEEPINESS termed NARCOLEPSY, which causes them to have impaired ALERTNESS during the day—a lifelong and incurable disorder.

sleep disorder specialist   A physician (M.D.) who is trained and knowledgeable in the practice of SLEEP DISORDERS MEDICINE. In the United States, the majority of sleep disorder specialists have undergone appropriate certification by passing the examination in sleep medicine that is given by the American Academy of Sleep Medicine. Most sleep disorder specialists have polysomnographic monitoring equipment available to assist in the diagnosis and management of sleep disorders. Sleep disorder specialists usually practice in a SLEEP DISORDER CENTER, which is a comprehensive diagnostic and treatment facility capable of diagnosing and treating all types of sleep disorders.

sleep drunkenness   Term applied to the condition of people who have difficulty awakening in the morning and who often awaken in a confused and disoriented state. Although originally proposed as a distinct disorder, sleep drunkenness is no longer thought to be a specific diagnostic entity. Instead, sleep drunkenness, or confusion and disorientation upon awakening, is a feature of many DISORDERS OF EXCESSIVE SOMNOLENCE, such as the OBSTRUCTIVE SLEEP APNEA SYNDROME, IDIOPATHIC HYPERSOMNIA, or CONFUSIONAL AROUSALS.

sleep duration   The time one spends sleeping varies according to age, and there are individual differences at any particular age. A number of factors can influence sleep duration, such as an individual's voluntary control of sleep duration (by going to bed earlier or later, or waking up earlier or later) and genetic determinants. Variation in sleep time may be determined by nighttime or daytime social or work commitments. When a short sleep episode persists on a regular basis it may impair daytime alertness and EXCESSIVE SLEEPINESS may occur. In such circumstances, the individual will have a tendency to fall asleep at inappropriate times and may take frequent daytime NAPS.

Sleep duration varies from approximately 16 hours in infancy (see INFANT SLEEP) to six hours in the elderly. In general, there is a gradual decline in the sleep duration as one ages. Sleep in infancy is characterized by short episodes of REM and non-REM sleep that alternate with short episodes of wakefulness. Approximately seven episodes of sleep occur throughout the 24-hour day. The number of episodes decreases, and the duration of the nocturnal sleep episode increases, so that by one year of age a child may be sleeping nine hours at night with two short naps of about two hours each during the rest of the 24-hour day. By age four years, the major sleep episode comprises about 10 hours in duration and there may or may not be one nap. Most prepubertal children have a nocturnal sleep duration of approximately 10 hours without a tendency for daytime naps, and this length of nocturnal sleep gradually reduces to six hours after 60 years of age.

Most young adults sleep 7.5 hours each night, with a slight increase in sleep duration on weekends by approximately one hour. However, there is a normal distribution of sleep length across each age group, with some individuals having less than five hours of sleep a night and others having more than nine hours. Recent research has indicated that adults who receive less than five hours of sleep on a regular basis, or more than nine hours of sleep, have an increased mortality (see DEATHS DURING SLEEP).

In addition to a reduction of total sleep duration as one gets older, there is also a change in the ratio of REM to non-REM sleep. In infancy, about 50% of all sleep is REM SLEEP, and this percentage decreases as one gets older so that by age two years, about 25% of the sleep period is REM sleep and at age 60 years, about 20% is REM sleep. In addition, the frequency and number of awakenings during the major sleep episode increases from childhood through adulthood to old age.

In some societies, the nocturnal sleep episode is of shorter duration because a daytime SIESTA is taken. Siestas that last four hours may be accompanied by a nocturnal sleep episode that is only four to six hours long. The total amount of sleep within a 24-hour period is usually normal, and is equivalent to that seen in societies without a siesta.

Research has demonstrated that sleep duration may be reduced voluntarily if one gradually cuts back on the amount of sleep at night. This sleep reduction is done at the expense of the lighter stages of sleep and REM sleep, which become reduced. If sleep duration is reduced below the physiological need for an individual then excessive sleepiness will result. Many people who report a long sleep duration often spend an excessive amount of time in bed awake at night. Reduction in hours spent sleeping will eliminate this wake time and lead to more consolidated and efficient nocturnal sleep. Although individuals have been reported to sleep as little as two hours per night, this is very rare. (Individuals who have a genetic predisposition to less sleep are termed SHORT SLEEPERS.) In order to confirm a short sleep duration, an individual must be studied in an environment free of time cues (see ENVIRONMENTAL TIME CUES) for at least seven days so that both nocturnal and daytime sleep can be recorded. Some individuals report the complete absence of sleep for months and even years. Such people, when studied in the sleep laboratory, are seen to be sleeping, yet upon awakening do not perceive that they slept. This disorder is called SLEEP STATE MISPERCEPTION or pseudosomnia.

Some persons have a genetic tendency for a prolonged nocturnal sleep episode (greater than nine hours of sleep per day). For others, very often prolonged nocturnal sleep episodes occur at the expense of consolidated sleep so that frequent or lighter stages of sleep occur throughout the sleep episode. Long sleep episodes may alternate with short sleep episodes; this is particularly seen with people who have mental disease characterized by manic-depressive stages. Rarely, some people can extend their nocturnal sleep for one or two nights for periods as long as 15 hours in total duration. When an episode of prolonged sleep occurs, there is usually a return of stage three or four sleep toward the end of the sleep episode. Awakening from this sleep can lead to a complaint of fatigue, tiredness and DROWSINESS for the remainder of the day. Such prolonged sleep durations in healthy people rarely occur for more than two nights at a time. However, a genetic predisposition to long sleep rarely occurs and those individuals are termed LONG SLEEPERS.

Many sleep disorders can affect sleep duration. Patients with insomnia typically report a short sleep duration at night, although recent studies have shown that sleep duration in insomnia patients is very similar to people without a complaint of insomnia. Disorders that affect the quality of nocturnal sleep may lead to a change in sleep duration; for example, OBSTRUCTIVE SLEEP APNEA SYNDROME and PERIODIC LIMB MOVEMENT DISORDER are two disorders commonly associated with an increased nocturnal sleep duration. In addition, patients with the disorder IDIOPATHIC HYPERSOMNIA typically have a rather prolonged nocturnal sleep episode.

sleep efficiency   The amount of sleep that occurs during a sleep episode in relation to the amount of time available for sleep. During POLYSOMNOGRAPHY it is usually expressed as a percentage of TOTAL SLEEP TIME according to the TOTAL RECORDING TIME. The sleep efficiency is an indication of how much wakefulness occurred during the time available for sleep. Usually a sleep efficiency of greater than 80% is regarded as normal in the sleep laboratory. Efficiencies greater than 95% are indicative of an abnormally high sleep efficiency and are typically seen in patients with NARCOLEPSY or IDIOPATHIC HYPERSOMNIA. Sleep efficiencies of less than 80% are typical of disorders that produce a complaint of INSOMNIA.

sleep enuresis   Also known as bed-wetting, this is a disorder that is characterized by urinating during sleep. See Chapter 9: Sleep Across the Life Cycle.

sleep exercises   Exercises prior to sleep at night are often recommended for patients who have an increase in muscle tension and a difficulty in relaxing that impairs the ability to fall asleep. The exercises are composed of relaxation techniques that lower arousal so that natural sleep can occur. They can be performed during the daytime (wakefulness) to assist in recognizing when muscle tension is high, and prior to the sleep episode to relax the tension and facilitate sleep onset. BIOFEEDBACK techniques have also been developed to aid in recognizing when muscle tension is high.

Typical relaxation exercises involve tensing and tightening up one or more muscles and then perceiving the sensation that occurs when they relax. Relaxation exercises can be performed while lying on the back with the eyes closed and the legs uncrossed. They should last at least 30 minutes; however, up to 60 minutes may be necessary if a great deal of muscle tension is present. Exercises of the legs involve bending both feet downward at the ankles and clawing the toes at the same time. The knees are straight and should not bend. The feet and toes are then allowed to go limp suddenly. Several minutes of relaxation should then occur before repeating the tension and relaxation phase of the feet. Following relaxation of the legs, the rest of the body, including the arms, should be relaxed. Similar exercises can be used for other muscles in the legs, arms, trunk, head and neck.

The muscle exercises proposed by Edmund Jacobson in 1983 have been found useful by many patients with increased muscle tension (see JACOBSONIAN RELAXATION).

sleep hygiene   A variety of different practices that are necessary in order to have normal, good quality nocturnal sleep and full daytime alertness. These practices ensure that a regular pattern of sleep and wakefulness will occur in association with a pattern of underlying circadian rhythms. ENVIRONMENTAL TIME CUES are an important component of ensuring that the sleep-wake cycle maintains a normal rhythm and timing; disturbances of these cues will lead to a weakening of the circadian rhythmicity with consequent disturbances of the sleep-wake pattern.

The strongest environmental time cues are those that occur around the time of awakening and involve the maintenance of a regular wake time with adequate exposure to light.

Practices that are associated with a normal sleep-wake pattern are: avoidance of napping during the daytime; regular wake and sleep onset times; ensuring that an appropriate length of time is spent in bed, which is neither too short nor too excessive; avoidance of stimulants such as CAFFEINE, NICOTINE and ALCOHOL in the period immediately preceding bedtime; avoidance of stimulating exercise before bedtime; an adequate relaxation period before bedtime; avoidance of emotionally-upsetting activities or conversations immediately before bedtime; avoidance of activities associated with wakefulness in bed, for example, watching television or listening to the radio; a pleasant sleep environment, which includes sleeping on a comfortable mattress with adequate bed covers, and ensuring that the bedroom environment is not too cold, too hot or too bright; avoidance of dwelling on mental problems in bed. (See also INADEQUATE SLEEP HYGIENE.)

sleep hyperhidrosis   Term for profuse sweating that occurs during sleep; also known as night sweats. The patient may have an excessive amount of sweating during daytime hours as well. This disorder can produce discomfort due to the excessive wetness of the bed clothes, which may need to be changed several times throughout the night. In some patients, the disorder can be relatively brief in duration, but in others it is a lifelong tendency. Excessive sweating can be exacerbated by chronic febrile (feverish) illness and a variety of other disorders, including diabetes insipidus, hyperthyroidism, pheochromocytoma, hypothalamic lesions, epilepsy, cerebral and brain stem strokes, cerebral palsy, chronic paroxysmal hemicrania, spinal cord infarction, head injury and spontaneous periodic hypothermia. Sleep hyperhidrosis can also be a feature of pregnancy and can be induced by the use of antipyretic medications.

There does not appear to be any gender difference in the presence of this disorder, and it can be seen at any age but most commonly is seen in early adulthood. Sleep hyperhidrosis can occur in older age groups in association with the development of the OBSTRUCTIVE SLEEP APNEA SYNDROME.

Treatment is dependent on the cause of the sweating. Some patients may respond to amitryptiline or clonidine given before sleep. However, for many patients no cause can be determined; for most patients, treatment is not required. (See also PREGNANCY-RELATED SLEEP DISORDER.)

sleep hypochondriasis   See SLEEP STATE MISPERCEPTION.

sleepiness   Difficulty in maintaining the alert state so that, if an individual is not kept active and aroused, he will readily fall into sleep. Sleepiness is not just a form of tiredness and fatigue, but a reflection of a true need for sleep. When sleepiness occurs in situations where sleep would be inappropriate, such as during the day, it is termed *excessive sleepiness*. A variety of disorders that affect the quantity or quality of nocturnal sleep can lead to excessive sleepiness; however, normal sleepiness occurs in relation to the major sleep episode at night. Although sleepiness may be predominant, the arousal system can allow the individual to maintain full alertness, despite there being a strong need for sleep. For example, this occurs in individuals working the night shift or in individuals staying up late at night because of work commitments or social interactions.

sleeping pills   See HYPNOTICS.

sleep latency   The amount of time from lights out, or bedtime, to the commencement of the first stage of sleep, either non-REM or REM sleep. The sleep latency is usually within 20 minutes in normal sleepers and is typically 30 minutes or longer in persons suffering from INSOMNIA. Short sleep latencies of less than 10 minutes are usually seen in disorders of EXCESSIVE SLEEPINESS, such as NARCOLEPSY or OBSTRUCTIVE SLEEP APNEA SYNDROME. This term is preferred over the term "latency to sleep."

sleep log   A written record for 24 hours or longer of a person's sleep-wake pattern. Sleep logs typically comprise information on sleep for at least two weeks. The information recorded includes the BEDTIME, SLEEP ONSET time, SLEEP DURATION, awake times, final wake-up, ARISE TIME and the timing and length of daytime NAPS. Other information can also be recorded, such as the use of sleep-inducing or STIMULANT MEDICATIONS, and the nature of wakeful activities. *Sleep log* is synonymous with the term *sleep diary*.

sleep mentation   The imagery and thinking experienced during sleep. Sleep mentation usually consists of a combination of thoughts and images that can occur during REM SLEEP. The imagery is most vividly expressed in DREAMS, which are clear representations of waking activity. This form of imagery is usually expressed during REM sleep, but it may occur less vividly during NON-REM-STAGE SLEEP, particularly during stage two sleep (see SLEEP STAGES). Sometimes mentation and dream imagery can occur at SLEEP ONSET and may be termed hypnagogic reverie.

sleep need   Like the need for air and water, sleep is a necessity for humans, not an optional activity or even a skill that has to be learned. About a third of our lives is spent sleeping. It is possible for a short while to get by on less sleep, or to put off sleeping, but the need to sleep will eventually force anyone to succumb (see SLEEP DEPRIVATION).

The question "Why do we need to sleep?" is one that has intrigued scientists over the centuries, ever since Aristotle, in the fourth century B.C., noted that afternoon sleepiness appeared to follow midday meals. Lucretius in 55 B.C. perceived a connection between sleep and wakefulness.

We know that all animals, and fish, sleep for part of the 24-hour day, yet there is little understanding about why sleep is necessary.

There are currently three main theories about why we need to sleep. The first, the Restorative Theory, hypothesizes that sleep restores some component of our physiology that is used up during wakefulness. This restoration may be of a physical, chemical or mental nature. However, no one has yet been able to determine exactly what might be lost during wakefulness that is restored during sleep.

Studies have centered around trying to determine if there is any direct association between daytime physical activity and nighttime sleep. But investigations into athletes who are well-trained have failed to show any association between increased daytime activity and improved quality or duration of nighttime sleep. Some studies, however, have tended to show that there is an increase in stage three/four sleep, particularly if the exercise is performed in the late afternoon. However, other studies have tended to show different results with delay and decrease in REM sleep. The means of analyzing electroencephalographic sleep may affect these results because more specialized forms of analysis (by means of spectral analysis, EEG frequency analysis) have given different information than studies that have been scored by more traditional methods. The spectral analysis studies have tended to give support to the restorative theory of exercise and SLOW WAVE SLEEP by demonstrating improved slow wave sleep.

A second theory, called the Cleansing Theory, was first proposed in 1958 by Hughlings Jackson, a neurologist. The Cleansing Theory suggests that sleep affects memory, it cleans away unwanted memories and allows consolidation of memories that are important and need to be retained. The theory has been extended by others, including Francis Crick in 1983, who has proposed that it is the REM sleep that is particularly valuable in cleaning out unwanted memories, perhaps by a mechanism that involves dreaming.

The third theory of sleep need is the Circadian Theory developed in the 1970s. This theory hypothesizes that sleep is necessary in order to maintain

CIRCADIAN RHYTHMS. It has been proposed that the interaction of the circadian rhythms is the most effective and efficient means of maintaining physiology in a state so that it can adequately adapt to changes in environmental or internal factors. A normal sleep-wake cycle has been shown to promote the maximal and ideal rhythm amplitude and phase relationships. Body temperature has its nadir during sleep and rises to a maximum amplitude 12 hours later. The strength of the cyclical pattern is diminished by a disrupted sleep pattern. (See also Chapter 9: Sleep Across the Life Cycle.)

sleep onset   The transition from wakefulness to sleep that usually comprises stage one sleep. In certain situations, particularly in infancy (see INFANT SLEEP) and in NARCOLEPSY, sleep onset may occur with REM SLEEP. Sleep onset is usually characterized by: a slowing of the ELECTROENCEPHALOGRAM (EEG); the reduction and eventual disappearance of ALPHA ACTIVITY; the presence of EEG vertex sharp transients; and slow rolling eye movements. Although an EPOCH (one page of a POLYSOMNOGRAM) of stage one sleep is usually required as documentation for sleep onset, some researchers prefer to take the first epoch of any stage of sleep other than stage one as being the criterion for sleep onset. The reason is that stage two sleep is more associated with subjective recall of sleep onset. Sometimes the sleep onset will be regarded as the onset of continuous sleep, which may comprise the beginning of three or more continuous epochs of stage one or other stages of sleep.

Sleep onset usually occurs within 20 minutes of the bedtime; however, people who complain of INSOMNIA may have a sleep onset that occurs 30 minutes or longer from the attempt to initiate sleep. Sleep onset may occur rapidly in disorders characterized by EXCESSIVE SLEEPINESS during the day or by hypersomnia, such as OBSTRUCTIVE SLEEP APNEA SYNDROME or narcolepsy. (See also SLEEP LATENCY, SLEEP STAGES.)

sleep onset association disorder   Primarily a disorder of childhood where a child typically needs to have a favorite object (teddy bear, stuffed toy, blanket or bottle) or behavior (rocking in a mother's arms, hearing lullabies) for SLEEP ONSET to occur. In adults, the associated behavior may be the use of a television or a radio. When the object or behavior is not present, sleep onset becomes more difficult, and awakenings may occur throughout the night.

The sleep onset association is often reinforced by a caregiver. A child may be put to bed with a pacifier or a bottle, and the pattern or association with sleep becomes fixed until the child reaches a level of independence when it can maintain its own sleep pattern without the use of the object. If the behavior is not spontaneously eliminated with increasing maturity, it may be necessary to actively limit the introduction of the object.

This form of sleep disorder can be present from the first few days of life, but most commonly it becomes set between six months and three years of age. The disorder can occur for the first time at any age, and it is frequently seen in adulthood to old age, when falling asleep to a television or radio is typical.

This sleep disturbance can also occur at any age in response to a household disturbance, such as a move to a new home, marital difficulties, sibling rivalries or other forms of emotional stress that necessitate getting a comforting object in order to initiate sleep.

Polysomnographic monitoring demonstrates essentially normal sleep patterns, particularly if the sleep onset association object is present. However, sleep onset difficulties and an increase in the frequency and duration of awakenings at night may occur if the object is unavailable.

This form of sleep disturbance needs to be differentiated from LIMIT-SETTING SLEEP DISORDER where inadequate limits on bedtimes and wake times are the primary cause of the sleep disturbance. It also needs to be distinguished from PSYCHOPHYSIOLOGICAL INSOMNIA in the adult, in which negative associations to sleep are developed rather than the positive associations seen in sleep onset association disorder.

Treatment involves a gradual withdrawal of the object so that positive associations are developed to sleep, in the sleeping environment, without the need for a specific object. During the time of withdrawal of the object, good SLEEP HYGIENE measures are essential in order to prevent a breakdown of the sleep pattern or the development of psychophysiological insomnia.

sleep onset insomnia   A form of insomnia characterized by difficulty in initiating sleep; there is an increased SLEEP LATENCY, but once sleep is initiated, little, if any, sleep disruption occurs. Sleep onset insomnia is typically seen in patients with the DELAYED SLEEP PHASE SYNDROME, where the timing of sleep is altered in relationship to the 24-hour day. There may be a prolonged sleep latency but, once sleep is initiated, sleep is normal in quality. Rarely, a sleep onset insomnia may be produced as a result of a PSYCHOPHYSIOLOGICAL INSOMNIA or an ANXIETY DISORDER; a pure sleep onset insomnia is also a rare feature of DEPRESSION. Some disorders, such as the RESTLESS LEGS SYNDROME or excessive SLEEP STARTS, may also be associated with a sleep onset insomnia.

sleep onset nightmares   See TERRIFYING HYPNAGOGIC HALLUCINATIONS.

sleep onset REM period (SOREMP)   Typically the onset of REM SLEEP is 90 minutes after sleep onset. But a sleep onset REM period is characterized by the initiation of REM sleep within 20 minutes of sleep onset. Sleep onset REM periods are a characteristic feature of NARCOLEPSY during the major sleep episode as well as during daytime NAPS. Two or more sleep onset REM periods seen during a daytime MULTIPLE SLEEP LATENCY TEST, in an individual who otherwise has a normal preceding night of sleep, may be diagnostic of narcolepsy. However, sleep onset REM periods may also be seen in other disorders of disrupted REM sleep, such as in severe OBSTRUC-TIVE SLEEP APNEA SYNDROME.

Most patients with narcolepsy will have three sleep onset REM periods during a five-nap multiple sleep latency test; however, not uncommonly five sleep onset REM periods will occur. A single sleep onset REM period, particularly on the first or second nap of the multiple sleep latency test, may be seen in normal individuals who otherwise do not have a sleep disorder. However, two or more sleep onset REM periods are regarded as being distinctly abnormal for people without a sleep disorder.

sleep palsy   A muscle weakness, present upon awakening, that is associated with pressure over nerves supplying a particular muscle or group of muscles. A sleep palsy is commonly experienced if the limb is not moved and pressure is sustained over the nerve for half an hour or longer.

sleep paralysis   A condition of whole body muscle paralysis that occasionally may be present at the onset of sleep, or upon awakening during the night or in the morning. It is a manifestation of the muscle atonia (loss of muscle activity) that occurs in association with the dreaming (REM) stage of sleep (see DREAMS). Dream activity can accompany the limb paralysis; however, the patient is usually awake and fully conscious during the phenomenon. Typically an individual will attempt to move a limb and, finding an inability to do so, will feel fear, panic and at times the sensation of impending death. Respiratory movements are usually unimpaired, but the sensation of an inability to breathe is common.

The episodes last from seconds to several minutes and usually terminate spontaneously. The individual may make some moaning sounds during the episode, which may attract the attention of the bed partner; being touched or some other stimulus will assist in terminating the episode.

The condition, when seen frequently in any individual, raises the possibility of the diagnosis of NARCOLEPSY and typically is associated with EXCESSIVE SLEEPINESS during the day and CATAPLEXY. Unless the condition is associated with narcolepsy, it usually does not warrant therapeutic intervention. Reassurance is often required, and the initial episodes are often those of most concern, since in time recognizing the benign nature of the episodes reduces the concern.

A familial form of the condition has been recognized that is unaccompanied by other abnormal neurological features.

Sleep paralysis can sometimes be seen where there has been insufficient or poor-quality nocturnal sleep, such as with patients who have been sleep deprived (see SLEEP DEPRIVATION) or who have OBSTRUCTIVE SLEEP APNEA SYNDROME.

If the treatment is indicated, a REM suppressant medication, such as one of the tricyclic ANTIDEPRESSANTS, may be useful.

sleep pattern   A person's routine of sleep and waking behavior that includes the clock hour of BEDTIME and ARISE TIME, as well as NAPS and time and duration of sleep interruptions. A typical 24-hour sleep pattern comprises eight hours of sleep at night, followed by 16 hours of wakefulness. A biphasic sleep pattern is seen in individuals who have a prolonged sleep episode in the late afternoon, such as a SIESTA, in association with a major sleep episode at night. (See also CIRCADIAN RHYTHMS, SLEEP DURATION, SLEEP INTERRUPTION.)

sleep-related abnormal swallowing syndrome   Disorder that occurs during sleep in which there is aspiration of saliva that produces coughing and choking episodes, due to inadequately swallowed saliva that collects in the pharynx and erroneously passes into the larynx and trachea. This choking and coughing can cause INSOMNIA.

This disorder was first described by Christian Guilleminault in 1976 as an unusual cause of insomnia. The patient described by Guilleminault had frequent episodes of coughing and gagging that were associated with "gurgling" sounds, probably due to the pooling of saliva in the lower part of the pharynx. Because of the frequent aspiration, patients with this disorder may be prone to respiratory tract infections that can be worsened by increased use of HYPNOTICS, which may be prescribed to help the insomnia.

Polysomnographic studies have demonstrated a very disturbed sleep pattern with frequent awakenings occurring throughout all the sleep stages; however, deep SLOW WAVE SLEEP does not occur. This disorder needs to be differentiated from other disorders that cause choking episodes during sleep, in particular, OBSTRUCTIVE SLEEP APNEA SYNDROME. Episodes of SLEEP-RELATED GASTROESOPHAGEAL REFLUX can also lead to coughing and choking during sleep, but daytime episodes of acid reflux associated with heartburn, chest pain and other features indicative of reflux are usually present in such patients. Patients with SLEEP-RELATED LARYNGOSPASM may appear to have a disorder similar to sleep-related abnormal swallowing syndrome; however, the episodes of laryngospasm are rare, and between episodes patients are typically asymptomatic.

The pathology of sleep-related abnormal swallowing syndrome is unknown; however, abnormalities in either the swallowing reflex, its motor component or the protective mechanism guarding the larynx are considered to be possible causes.

Treatment is largely symptomatic, and one can consider the use during sleep of anticholinergic agents, such as amitriptyline (see ANTIDEPRESSANTS), which reduce upper airway secretion.

sleep-related asthma   Frequent asthmatic attacks that occur during sleep. Typically these episodes will lead to an arousal or an awakening from sleep. The awakenings are characterized by difficulty in breathing, wheezing, coughing, gasping for air and chest discomfort. Often there may be excessive mucus produced during these episodes. Typically the patient will use a medication, such as a bronchodilator, that relieves the acute episodes.

Asthma attacks during sleep appear to be more common in children, and it is reported that up to 75% of asthmatic patients have some night-time episodes. Generally the severity of the sleep-related asthma parallels the severity of daytime asthma.

The cause of sleep-related asthma is unknown; however, circadian factors are thought to play a part. There is a circadian variation in bronchial resistance, which tends to be increased in the early morning hours, and there may also be a circadian change in the intensity of airway inflammation at night. There are also nighttime reductions in the serum level of epinephrine (chemical produced by the adrenal gland) and CORTISOL (hormone produced by adrenal gland) that may predispose an individual to an asthmatic attack. In addition, the effect of medications during the daytime may wear off during the nocturnal sleep episode.

Polysomnographic evaluation of persons with sleep-related asthma tends to show that episodes are more likely to occur during the second half of the sleep episode. However, there does not appear to be a specific sleep stage relationship.

Episodes of acute difficulty in breathing at night need to be differentiated from a variety of other SLEEP-RELATED BREATHING DISORDERS, as well as SLEEP-RELATED GASTROESOPHAGEAL REFLUX, SLEEP-RELATED LARYNGOSPASM or the SLEEP CHOKING SYNDROME.

Treatment of sleep-related asthma involves appropriate management of daytime asthma. Appropriate treatment of the acute sleep-related attacks is also required. In addition, elimination of any potential bedroom allergens may reduce the frequency of sleep-related asthma.

sleep-related breathing disorders   This term applies to breathing disorders that are induced or exacerbated during sleep. Although many different respiratory disorders are affected by sleep, the three main syndromes associated with sleep are the OBSTRUCTIVE SLEEP APNEA SYNDROME, CENTRAL SLEEP APNEA SYNDROME and the CENTRAL ALVEOLAR HYPOVENTILATION SYNDROME.

The sleep-related breathing disorders can occur at any age, from infancy through old age, and can have a spectrum of severity ranging from very mild to life threatening.

Treatment varies depending upon the primary cause of the respiratory disturbance but can range from behavioral techniques, such as weight loss, the use of RESPIRATORY STIMULANTS, the use of mechanical devices to prevent upper airway obstruction, or assisted ventilation, to surgical treatments (see SURGERY AND SLEEP DISORDERS) ranging from TONSILLECTOMY to TRACHEOSTOMY, in order to relieve the upper airway obstruction.

sleep-related cardiovascular symptoms   Symptoms that arise from a variety of cardiac disorders, including those that affect cardiac rhythm and cardiac output. The symptoms are primarily discomfort or pain in the chest, or respiratory difficulty.

One of the most common symptoms related to cardiovascular disease is PAROXYSMAL NOCTURNAL DYSPNEA, which is shortness of breath related to recumbency (lying down), which is usually associated with sleep. This symptom is indicative of heart failure as a result of either myocardial or valvular disease and features difficulty in breathing and a sensation of suffocation that induces the patient to sit up or get out of bed. There may be a sensation of needing air, "air hunger," and persons may need to open a window in order to inspire cooler air. Due to the difficulty in breathing when lying down, a large proportion of the night may be spent sleeping in a semi-reclining or sitting position. The shortness of breath while lying flat is called ORTHOPNEA.

Chest pain may occur during sleep. The terms "nocturnal angina" or NOCTURNAL CARDIAC ISCHEMIA have been used to describe the chest pain that occurs in sleep at night. Precipitation of chest pain during sleep may be the result of REM sleep features, such as variability in blood pressure and heart rate. It is also possible that the lowering of blood pressure during SLOW WAVE SLEEP may precipitate coronary artery insufficiency, leading to angina.

Sleep disorders, such as the SLEEP-RELATED BREATHING DISORDERS, in particular the OBSTRUCTIVE SLEEP APNEA SYNDROME, are also believed to be a cause of nocturnal angina and cardiac ischemia during sleep. Cardiac ARRHYTHMIAS may also be precipitated by sleep-related breathing disorders and may induce symptoms of chest discomfort or shortness of breath.

Some cardiovascular disorders during sleep are essentially asymptomatic; for example, REM SLEEP-RELATED SINUS ARREST generally does not have any sleep-related symptoms. Individuals who die from SUDDEN UNEXPLAINED NOCTURNAL DEATH SYNDROME (SUND) are asymptomatic prior to the terminal event.

Patients with sleep-related cardiovascular symptoms need to undergo electrocardiography throughout sleep, in association with POLYSOMNOGRAPHY, to determine oxygen saturation levels and the presence of sleep-related breathing disorders. Correction of the sleep-related breathing disorders can reduce symptoms during sleep and reduce the likelihood of a catastrophic cardiovascular event. Patients with REM sleep-related sinus arrest may require the insertion of a permanent pacemaker as a preventative measure.

Chest discomfort during sleep may be due to a number of different sleep disorders. SLEEP-RELATED GASTROESOPHAGEAL REFLUX commonly produces chest discomfort that may be difficult to distinguish from that of a cardiac cause. Difficulty in breathing at night is commonly produced by the sleep-related breathing disorders, such as obstructive sleep apnea syndrome, CENTRAL SLEEP APNEA SYNDROME and CENTRAL ALVEOLAR HYPOVENTILATION SYNDROME. Occasional awakening with the sensation of the heart having stopped is not uncommon in patients who have ANXIETY DISORDERS, PANIC DISORDER or SLEEP TERRORS. Choking episodes during sleep can also be seen in patients with the SLEEP CHOKING SYNDROME or SLEEP-RELATED LARYN-GOSPASM.

sleep-related enuresis   See SLEEP ENURESIS.

sleep-related epilepsy   Epilepsy is a disorder characterized by the sudden occurrence of an excessive cerebral electric discharge. Epilepsy has a very specific relationship with the sleep-wake cycle, which can lead to epilepsy being exacerbated during sleep.

The generalized seizures (grand mal), the partial or focal motor seizures, and complex partial seizures are three forms of epilepsy that can occur during sleep. Although epilepsy can produce sleep disruption and lead to a complaint of INSOMNIA, in general the primary complaint is of abnormal movement activity during sleep. Episodes of sudden awakening with movements or walking raise a possibility that the episode is due to epilepsy, particularly if there is associated confusion.

Because sleep is a powerful activator of epilepsy, sleep is used for diagnostic purposes.

Electroencephalography (see ELECTROENCEPHALOGRAM) is often performed after a night of SLEEP DEPRIVATION so that the effects of either sleep loss or the subsequent sleep episode can be utilized to enhance detection of abnormal epileptic activity. Sometimes HYPNOTICS such as chloral hydrate are given to the patient, when epilepsy is suspected, to enhance the detection of epileptic discharges during sleep.

The form of epilepsy that causes the most difficulty in its differentiation from other sleep disorders, such as SLEEPWALKING, is the partial complex seizure. In this particular seizure type, a patient may awaken from sleep, pick at the bedclothes, have lip-smacking, get out of bed and walk around and appear to be unaware of other people in the environment. Usually the walking is performed in a semi-purposeful manner; however, the individual may be difficult to awaken and may go back to bed without assistance. If the person does awaken there is generally confusion followed by lethargy. What distinguishes this seizure disorder from sleepwalking episodes is the presence of the automatic and repetitive type of limb movements and lip-smacking behavior.

In generalized tonic-clonic seizures that occur during sleep, there is little difficulty in diagnosis because of the repetitive jerking of the limbs and associated urinary or fecal incontinence. The patient is also typically confused following the episode.

A focal epilepsy characterized by small jerking movements of one part of the body needs to be distinguished from other forms of movement disorder, such as PERIODIC LIMB MOVEMENT DISORDER. Sometimes a whole body jerk can occur at SLEEP ONSET, due to epilepsy, that is difficult to differentiate from SLEEP STARTS; however, such episodes usually recur during sleep, whereas sleep starts are present only at sleep onset.

A patient who presents with a single epileptic seizure during sleep may not proceed to have further episodes; however, most patients will develop not only sleep-related epileptic seizures but also daytime episodes. In the initial stages, a daytime electroencephalogram may help diagnose epilepsy. Polysomnographic monitoring with extensive electroencephalographic recording during sleep is necessary in some patients to confirm the diagnosis.

Sometimes epileptic seizures are heralded by a loud cry, followed by a generalized tremor, and such an episode may be difficult to differentiate from sleep terrors. However, other behavioral manifestations of epilepsy are usually present, such as repetitive movements like lip-smacking or jerking of the limbs, and there is the absence of the intense fear and panic that is characteristic of sleep terrors.

The diagnosis of epilepsy is confirmed if a specific electroencephalographic pattern is seen during the behavioral event. For tonic-clonic epilepsy, generalized spike and wave activity occurring bilaterally and in a synchronous manner is diagnostic. These spike and wave episodes occur with a frequency that is generally in the delta range (2 to 4 Hz), lasting up to five seconds in duration in the interictal period. Repetitive spike activity, called polyspikes, is also frequently seen during non-REM sleep in patients with generalized seizure disorders. Abnormal EEG activity is often suppressed during REM sleep. Polysomnographic monitoring of patients for seizure disorders is aided by using an extensive electroencephalographic array (arrangement or montage) with 12 to 16 channels of information, coupled to simultaneous audiovisual monitoring.

Treatment of the epilepsy depends upon the underlying type of epilepsy, and usually one or more anticonvulsant medications are required. (See also RHYTHMIC MOVEMENT DISORDER.)

sleep-related gastroesophageal reflux   A disorder characterized by a reflux (backward flow) of acid from the stomach into the esophagus during sleep. Usually this disorder will cause the patient to awaken with a discomfort or pain in the chest or an awareness of a sour, acid taste in the mouth. The pain that is experienced is usually in the mid-chest behind the sternum and is often associated with a general tightness in the chest.

Gastroesophageal reflux can cause pharyngitis (inflammation of the throat), laryngospasm and difficulty in swallowing because of the acid irritation. Although episodes of gastroesophageal reflux can occur during the day, episodes occur more frequently at night. Ulcers and inflammation of the esophageal mucosa can occur that may progress to a complete constriction of the esophagus. Long-standing gastroesophageal reflux may lead to the development of an abnormal lining to the lower esophagus, which may be a premalignant condition.

Approximately 7% to 10% of the general population has HEARTBURN due to gastroesophageal reflux. It is a more common disorder in persons over the age of 40 years.

Gastroesophageal reflux may be precipitated by the OBSTRUCTIVE SLEEP APNEA SYNDROME, which causes an increased intra-abdominal pressure due to the increasing respiratory muscle activity. Reflux of acid may lead to pulmonary aspiration with subsequent pneumonia.

Sleep-related gastroesophageal reflux can be demonstrated by 24-hour esophageal acid (pH) monitoring. An acid-sensitive probe is placed through the nose and into the lower esophagus where changes in the acid content of the lower esophagus are detected. Concurrent polysomnographic monitoring demonstrates whether a physiological event, such as an obstructive sleep apnea, is associated with the precipitation of an episode of sleep-related gastroesophageal reflux.

Treatment of gastroesophageal reflux is primarily by weight reduction in those patients who are overweight. Prilosec is the drug of choice. Antacids and inhibitors of acid secretion such as rantidine (Zantac) or cimetidine (Tagamet) may be prescribed. Small meals taken at two- to three-hour intervals during the day may be useful in reducing gastroesophageal reflux; large meals should be avoided before going to bed at night. (See also OBESITY.)

sleep-related headaches   The headache forms that are most likely to occur during sleep are MIGRAINE, cluster headache and chronic paroxysmal hemicrania.

These three headache forms appear to have a common pathophysiological basis in that they are all associated with autonomic (involuntary neurological system concerned with involuntary functions) features, especially cluster headache and chronic paroxysmal hemicrania. Polysomnographic monitoring has demonstrated that these headache forms are more likely to occur in REM SLEEP, and chronic paroxysmal hemicrania is more closely tied to REM sleep than the other two.

These headaches need to be differentiated from the group of headaches termed muscle contraction or tension headaches, which may be associated with ANXIETY or HYPERTENSION. Tension headaches typically occur upon awakening in the morning and do not usually cause an abrupt awakening from sleep.

Treatment of sleep-related headaches depends upon the particular headache form involved and may require the use of medications such as cafergot, Midrin, beta-blockers, calcium channel blockers or morphine derivative analgesics, in the case of migraine headaches. Cluster headaches may be treated by steroids, methysergide or oxygen therapy.

Muscle contraction headaches that occur upon awakening in the morning may be helped by relaxation therapy, amitriptyline (see ANTIDEPRES-

SANTS) or anxiolytic agents. Muscle contraction headaches need to be differentiated from headaches that occur upon awakening in the morning due to the OBSTRUCTIVE SLEEP APNEA SYNDROME, which respond to specific treatment for that syndrome.

sleep-related laryngospasm   Condition characterized by an abrupt awakening from sleep with an intense inability to breathe and the development of stridor (a high-pitched inspiration sound). Stridor is characterized by a high-pitched sound made when trying to inspire through a partially closed upper airway. Patients with this disorder are abruptly awakened from sleep and typically will jump out of bed in intense fear and panic of dying. The patient will clutch his throat and try to inspire and often produce a loud and rather frightening gasping sound. Bed partners are always awoken by the event, which is very dramatic, and the patient may be seen to be slightly cyanotic (blue in color). Typically the episode will subside within five minutes; sometimes the individual requires a drink to speed the resolution of the episode. Following the episode of stridor, there may be hoarseness of the voice, and the anxiety and panic gradually subsides and the individual returns to sleep. Episodes usually occur only once a night and are very rare, recurring only two to three times a year.

In most patients, the cause of the episodes is unknown. However, episodes can occur with gastroesophageal reflux of acid. Sleep-related laryngospasm is also known to occur in patients who have the OBSTRUCTIVE SLEEP APNEA SYNDROME, usually as a result of associated gastroesophageal reflux. Patients with gastroesophageal reflux and laryngospasm will usually be aware of an acid taste in the mouth at the time of the awakening.

The cause of the stridor is believed to be vocal cord spasm; however, endoscopic evaluations immediately following the episodes have failed to show any abnormality of this laryngeal region.

The episodes of inability to breathe need to be distinguished from other causes of respiratory difficulty during sleep, such as the obstructive sleep apnea syndrome. The intense panic and anxiety associated with the episode requires one to distinguish it from SLEEP TERRORS or a panic attack due to a PANIC DISORDER. The SLEEP CHOKING SYNDROME is characterized by a sensation of an inability to breathe, but stridor and cyanosis do not occur in sleep choking syndrome, nor do episodes of the sleep choking syndrome disrupt the bed partner. Episodes of sleep choking syndrome, unlike sleep-related laryngospasm, occur on numerous occasions, often more than once at night. The SLEEP-RELATED ABNORMAL SWALLOWING SYNDROME, which is also associated with choking during sleep, can be differentiated by its typical clinical features, which include "gurgling" sounds during sleep.

Many patients with daytime stridor have been demonstrated to have the stridor as a result of psychogenic factors. Such patients can voluntarily induce stridor during wakefulness. The occurrence of stridor during sleep in such patients has not been reported to occur. Treatment of the sleep-related laryngospasm is dependent upon the discovery of an underlying cause, if one can be established. Usually sleep-related laryngospasm does not require treatment due to its very infrequent occurrence.

sleep-related neurogenic tachypnea   Disorder characterized by a sustained increase in respiratory rate that occurs during sleep as compared with wakefulness. The respiratory rate increase is not due to alterations in blood gases that might result from cardiac or respiratory factors; it appears to be of central nervous system origin. Some patients with sleep-related neurogenic tachypnea have been reported to have EXCESSIVE SLEEPINESS during the day that appears to be related, at least in part, to the underlying tachypnea.

Neurological disorders have been associated with sleep-related neurogenic tachypnea, particularly lesions of the brain stem, such as the lateral medullary syndrome and multiple sclerosis. An idiopathic (without a known cause) form of the disorder can occur.

There have been only a few reports of this disorder and its exact cause is not understood. Polysomnographic monitoring has demonstrated sleep fragmentation, which appears to be related to the respiratory rhythm. Although excessive sleepiness would be expected, sleep latency testing has not been reported in this disorder.

Sleep-related neurogenic tachypnea must be differentiated from other SLEEP-RELATED BREATHING DISORDERS, such as OBSTRUCTIVE SLEEP APNEA SYNDROME, CENTRAL SLEEP APNEA SYNDROME and CENTRAL ALVEOLAR HYPOVENTILATION SYNDROME. These disorders can all produce an increase of respiratory rate during sleep. Left-sided heart failure and PAROXYSMAL NOCTURNAL DYSPNEA can result in an increase of respiratory rate during sleep.

No specific treatment is known for this disorder.

sleep-related painful erections   Condition where penile erections occurring at night are very painful. All males, from infancy to old age, have erections during REM sleep, and the occurrence of a partial or full erection may be associated with intense pain that awakens the person during sleep. The frequent interruptions of sleep can cause the sufferer to have daytime tiredness and fatigue.

Typically erections during wakefulness are not painful.

This disorder is rare and typically will occur in the age group over 40, although it can occur at an earlier age. It tends to become more severe with increasing age. No clear penile pathology has been shown to explain this disorder.

Polysomnographic studies will demonstrate an awakening during an episode of sleep-related penile tumescence accompanied by the complaint of penile pain.

Treatment of the disorder is usually symptomatic, although medications such as tricyclic ANTIDEPRESSANTS, which impair sleep-related erections, may be effective. (See also IMPAIRED SLEEP-RELATED PENILE ERECTIONS.)

sleep-related penile erections   All healthy males from infancy to old age have penile erections during sleep. The erections occur with each REM sleep episode, that is, approximately five times in a night, each erection lasting about 30 minutes in duration. The total amount of time that the penis is erect decreases slightly with age to a total of approximately 100 minutes in the elderly.

Erections during sleep have their onset in infants between three and four months of age. They are usually not produced by sexual excitement, but are an automatic response generated by the nervous system. However, some erections during sleep occur in association with sexual dreams, and NOCTURNAL EMISSIONS ("wet dreams") during sleep are always associated with sexual dreaming.

An assessment of normal penile erectile ability during sleep can be used to determine whether a complaint of IMPOTENCE has an organic or psychological cause. Patients with an organic cause of the impotence have an inability to obtain adequate erections during sleep. This form of testing, termed NOCTURNAL PENILE TUMESCENCE TESTING, is often used to determine the cause of the impotence before the patient is referred either for implantation of an artificial penile prosthesis or for psychiatric or sex therapy. (See also IMPAIRED SLEEP-RELATED PENILE ERECTIONS, IMPOTENCE, SLEEP-RELATED PAINFUL ERECTIONS.)

sleep-related penile tumescence   See SLEEP-RELATED PENILE ERECTIONS.

Sleep Research Online (SRO)   A sleep research journal published online by the SLEEP RESEARCH SOCIETY. For further information, contact Sleep Research Online, c/o WebSciences, 10911 Weyburn Avenue, Suite 348, Los Angeles, California 90024. E-mail: sro@sro.org; Web: http://www.sro.com.

Sleep Research Society (SRS)   Originally founded in Chicago in 1961 as the ASSOCIATION FOR THE PSYCHOPHYSIOLOGICAL STUDY OF SLEEP. In 1983, the association changed its name to the Sleep Research Society, in part because the society no longer primarily concerned itself with the psychophysiological aspects of sleep research.

The Sleep Research Society joined with the American Sleep Disorders Association (see AMERICAN BOARD OF SLEEP MEDICINE) to form the federation called the Association of Professional Sleep Societies, which holds a combined annual meeting of sleep research.

sleep restriction therapy   A treatment for patients with INSOMNIA based upon the recognition that excessive time spent in bed often perpetuates insomnia. Typically, patients with insomnia go to bed on some nights earlier than usual in order to obtain more sleep, or to counteract feelings of daytime tiredness and fatigue. In addition, patients may stay in bed longer in the morning to make up for lost sleep at night, or because of feelings of tiredness or fatigue. Because sleep is often spread out over a longer portion of the 24-hour day, often as much as 12 hours, sleep becomes fragmented, with frequent intervals of wakefulness. Maintaining a consolidated nighttime sleep and a full episode of wakefulness for the rest of the day is most helpful in promoting normal and strong circadian rhythms.

Sleep restriction therapy involves reducing the amount of time spent in bed by one or more hours and ensuring that sleep occurs only during the set BEDTIME and awake times. In that way, sleep becomes more consolidated after one or two days on the new pattern. In some cases, the total time recommended for sleep may be as little as 4.5 hours, but typically it is on the order of 6 to 7.5 hours. Once the sleep restriction produces an increased consolidation of sleep with less wakefulness and more continuous and longer durations of sleep, the total time available for sleep may be increased slightly by 15 or 30 minutes. In this manner, an initial restricted pattern of 4.5 hours may be increased to 5 hours after one week, and then to 5.5 hours one week later, with sequential increases until a point is reached where allowing additional time contributes only to increased wakefulness at night.

People who undergo sleep restriction therapy may notice an increased tendency for sleepiness in the first few days, often because the reported TOTAL SLEEP TIME is less than the actual sleep and therefore there may be an element of SLEEP DEPRIVATION. However, as sleep fills the available time for sleeping, and the time for sleeping is extended, the tendency for daytime sleepiness reduces.

This therapy improves sleep by consolidating sleep and also by reducing the number of disrupting factors associated with sleep disturbance. Maintaining regular SLEEP ONSET and wake times and the occurrence of sleep at the time of the maximum circadian phase for sleep are some of the features that make sleep restriction therapy effective. (See also CIRCADIAN RHYTHMS, FATIGUE, SLEEP PATTERN as well as Chapter 3, Insomnia, pages 29–30.)

sleep schedule   The pattern of sleep that occurs within a 24-hour day. Typically, the sleep schedule involves the sleep onset and awake times in relationship to the 24-hour clock time. The sleep schedule may vary if the times for sleep change, in which case an irregular sleep schedule may occur. However, a typical sleep schedule is one that has a regular sleep onset time at night and a regular awake time in the morning. (See also CIRCADIAN RHYTHMS, IRREGULAR SLEEP-WAKE PATTERN, NREM-REM SLEEP CYCLE, TOTAL SLEEP TIME.)

sleep spindles   A pattern of electrical activity occurring during sleep that appears in an electroencephalographic recording. Sleep spindles are an identifying feature of stage two sleep. A sleep spindle consists of a spindle-shaped burst of 11 to 15 Hz waves that lasts for 0.5 to 1.5 seconds. Spindles can occur diffusely over the head and are of highest voltage over the central regions, with an amplitude that is usually less than 50 microvolts in adults. Sleep spindles, although characteristic of stage two sleep, may persist into deeper stages three and four sleep but usually are not seen in REM sleep. Reduction of spindle activity may be seen in the elderly, and an increase can be seen in association with disorders of the basal ganglia of the brain, such as dystonia, or as a result of medications, such as the BENZODIAZEPINES. Sleep disruption, if severe, can cause spindle activity to occur in other sleep stages, including REM sleep. (See also ELECTROEN-CEPHALOGRAM, HYPNOTICS, SIGMA RHYTHM, SLEEP STAGES.)

sleep stage episode An interval of sleep that represents a specific sleep stage in the non-REM/REM cycle. For example, the first REM sleep episode is the first interval of REM sleep that occurs in the major sleep episode and will comprise a part of the NREM-REM SLEEP CYCLE. Typically, four to six recurring cycles of non-REM-REM sleep occur, therefore four to six discrete stage episodes of non-REM and REM sleep will occur. (See also SLEEP STAGES.)

sleep stage period See SLEEP STAGE EPISODE.

sleep stages Following the development of the ELECTROENCEPHALOGRAM (or EEG) in 1930 by Hans Berger, sleep was recognized to consist of changes in the electroencephalographic activity of the brain. Based on these electroencephalographic patterns, sleep was originally classified into four stages, sometimes characterized by letters of the alphabet, excluding REM sleep, which was not discovered for another two decades. With the discovery of REM sleep in 1953 by NATHANIEL KLEITMAN, Eugene Aserinsky and WILLIAM DEMENT, sleep was recognized to be a continuous state of alternating rhythm with very pronounced physiological changes. REM sleep was occasionally termed stage five sleep, or D sleep. The electroencephalographic pattern of REM sleep was also termed desynchronized sleep, compared with the synchronized EEG activity of non-REM or SLOW WAVE SLEEP.

In 1968 a group of researchers headed by Alan Rechtschaffen and Anthony Kales developed a standardized method of sleep scoring, and sleep was divided into four stages, plus REM sleep. The four stages of sleep came to be called NREM or non-REM sleep. In order to standardize the scoring of sleep, the record was divided into epochs of 20 or 30 seconds in duration. The electroencephalogram is performed at a slower rate of 10 or 15 millimeters per second than the more typical EEG speed of 30 millimeters per second. In addition to the electroencephalogram, electrodes placed to record eye movements and muscle tone are required to more adequately determine sleep stages.

The electroencephalogram electrode placement is at either C3 or C4 position. Eye movements are detected by electrodes placed at the outer CANTHUS of each eye and referred to a reference electrode, and the ELECTROMYOGRAM is typically recorded by electrodes placed over the muscles at the tip of the chin.

Stage One Sleep

Stage one sleep occurs right after the awake stage and comprises 4% to 5% of TOTAL SLEEP TIME. It is characterized by medium amplitude, mixed frequency activity that is mainly theta and comprises more than 20% of an epoch. During this stage there may be SLOW ROLLING EYE MOVEMENTS in contrast to the RAPID EYE MOVEMENTS seen during wakefulness. There are no SLEEP SPINDLES, K-COMPLEXES or REMs.

Stage Two Sleep

Stage two sleep is characterized by sleep spindles and K-complexes; it accounts for 45% to 50% of total sleep time. The sleep spindles are 11 to 15 Hz activity occurring in episodes greater than .5 second in duration and reaching 25 microvolts in amplitude. K-complexes consists of a negative vertex, sharp wave followed by a positive slow wave and are frequently seen accompanied by sleep spindles.

Electrode EEG studies, in which the electrodes are inserted directly through the scalp into the brain, performed concurrently with scalp electrode recordings suggest that spindle activity appears first in the thalamic nucleic of the brain and undergoes a certain degree of synchronization before it is detectable at the scalp EEG electrodes. Superior frontal regions appear to be the starting point for the spindle activity.

Stage Three Sleep

A deep level of sleep that comprises 4% to 6% of total sleep time. This stage is sometimes combined with stage four into NREM stages three and four because of the physiological similarities between the two stages, and called slow wave sleep. Stage three is present when between 20% and 50% of the epoch contains delta waves of .5 to 2.5 Hz, which are 75 microvolts or greater in amplitude. Typically eye movement activity is absent during this stage.

Stage Four Sleep

Stage four sleep is scored when over 50% of the epoch contains delta waves of the same frequency and amplitude as those seen in stage three sleep. Although rarely, sleep spindles may occur in stage four sleep. This stage, the deepest sleep of the four non-REM stages, is synonymous with slow wave sleep and usually comprises 12% to 15% of total sleep time. It is during this stage that SLEEP TERRORS or SLEEPWALKING may occur. Sometimes stage four is combined with stage three into NREM stages three and four because the stages are so similar.

Rapid Eye Movement Sleep (REM)
REM sleep is characterized by rapid eye movement (hence its name, REM), loss of muscle tone (or REM ATONIA) and a mixed frequency, low voltage EEG pattern with occasional bursts of "sawtooth" theta waves of 5 to 7 Hz. Dreaming occurs during REM sleep. (See also DREAMS, POLYSOMNOGRAPHY.)

sleep starts   Also known as hypnagogic jerks, predormital myoclonus or hypnic jerks. Sleep starts are sudden, shocklike sensations that involve most of the body, particularly the lower limbs. They usually consist of a solitary, generalized contraction that occurs spontaneously or is caused by a stimulus. Sleep starts bring the individual to wakefulness, and a sensation of falling or a visual flash, dream or hallucination may be experienced at this time. Rarely the individual may call out with the acuteness of the episode. Multiple episodes can occur at SLEEP ONSET, and SLEEP ONSET INSOMNIA may develop. Not infrequently, individuals will have multiple episodes that do not induce a full awakening. Such episodes may not be remembered by the individual but will be reported by a bed partner.

It is thought that most people experience sleep starts at some time in their life, and only a few have frequent episodes. There is some evidence to suggest that the ingestion of stimulant agents, such as CAFFEINE, or the use of NICOTINE may exacerbate the occurrence of sleep starts. Physical exercise and emotional STRESS have also been reported to be associated with such episodes.

Sleep starts may occur at any age, although most typically they are reported in adulthood. There does not appear to be any gender or familial tendency.

Polysomnographic monitoring of sleep starts demonstrates a brief (generally 75–250 millisecond), high amplitude muscle potential that can be associated with an arousal pattern seen on the EEG. There may be accompanying increased heart rate following an episode, but usually the heart rate returns to normal and sleep resumes rapidly.

Sleep starts must be distinguished from hyperexplexia syndrome in which a generalized body jerk can occur during wakefulness or during sleep. The association of hyperexplexia with full wakefulness differentiates that disorder from sleep starts. An epileptic form of myoclonus can produce similar generalized body jerks; however, abnormal EEG activity can help differentiate that disorder. RESTLESS LEGS SYNDROME is not likely to be confused because the leg movements are slower and not associated with a whole body jerk. PERIODIC LEG MOVEMENTS, as with restless legs syndrome, generally have more prolonged muscle episodes and do not have the shocklike, brief character of the sleep start. Periodic movements occur in a repetitive manner during sleep and do not usually occur solely at sleep onset.

Treatment of sleep starts is usually unnecessary as they are an infrequent occurrence and usually are not associated with any great concern.

However, in some individuals sleep starts may be a cause of sleep onset insomnia, in which case benzodiazepine muscle relaxants (see BENZODIA-ZEPINES), such as triazolam, may be useful in suppressing episodes and in allowing sleep onset to be initiated.

sleep state misperception   A disorder where there is a complaint of insomnia, yet the major sleep episode is objectively normal. This disorder has also been called "subjective DIMS complaint without objective findings," "pseudoinsomnia" or "sleep hypochondriasis," but sleep state misperception is the preferred term. Patients with this disorder present a very convincing history of sleep disturbance and insomnia and typically will awaken feeling unrefreshed. When studied polysomnographically in the sleep laboratory, sleep is normal in duration, sleep stages and sleep efficiency, yet the patient will awaken and report having had no sleep at all.

The cause of the misperception of sleep is unknown; however, it does appear to be an exaggeration of a normal phenomenon. Healthy individuals who have been asleep for only a few minutes often will report not having slept at all. As the duration of sleep increases, the awareness of having slept also increases. However, patients with sleep state misperception, despite having prolonged periods of good quality sleep, misperceive sleep as being a time of no sleep.

This disorder must be differentiated from individuals who report a lack of sleep in order to obtain MEDICATIONS. Such patients are often drug abusers, and the report of no sleep is usually not a convincing or honest report. This disorder also needs to be differentiated from other causes of insomnia, such as PSYCHOPHYSIOLOGICAL INSOMNIA or insomnia related to a mental disorder. Sleep fragmentation, reduced total sleep time and reduced sleep efficiency are characteristically seen in patients with insomnia due to these other causes. (See also DISORDERS OF INITIATING AND MAINTAINING SLEEP, PSYCHIATRIC DISORDERS.)

sleep surface   The sleep surface has been subject to investigation over the years to determine its role in the maintenance of good quality sleep. Most of the research has tended to demonstrate that the quality of sleep is independent of the surface on which a person sleeps; however, a change in the sleeping surface can disrupt sleep. The inhabitants of some countries typically sleep on a hard surface yet appear to sleep as well as people who sleep on soft, innerspring mattresses. Adaptation to the new surface needs to occur if someone changes from a hard to a soft surface, or vice versa. Many different sleeping surfaces have been produced; hard mattresses have been marketed particularly for people who have back complaints, whereas softer surfaces, such as water BEDS, appear to have more appeal to young adults.

Whether to change the sleeping surface should depend solely on comfort. If a mattress is too soft or too hard, a change may be beneficial to sleep. For most people, however, the sleeping surface plays a small role in the cause or maintenance of sleep disturbance. (See also INSOMNIA.)

sleep talking   Also known as somniloquy. Sleep talking is the production of utterances of speech or other sounds during a sleep episode. Typically, individuals suffering from sleep talking are unaware of the content of their speech, which is reported afterward. The utterances may take the form of comprehensible speech, isolated words, parts of sentences, moans or other nonverbal sounds. Typically sleep talking is devoid of emotional content; however, it can be associated with intense emotional stress, at which time calling out, crying, screaming or cursing may occur.

Sleep talking is often a temporary phenomenon, although it may be a repetitive occurrence in those who suffer from SLEEP TERRORS or somnambulism (see SLEEPWALKING). It also is seen in individuals who have significant psychopathology, emotional stress or medical illness, such as febrile (feverish) illness, in which case it is related to that illness. It appears to be more common in males than females and a slight familial tendency is reported.

Sleep talking has been demonstrated to occur during all stages of sleep, including REM SLEEP. The majority of episodes, in fact, have been reported out of REM sleep, with the next most common being sleep stage two, followed by slow wave sleep. Individuals who have somnambulism or sleep terrors are more likely to have sleep talking out of slow wave sleep, whereas individuals who have the REM SLEEP BEHAVIOR DISORDER are more likely to have episodes out of REM sleep. (See also CONFUSIONAL AROUSALS, SLEEP STAGES.)

sleep terrors   Considered one of the disorders of arousal as described by Roger J. Broughton in 1968. These episodes also go under the name of night terrors and they have occasionally been called pavor nocturnus (derived from the Latin *pavor,* for "terror," and *nocturnus,* for "at night") in children and incubus in adults.

Sleep terror episodes are characterized by an arousal during the first third of the night from deep stage three/four sleep (see SLEEP STAGES), and are heralded by a loud, piercing scream along with intense fear and panic. An individual experiencing a sleep terror will typically sit up abruptly in bed with an agitated and confused expression. Following the intense and loud scream, there may be other features of panic and fear, such as rapid breathing, rapid heart rate, dilation of the pupils and profuse sweating. The individual will usually flee from the bedroom in an intense panic and is often inconsolable until the episode subsides. Most episodes last less than 15 minutes; sleep usually follows very rapidly, and the individual is unable to recall the episode the next morning.

The cause of the episodes is unknown, but it appears to be a benign and maturational behavior frequently seen in children. Up to 6% of prepubescent children will have recurrent episodes of night terrors, with the peak frequency of the behavior being around six years of age. Episodes then decrease in frequency and generally cease in early adolescence.

The frequency in adults is typically less than 1% and episodes usually persist from childhood, although episodes may occur for the first time in adulthood. Episodes occur equally in males and females, and there are no racial or cultural differences in the prevalence. However, there is a marked familial incidence of the disorder, with up to 96% of individuals having a family history of the disorder.

Episodes may be precipitated in susceptible individuals by fatigue, emotional stress and febrile illness. Adults with the disorder may also have evidence of psychopathology characterized by psychoasthenia (weakness and reduced motivation), DEPRESSION and schizophrenia.

Children with sleep terror episodes either concurrently have SLEEP-WALKING episodes or develop sleepwalking episodes subsequently. Sleep terror episodes rarely occur in adulthood after the fifth decade.

Because of the intense fear and anxiety, sleep terror episodes are differentiated from more typical NIGHTMARES or DREAM ANXIETY ATTACKS. Nightmares usually occur in the later half of the night, more typically during REM sleep. Nightmares also have a less intense scream at their onset than sleep terrors, and usually the individual comes to full alertness, whereas the sufferer of night terrors does not usually become fully awake during an episode. Rarely does an epileptic seizure produce an episode similar to sleep terror; other features of epilepsy would typically be present in such individuals. Since injuries might occur during the intense fleeing from the bedroom, objects liable to cause injury should be removed and appropriate steps made to secure the bedroom. (See also ANTIDEPRESSANTS, BENZODIAZEPINES, CONFUSIONAL AROUSAL.)

sleep therapy   Term related to a treatment that employs the inducement of sleep in order to treat various medical disorders. In its simplest form, sleep therapy can be viewed as treatment by rest—required by situations that promote fatigue. Sleep therapy may also involve the inducement of sleep by MEDICATIONS and drugs, the use of HYPNOSIS to induce prolonged sleep, or the application of electrical current, which has been termed electrosleep, electronarcosis or electroanesthesia.

Sleep therapy has been used to treat a variety of disorders, most commonly the mental disorders, but also cardiovascular, gastrointestinal, central nervous system and infective disorders.

The majority of studies on sleep therapy occurred around the turn of the century, and little objective documentation of their effectiveness has been presented. Electrosleep is still performed in some European countries and is administered in a variety of different manners. Electrodes may be applied to the forehead and a limb, and then the electrical current gradually increased to the amount of approximately three-quarters of a milliamp, at which time the patient can feel a tingling sensation through his head, which is believed to induce sleep. The majority of publications on electrosleep come from the Russian literature.

The usefulness of sleep therapy is believed to be limited at best. There is a need for more research and documentation of its effectiveness before it can be widely recommended.

sleep-wake cycle   See NREM-REM SLEEP CYCLE.

sleep-wake disorders center   This term is occasionally used to describe a facility that evaluates patients who have disorders of sleep and wakefulness. The hyphenated term was used initially to emphasize the importance of disorders of both sleep and wakefulness, such as the disorders that produce EXCESSIVE SLEEPINESS. The shorter term, SLEEP DISORDER CENTERS, is more commonly used. (See also ACCREDITATION STANDARDS FOR SLEEP DISORDER CENTERS.)

sleep-wake schedule disorders   See CIRCADIAN RHYTHM SLEEP DISORDERS.

sleep-wake transition disorders   A subgroup of the PARASOMNIAS, as listed in the INTERNATIONAL CLASSIFICATION OF SLEEP DISORDERS, consisting of RHYTHMIC MOVEMENT DISORDER, SLEEP STARTS, SLEEP TALKING, and NOCTURNAL LEG CRAMPS. These disorders occur mainly during the transition from wakefulness to sleep, or during the transition from one SLEEP STAGE to another. Some of these disorders may occur during sleep, but the predominant activity occurs in the transition to and from sleep.

sleepwalking   Episodes characterized by movement that occurs while the subject is still asleep and in a partially aroused state. This disorder, which is also known as somnambulism, typically occurs during deep SLOW WAVE SLEEP in the first third of the night. The behavior is often seen in prepubescent children, although it can persist or start anew in adulthood.

A typical sleepwalking episode is characterized by the individual sitting up in bed, usually with a vacant and unresponsive look. Repetitive movements, such as picking at the bedclothes, may occur prior to the individual rising from the bed and walking around the room. Episodes last minutes or hours at most. Frequently the individual will open doors and walk out of the bedroom, or sometimes walk out of the house. During the sleepwalking episode, there is a limited capacity to appreciate environmental stimuli, and there is an impaired ability to fully awaken. Occasional utterances may occur during sleepwalking, but verbalizations usually do not occur, and rarely is any cognitive or mental content expressed. Although unresponsive to environmental stimuli, the individual is able to negotiate objects without difficulty, although occasional stumbling or banging into walls or furniture may occur. Attempts at restraining a sleepwalker are usually met with some resistance. Sleep-walking episodes may involve dangerous activities, such as opening windows and climbing onto fire escapes, and serious falls have been reported. There are occasional reports of violent behavior during sleepwalking being directed toward a specific individual. Following a period of ambulation, the sleepwalker usually returns to bed and rapidly returns to sleep. The next morning, the individual is typically unable to recall the episode and is often surprised by the accounts of others.

Sleepwalking episodes usually occur in children in the prepubescent age group, and the peak frequency is around 10 years of age. According to Anthony Kales et al., up to 30% of healthy children are said to have sleep-walked at least once in their lives, and up to 5% of healthy children are reported to have frequent episodes.

Following puberty, episodes decrease in frequency, and usually children have outgrown them by the age of 15. It is estimated that approximately 1% of adults sleepwalk, the majority having done so since childhood. Usually, episodes in adulthood resolve by the fifth decade.

Elderly persons who walk around a house at night may be mistaken for sleepwalkers. They may be suffering from a brain dysfunction, such as DEMENTIA, and are typically awake when they walk about, although confused about their behavior.

Sleepwalking occurs equally in males and females, and there is little evidence for any cultural or racial differences in the tendency to sleep-walk. However, there is a strong pattern of inheritance, with a high rate of sleepwalking activity seen in relatives of sleepwalkers.

The cause of sleepwalking is unknown; however, sleepwalking can be provoked by arousing sleepwalking-prone individuals and standing them on their feet when they are in a deep sleep. Excessive fatigue can precipitate episodes as can febrile (feverish) illness. Episodes of sleepwalking behavior have been reported in association with mediations such as LITHIUM and triazolam (see BENZODIAZEPINES), or other HYPNOTICS.

Polysomnographically, the episodes are characterized by an abrupt arousal that occurs during the deep stage three/four sleep (see SLEEP STAGES). The slow wave activity appears to persist throughout the walking episode with some faster rhythms, such as theta and alpha activity. Individuals who sleepwalk may demonstrate abrupt arousals from deep sleep in the absence of full sleepwalking episodes.

Sleepwalking in children is not associated with any psychopathology, but Anthony Kales has reported a clear association between psychopathology and sleepwalking episodes in adults. Such individuals are reported to be more aggressive, hypomanic and have a tendency for acting out.

Sleepwalking episodes may be very similar to episodes of psychomotor epilepsy with ambulation. However, repetitive automatisms are more common during epileptic seizures and there is more confusion upon awakening.

Recently a form of episodic nocturnal wandering has been reported to occur in young adults in association with abnormal electroencephalographic activity on a daytime, awake ELECTROENCEPHALOGRAM. Such patients respond to anticonvulsant therapy, which may suggest that these individuals have a form of epilepsy and not true sleepwalking.

Sleepwalking episodes can be differentiated from psychogenetic fugues, which usually occur in individuals with severe psychopathology. Fugues consist of episodes of wandering that usually last for hours and days and are often associated with complex behaviors that are more typically seen during wakefulness. REM SLEEP BEHAVIOR DISORDER has similarities to sleepwalking in that motor activity can occur during sleep, but such individuals are usually elderly and the activity more clearly represents acting out of dream content. In addition, in REM sleep behavior disorder the abnormal features are seen during REM sleep and not slow wave sleep. OBSTRUCTIVE SLEEP APNEA SYNDROME can produce nocturnal wanderings that may simulate sleepwalking, although other typical features of obstructive sleep apnea, such as snoring and episodes of cessation of breathing, usually allow an easy differentiation from more typical sleepwalking episodes.

The child who infrequently sleepwalks requires no specific treatment other than making sure that the bedroom is secure to prevent the child from injury. It may be necessary to place locks on windows or doors for the child who walks excessively at night. The older individual and adult should be evaluated for underlying psychopathology, and the appropriate psychiatric treatment should be instituted. There have been good reports of response to psychotherapy and psychiatric management. In many situations sedatives, including imipramine, diazepam or flurazepam, can be helpful in suppressing episodes, particularly if an individual sleeps away from home.

Case History

A 26-year-old woman sought help at a SLEEP DISORDER CENTER because of sleepwalking episodes that had been occurring since she was 10 years of age. When the episodes began, they were infrequent and were regarded as being typical for childhood sleepwalking in that she would be found by her parents walking in the corridor and returned to her bedroom where she would go back to sleep without any difficulty. During the walking episodes, she was unaware of the environment although she did not walk into objects or injure herself.

At age 13, the episodes became less frequent until age 16, when they again increased in frequency. Over the following years, she would have episodes of sleepwalking that caused her considerable embarrassment, particularly when staying at the homes of friends. She would often have some DREAM CONTENT along with the episodes and get up and start to walk around the house. On one occasion she picked up some keys, put them in her pocket and walked out the front door. She was found by a friend sleepwalking outside the house.

With some of the episodes, she would awaken and become aware of having been sleepwalking. On other occasions, she would be returned to her bedroom by friends or family only to be told about the episodes the next morning.

The sleepwalking episodes appeared to occur less often when she was not in her usual environment. There was an increase in the frequency of the episodes if she became very tired, fatigued or was ill with a fever. There was no evidence of underlying psychopathology except for one short-lasting episode of DEPRESSION that had occurred several years prior to her presentation at the sleep disorder center. She would see a psychologist intermittently in order to help her cope with everyday stress, but not because of any psychiatric disturbance. She was successful in her occupation as a clerical administrator and outwardly was a bright and energetic woman who was involved in many social activities.

Polysomnographic evaluation during sleep did not reveal any sleepwalking episodes, and there was no evidence of any epileptic activity. However, she had frequent, abrupt awakenings from stage four sleep.

She was commenced on triazolam, 0.25 milligram taken on a nightly basis, and this completely suppressed the episodes. After six months, she attempted to gradually withdraw from the medication in the hope that the episodes would no longer occur. However, as the dose was reduced she had a return of the sleepwalking episodes and then recommenced the medication for a longer period of time. Five years after being placed on medication, she was free of sleepwalking episodes so long as she continued to take the medication. However, several additional attempts to withdraw from the medication were associated with a recurrence of episodes. She no longer had embarrassment or fear at staying over at other people's homes, and she felt more secure and confident of having a sound night of sleep.

If she ever decides to raise a family, she will need to consider coming off the medication prior to and during pregnancy. The decision to continue medication in the pregnancy will need to be balanced against her potential for harm from the sleepwalking episodes at that time. It is likely that her tendency for sleepwalking will gradually lessen in time.

slow rolling eye movements   Movements that occur with the entrance into stage one non-REM sleep (see SLEEP STAGES). The eye movements begin a slow sinusoidal (cyclical) pattern of movement on a horizontal plane while other EEG (ELECTROENCEPHALOGRAM) and EMG (ELECTROMYOGRAM) features of stage one sleep are present. As the individual passes from stage one into deeper stage two and three sleep, the eye movements become less active. The presence of slow eye movements marks the onset of sleep from the rapid eye movements that are typically seen during wakefulness and helps distinguish stage one sleep from REM SLEEP, which is also characterized by rapid eye movements. Chin muscle activity is usually lower in stage one sleep than in wakefulness but is much higher than the muscle activity seen during REM sleep.

slow wave sleep (SWS)   Sleep that is characterized by electroencephalographic waves of a frequency less than 8 Hz; typically comprises stages three and four sleep combined. Slow wave sleep usually comprises approximately 20% of the sleep of the young adult; however, greater percentages are seen in prepubertal children. Gradual reduction in the total amount of slow wave sleep is seen with aging so that after the age of 60 years, there is little slow wave sleep. Slowing of the EEG (see ELECTROENCEPHALOGRAM), with increased amounts of slow wave sleep, can be seen in several situations.

During partial SLEEP DEPRIVATION, the amount of stage three/four sleep (see SLEEP STAGES) is usually reduced. Following the sleep deprivation, slow wave sleep rebounds so that a greater percentage of slow wave sleep can be seen on the subsequent sleep episode. In addition, disorders that affect the cerebral hemispheres, such as a cerebral vascular accident, can be associated with an increased amount of slowing and therefore an increased amount of slow wave sleep. Drug effects, such as the use of HYPNOTICS or other central nervous system depressants, can also increase EEG slowing and lead to a greater amount of slow wave sleep. Lithium is a known cause of increased slow wave sleep.

smoking   Smoking cigarettes can have an important effect upon INSOMNIA and the OBSTRUCTIVE SLEEP APNEA SYNDROME. Cigarettes contain NICOTINE, a stimulant that causes central nervous system arousal and therefore can contribute to difficulty in initiating sleep. People who suffer from insomnia are advised not to smoke prior to bedtime, and it is counterproductive to smoke cigarettes during nighttime awakenings. (See also SLEEP HYGIENE, STIMULANT MEDICATIONS.)

snoring   A noise produced by vibration of the soft tissue of the back of the mouth. Most typically the soft palate and the anterior and posterior pillar of fauces, which surround the tonsil, vibrate, causing the sounds. Snoring is associated with obstruction of the upper airway that occurs during sleep. Some snorers have only a very slight degree of UPPER AIRWAY OBSTRUCTION, and snoring will be rhythmical and regular on a breath to breath basis; lung ventilation is not compromised. Alternatively, if the upper airway obstruction is more severe, there may be a complete inability to inspire air, and consequently the oxygen in the lung will decrease, causing blood HYPOXEMIA. When snoring is severe, with associated hypoxemia, the disorder of OBSTRUCTIVE SLEEP APNEA SYNDROME most likely is present. This disorder is characterized by repetitive episodes of upper airway obstruction, loud snoring and EXCESSIVE SLEEPINESS during the day. Individuals with obstructive sleep apnea syndrome are at risk of developing cardiac irregularity during sleep and sudden death.

There is some evidence to suggest that snoring may be associated with elevated blood pressure, even in the absence of obstructive sleep apnea syndrome. Other epidemiological studies, which have not differentiated simple snoring from that associated with the obstructive sleep apnea syndrome, have shown a correlation of snoring with ischemic heart disease and stroke.

In addition to the direct cardiorespiratory consequences of snoring, the noise of snoring may be a social annoyance and handicap. A spouse's snoring may be the cause of marital discord that leads to the snorer having to sleep in a separate bed, or even in another room. Not only can snoring affect a spouse, it can also affect other people who are sleeping nearby. Snoring can be particularly disturbing to roommates who have to share rooms, such as on business trips, in the armed forces or at summer camp. Snoring has been measured at up to 80 decibels, a level that can be potentially harmful to hearing.

Some 300 mechanical devices have been patented in the United States to reduce or eliminate snoring. However, the majority are ineffective. Very few effective treatments are available for snoring, and, because most loud snorers will tend to have some degree of obstructive sleep apnea syndrome, a medical evaluation may be necessary.

Snoring may be affected by a number of factors, such as increased body weight, alcohol consumption, body position, respiratory tract infections and central nervous depressant medications, such as HYPNOTICS. Sleeping on the back is liable to induce snoring in a person who otherwise does not snore when sleeping on the side or stomach. However, most loud snorers will tend to snore in any position.

Treatment of snoring, if required, may encompass weight reduction, avoidance of alcohol, avoidance of depressant medications and training to sleep on the side rather than on the back. When these measures are ineffective, or if obstructive sleep apnea syndrome is present, then other forms of treatment may be necessary, such as surgical or mechanical treatment (see SURGERY AND SLEEP DISORDERS).

The most effective surgical treatment for loud snoring is removal of the upper airway obstructive lesion. Children who can be loud snorers with severe obstructive sleep apnea syndrome most typically will have upper airway obstruction due to enlarged tonsils or adenoids, which, when surgically removed will eliminate the snoring (see TONSILLECTOMY AND ADENOIDECTOMY). However, enlarged tonsils or adenoids are rarely the cause of snoring in adults, who more typically have an increase in the soft tissues of the pharynx, such as an elongated soft palate and excessive pillars of fauces. An operative procedure termed UVULOPALATOPHARYN-GOPLASTY (UPP) is usually very effective in reducing the sound of snoring. UPP consists of the removal of the uvula and the lower portion of the soft palate as well as the removal of the tissue associated with the pillar of fauces. In general, this operation is not indicated for people who have snoring in the absence of obstructive sleep apnea syndrome because of the very slight risk that general anesthesia presents. However, this procedure may be performed on some snorers, but more commonly is performed on patients with obstructive sleep apnea syndrome in whom the snoring is associated with medically important upper airway obstruction. Two new forms of uvulopalatoplasty have been developed: LASER UVULOPALATOPLASTY and radiofrequency uvulopalatoplasty (see SOMNOPLASTY). Laser uvulopalatoplasty is a procedure that can be performed within 20 minutes in a physician's office. It is primarily done to eliminate snoring. Radiofrequency uvulopalatoplasty involves inserting a needle into the tissues of the soft palate and exposing the tissues to high-frequency radio waves. It is a less painful procedure than laser uvulopalatoplasty. Careful polysomnographic documentation of the presence and severity of the sleep apnea is essential before surgery is undertaken.

Alternative treatments of snoring can involve the use of mechanical devices, such as CONTINUOUS POSITIVE AIRWAY PRESSURE (CPAP) devices or airway patency devices such as the TONGUE RETAINING DEVICE (TRD) or other ORAL APPLIANCES. These appliances may be useful in treating some patients who have snoring; however, with the exception of the CPAP, these other mechanical devices have generally not been effective for the treatment of obstructive sleep apnea syndrome.

socially or environmentally induced disorders of the sleep-wake schedule   This term has been applied to the CIRCADIAN RHYTHM SLEEP DISORDERS, which are induced by external or behavioral factors such as TIME ZONE CHANGE (JET LAG) SYNDROME and SHIFT-WORK SLEEP DISORDER. It can be applied to DELAYED SLEEP PHASE SYNDROME, ADVANCED SLEEP PHASE SYNDROME, and NON-24-HOUR SLEEP-WAKE SYNDROME when the cause of the disorder is induced by social or environmental factors. Examples of social or environmental factors include social isolation, extremes of light exposure such as that seen in the polar regions, or excessive activity late at night.

somniferous   Term meaning "causing or inducing sleep." The word is derived from the Latin word *somnus*, for "sleep."

somniloquy   See SLEEP TALKING.

somnolence   See EXCESSIVE SLEEPINESS.

somnologist   Term applied to sleep specialists. The word is derived from the Latin *somnus*, for "sleep." The term SLEEP DISORDER SPECIALIST is preferred. (See also SLEEP DISORDERS MEDICINE.)

somnology   Word meaning the study of sleep, derived from the Latin *somnus*, for "sleep," and *ology*, meaning "the study of."

somnoplasty   A surgical method that uses radiofrequency heating to create targeted tissue ablation to reduce tissue volume; also known as radiofrequency thermal ablation. The procedure uses very low levels of radiofrequency energy to create small, finely necrotic lesions in soft tissue structures. The necrosis leads to scar formation and retraction of tissue. This method has been applied to the soft palate of snorers to reduce soft palate tissue and thereby reduce SNORING. The procedure has been used successfully in clinical trials; patients experience a minimal amount of pain, mainly from the insertion of the needle into the soft palate to administer the local anesthesia. The procedure uses temperatures of less than 100 degrees centigrade, much less than those used in laser surgery (over 600 degrees centigrade).

The effectiveness of radiofrequency ablation has not been reported in patients with OBSTRUCTIVE SLEEP APNEA SYNDROME; however, the procedure appears to be effective in reducing tongue-based soft tissue in animal studies and therefore could be an effective treatment for human obstructive sleep apnea syndrome. Further research is required. (See also LASER UVULOPALATOPLASTY, SURGERY AND SLEEP DISORDERS, UPPER AIRWAY OBSTRUCTION, UVULOPALATOPHARYNGOPLASTY.)

Somnus   The ancient Roman god of sleep, who was the son of night and the brother of death. The words "somnambulism" (SLEEPWALKING) and "somnolent" (sleepy) were derived from the Latin *somnus*. (See also HYPNOS.)

Sonata   See HYPNOTICS.

soporific   Term derived from Latin *sopor*, meaning "a deep sleep," and *ferre*, "to bring," that refers to the induction of a deep sleep, typically by the use of drugs. MEDICATIONS that can induce a deep sleep-like state are the HYPNOTICS and anesthetic agents, which include the BENZODIAZEPINES, BARBITURATES and opiate derivatives. These agents in high doses will produce a slowing of the ELECTROENCEPHALOGRAM and the patient will be difficult to arouse. (See also COMA, NARCOTICS.)

SOREMP   See SLEEP ONSET REM PERIOD.

Stanford Sleepiness Scale (SSS)   A subjective measure of alertness developed at Stanford University in 1973. Individuals rate themselves according to one of several statements that most closely describes their level of ALERTNESS or SLEEPINESS. In order to achieve a spectrum of sleepiness across a day, the Stanford Sleepiness Scale is administered at two-hour intervals, most commonly across the waking part of the day. It is often completed immediately before and after the NAPS during a MULTIPLE SLEEP LATENCY TEST.

The Stanford Sleepiness Scale is as follows:

1. Feeling active, vital, alert, wide awake.
2. Functioning at a high level but not at peak. Able to concentrate.
3. Relaxed, awake, but not fully alert, responsive.
4. A little foggy, let down.
5. Foggy, beginning to lose track. Difficulty in staying awake.
6. Sleepy, prefer to lie down, woozy.
7. Almost in reverie, cannot stay awake, sleep onset appears imminent.

status cataplecticus   Continuous state of CATAPLEXY that occurs in a patient with NARCOLEPSY. The continuous cataplectic state can be induced by a persistence of the stimulus causing cataplexy, such as laughter, elation or anger. During the state of cataplexy the individual generally is paralyzed and, at most, can make moaning sounds. The episode may last several minutes and rarely can last up to one hour. The condition can also be precipitated by a sudden withdrawal of anticataplectic medications, such as the tricyclic ANTIDEPRESSANTS, in an individual with a diagnosis of narcolepsy.

stimulant-dependent sleep disorder   Disorder characterized by a reduction in the ability to fall asleep at night, produced by the use of central nervous system stimulants, or an increase in drowsiness during the day, following drug abstinence. The central nervous system stimulants encompass a wide variety of medications that include amphetamines (see STIMULANT MEDICATIONS), COCAINE, thyroid hormones, CAFFEINE, methylxanthines (see RESPIRATORY STIMULANTS), bronchodilators and antihypertensives. Many over-the-counter medications also contain stimulants such as decongestants, cough mixtures or diet suppression medications. Typically these medications are associated with difficulty in the ability to fall asleep, especially when treatment with the medications is first started. After a period of time, tolerance to this effect develops so that sleep initiation difficulties are less frequent. However, upon withdrawal of the medication, symptoms of sleepiness, irritability, tiredness and fatigue are common. The recurrence of daytime symptoms on withdrawal of the stimulant medications often leads to a cyclical pattern of administration. This can lead the individual to believe that the medication is required in order to maintain full daytime ALERTNESS.

Individuals can be oblivious to the pattern of medication use because it is not regarded as a problem. However, others may become aware of the relationship of the stimulant medication to changes in behavior that include periods of excessive acting out with high activity, sometimes with paranoid ideas and repetitive behaviors. In the case of high doses of cocaine, for example, generalized convulsions can occur; with the amphetamines, a severe psychiatric state of psychosis may develop. Abnormal movement disorders can also occur with toxic levels of amphetamines. Addiction to stimulant medications can develop, with severe DEPRESSION and often suicidal ideation and hallucinations.

The pattern of behavior associated with excessive stimulant ingestion often leads to denial of drug use, which may be detected only by means of urinary and screening tests.

Severe addiction to stimulants may lead to intravenous administration, which increases the possibility of contacting infectious hepatitis, acquired immune deficiency syndrome (AIDS) or a systemic arteritis. Infection with the AIDS virus is a real possibility for intravenous stimulant abusers. Acute severe toxicity of the medications may result in death from cardiac ARRHYTHMIAS, brain hemorrhages, convulsions and respiratory arrest.

Stimulant abuse is most common in adolescents and young adults, and it appears to be equal among the sexes. The effects of stimulant abuse may be seen on polysomnographic testing as a prolonged SLEEP LATENCY, reduced TOTAL SLEEP TIME and an increased number of awakenings. REM SLEEP is often reduced and fragmented. Upon withdrawal of the stimulants, there may be a REM REBOUND, with an increased amount of REM sleep. The chronic use of stimulants may give a picture on the MULTIPLE SLEEP LATENCY TEST suggestive of NARCOLEPSY. A one- to two-week withdrawal period from all medications may need to be documented before an accurate diagnosis of EXCESSIVE SLEEPINESS can be given.

Stimulant abusers may attempt to obtain stimulant medications from physicians by falsely giving a history of another sleep disorder, such as narcolepsy. Polysomnographic monitoring of patients to confirm a bona fide diagnosis of a sleep disorder is necessary prior to the long-term administration of stimulant medications.

Patients who have stimulant dependency should embark upon a program of drug withdrawal under medical supervision and, if necessary, appropriate psychiatric therapy. Individuals who suffer from severe drug dependency may require treatment in a specialized drug detoxification clinic.

stimulant medications   This term applies to drugs that stimulate the central nervous system. It includes methylxanthines, the amphetamines and the RESPIRATORY STIMULANTS, such as doxypram and nikethimide, as well as other miscellaneous medications, such as pemoline and methylphenidate hydrochloride.

In sleep disorders medicine, the stimulant medications are primarily used for the improvement and relief of EXCESSIVE SLEEPINESS, and the most commonly used medications are the amphetamines, methylphenidate and pemoline.

The major disadvantage of the stimulant medications is that they produce general body stimulation and therefore can induce ANXIETY and cardiac stimulation, leading to HYPERTENSION or tachycardia (abnormally rapid heartbeat). There may also be gastrointestinal stimulation with resulting diarrhea.

Amphetamines

Stimulant medications that are derived from the sympathomimetic amines and consist of a benzene and an ethylamine group. The amphetamines have powerful central nervous system stimulant effects, and therefore are used to produce ALERTNESS in disorders associated with excessive sleepiness during the day. Most often, they are used for the treatment of NARCOLEPSY and related conditions. Due to their stimulant effects, these drugs can also be abused and illegally used for recreational purposes to provoke central nervous system excitement.

Amphetamines were first used for the treatment of narcolepsy in the 1930s and were found to be an effective agent for improving daytime sleepiness. However, the powerful side effects were also recognized, such as elevated blood pressure and greater incidence of cardiac ARRHYTHMIAS. The central nervous system effects can also provoke agitation, confusion, anxiety, irritability, delirium and DEPRESSION. However, in appropriate doses, amphetamines are very helpful in the treatment of narcolepsy, improving patients' functioning during the daytime.

Other forms and derivatives of amphetamines have been used more recently in the treatment of narcolepsy because they have less tendency for adverse reactions. Methamphetamine (Desoxyn) was also used to improve alertness but, like amphetamine, caused side effects and has largely been replaced by dextroamphetamine sulfate (Dexedrine).

Dextroamphetamine is available in 5-, 10- and 15-milligram tablets, a 5 milligram per 5 milliliter Elixir, and in 5-, 10- and 15-milligram slow-release spansules. Initial doses are typically 5 milligrams, three times a day, but may need to be increased to as much as 100 milligrams per day. The tablets have a duration of action of three to four hours, whereas the spansules have a duration of action up to 12 hours. Some patients find that a background dose of the longer-acting form of the medication, such as a 15-milligram Dexedrine spansule, can be used with the extra stimulant effect of the shorter-acting tablets.

The adverse effects of dextroamphetamine are similar to those of the other amphetamines except there is less peripheral stimulant effect. But because of the potential for cardiac and mental stimulation, disorders of daytime sleepiness, such as narcolepsy, are now more frequently treated with methylphenidate hydrochloride (Ritalin) or pemoline (Cylert).

Amphetamine users develop a tolerance to the drug; consequently, prescribed dosages are increased in order to maintain improved alertness.

Sudden cessation of medication will induce a level of sleepiness that is greater than baseline levels, thereby promoting the continued use of the medication. An amphetamine psychosis and abnormal movements have been reported to be associated with toxic doses of amphetamines.

Anorectics

Anorectics are the appetite suppressant medications. Anorectics typically are comprised of two groups, amphetamines and the non-amphetamines. As the amphetamines have stimulant effects, they are also used for the treatment of excessive sleepiness. When prescribed in appropriate dosages, they can be useful for the treatment of narcolepsy or IDIOPATHIC HYPERSOMNIA. However, some disorders that can produce daytime sleepiness, such as the OBSTRUCTIVE SLEEP APNEA SYNDROME, may be adversely affected by the use of amphetamines. These medications can be dangerous in the sleep apnea syndromes due to their cardiac stimulant effect. Also, the amphetamine anorectic medications are liable for abuse because of their general stimulant properties.

Anorectics, because of their stimulant effects, can produce an impaired ability to sleep at night. SLEEP ONSET and sleep maintenance difficulties are common. A STIMULANT-DEPENDENT SLEEP DISORDER may result from their chronic ingestion. They can also produce a feeling of fatigue or sleepiness when not taken, thereby leading to repeated ingestion to maintain full alertness.

Some non-amphetamine anorectic agents are available, such as phentermine, mazindol or diethylpropion. These agents are generally less effective than the amphetamines in producing weight reduction. Mazindol (see below) can be helpful in improving alertness in some patients with narcolepsy.

Methylphenidate Hydrochloride

This agent, a piperidine derivative, was first introduced by Dan Daly and Robert Yoss in 1956 as the treatment of choice for narcolepsy. The reduced tendency for central nervous system stimulation and peripheral stimulation, compared to amphetamines, was considered advantageous for the treatment of sleepiness in narcolepsy. Methylphenidate is still the treatment of choice for patients with severe narcolepsy, although patients with mild cases of narcolepsy are more typically treated with pemoline.

Methylphenidate is usually given in divided doses, two to three times a day. It has a relatively short duration of action, from four to six hours. Although most patients can be controlled with a dose of about 20 milligrams per day, doses of up to 60 milligrams may be required in some patients. Due to its poor absorption when taken with food, patients are instructed to take the medication on an empty stomach.

This drug is available in 5-, 10- and 20-milligram tablets and is also available in a sustained-release form of 20 milligrams (Ritalin-SR). Ritalin is the trade name for methylphenidate. Although some patients find the sustained-release form effective, others prefer the intermittent use of the shorter-acting form of the medication.

Pemoline

This is an oxizolidinone derivative stimulant that is quite different structurally from the amphetamines or methylphenidate hydrochloride. It is used for central nervous system stimulation to improve arousal in patients with narcolepsy or other disorders of excessive daytime sleepiness. It has fewer peripheral stimulant effects than the amphetamines or methylphenidate. It also has a longer duration of action, approximately 12 hours. It is available in 18.75-, 37.5- and 75-milligram tablets. Cylert is the trade or pharmaceutical name for pemoline.

Pemoline has a slow onset of action over several hours; initially, soon after ingestion, some patients may notice a worsening of their excessive sleepiness, which then dissipates. The clinical effects of pemoline may take several days or even weeks to occur. Because of its slow onset of action, and long half-life, there can be a tendency for drug buildup, with a consequent development of excessive central nervous system stimulation.

There is less tendency for tolerance with pemoline than with other central nervous system stimulants. Objective studies have shown that pemoline does not reduce the tendency or the ability to fall asleep; however, it does improve the ability to remain awake. This effect is demonstrated by an individual's ability to fall asleep in a situation conducive to sleep after having taken pemoline. However, tasks requiring alertness are improved when the individual tries to remain awake.

Pemoline can produce liver impairment, and therefore intermittent monitoring of blood liver enzymes is required for patients who chronically take the medication.

Over-the-Counter Medications

A number of nonprescription over-the-counter medications are available for weight reduction or stimulant purposes. These include phenylpropanolamine, which is sometimes given in combination with CAFFEINE. The use of these medications is controversial as they may be ineffective yet dangerous to individuals, particularly those with hypertension or cardiac disease.

stimulus control therapy   BEHAVIORAL TREATMENT of INSOMNIA that counteracts the development of negative conditioning in someone who lies in bed awake at night, allowing the insomnia to persist. (Lying in bed awake at night heightens the ANXIETY for insomnia patients and further disrupts sleep and prevents its onset.)

Stimulus control instructions, ensuring that wakeful activities are kept away from the bedroom, are as follows: 1) go to bed only when sleepy; 2) if not asleep within 10 minutes of getting into bed, get out of bed and, after returning to bed, if sleep does not occur within 10 minutes, again leave the bed; 3) an alarm should be set so that awakening occurs at the same time every morning and the taking of NAPS should be avoided; 4) the bed should not be used for wakeful activities other than sexual activity. (See also SLEEP RESTRICTION THERAPY.)

strain gauge   A mercury-filled tube that acts as a transducer for movement; most commonly used for the measurement of respiratory movements or penile tumescence (erection) during sleep. Strain gauges may be applied to the chest or abdomen in several places in order to detect respiratory movement. (See also NOCTURNAL PENILE TUMESCENCE TEST, POLYSOMNOGRAPHY.)

stress   Term applied to the body's physical or psychological response to an unexpected or unpleasant environmental or emotional stimulus, such as marital problems, pressure at work, upcoming examinations, or even changes in everyday patterns, such as spending the night away from home or having to make a public speech. The term is most commonly used in SLEEP DISORDERS MEDICINE for the cause of a disturbed sleep pattern that occurs due to a marital, financial or employment situation. Typically, the sleep disorder, termed ADJUSTMENT SLEEP DISORDER, is a result of the psychological stress produced by such events. When the event produces a greater degree of stress, an overt ANXIETY DISORDER may result. (See also INSOMNIA, SHORT-TERM INSOMNIA.)

stupor   A state of altered consciousness characterized by unresponsiveness to strong stimuli. Such patients are usually perceived as being in a deep sleep, and electroencephalographic studies may indicate slow wave activity. However, unlike in COMA, individuals can be awakened and become aware of the environment, but they usually return rapidly to the unresponsive state.

Stupor may be produced by metabolic or pharmacologic insults to the central nervous system. However, this condition can also be seen in severe psychiatric illness, such as that seen with catatonic schizophrenia or severe DEPRESSION.

sudden infant death syndrome (SIDS)   The term used for the death of an otherwise healthy infant who dies suddenly and in whom a post-mortem examination fails to reveal a cause of death. The majority (over 80%) of SIDS infants die during sleep.

Less than 5% of children who die of sudden infant death syndrome have been known to have some respiratory disturbance during sleep. However, the cause of the sudden infant death syndrome is unknown. Recent evidence suggests that it is not directly related to any prior respiratory irregularity.

There appear to be some predisposing factors, derived from epidemiological studies, that indicate that premature infants, infants with low birth weight, infants that are twins or of a multiple birth, and siblings of another child who has died of SIDS are at greater risk. Sleeping on the stomach is also a major factor. In addition, there are a number of maternal factors that appear to predispose some children to the development of SIDS: for example, infants born to mothers who are substance abusers of agents such as COCAINE or heroin. It does appear that SIDS is more common in lower socioeconomic and minority groups, such as American blacks and American Indians. Sudden infant death syndrome has a prevalence of between one and two per 1,000 live births, with the peak onset around three months of age, and up to 90% of cases occur before the sixth month of age. There is a slightly increased male to female ratio.

After death, autopsy examinations have demonstrated a number of features that suggest that the infant may have suffered from an acute upper respiratory tract obstruction. There are petechiae and evidence of pulmonary congestion and edema. Also, pathological abnormalities have been reported in the brain stem, suggesting a prior central nervous system insult, such as HYPOXIA.

Polysomnographic investigations are rarely useful. Although originally there was some suggestion that short apneic episodes may be predictive of SIDS, subsequent research has not confirmed this finding. Infants who have significant apneic events, such as those with apnea of prematurity, or infants requiring assisted ventilation following an apneic event, do have a higher risk for sudden infant death syndrome, although this risk is less than 5%.

Having an infant sleep on the back is the most effective preventative measure a parent or caregiver can take. (See also CAHS [CENTRAL ALVEOLAR HYPOVENTILATION SYNDROME], CENTRAL SLEEP APNEA SYNDROME, INFANT SLEEP APNEA, INFANT SLEEP DISORDERS, OBSTRUCTIVE SLEEP APNEA SYNDROME.)

sudden unexplained nocturnal death syndrome (SUND)   Syndrome primarily recognized in people of Southeast Asian descent who die unexpectedly during sleep. It occurs in healthy young adults without any prior history of cardiac or respiratory disease. Typically there will be a sudden awakening with a choking or gasping sensation and difficulty in breathing. Cardiorespiratory arrest occurs with a fatal outcome. In very rare situations, patients have been successfully resuscitated and found to have cardiac irregularity called ventricular arrhythmias.

This rare and unusual syndrome primarily affects persons between the ages of 25 and 45 who are of Laotian, Kampuchean (Cambodian), or Vietnamese origin. It is primarily a male disorder, although rare cases have been reported in females, and most of the reported cases have been described in refugees who have immigrated to the United States. However, the disorder has been recognized for a long time, and the Laotian term for the disease is *non-laita*, in Tagalog, *bangungut*, and in Japanese, *pokkuri*.

Investigations have failed to reveal any specific cause for the disorder either clinically or by autopsy. There has been no evidence of exposure to either biological or chemical toxins, or the use of drugs or alcohol.

Many of the victims of SUND have been reported to have had prior SLEEP TERROR episodes with a sudden awakening and screaming. It has been suggested that the sudden death during sleep may be due to a severe form of terror episode in which the heart is so stimulated that it goes into a fatal arrhythmia.

Most of the reported cases in the United States have been in the ethnic subgroup called the Hmong, from the highlands of northern Laos. The incidence of the disorder in the Hmong refugees in the United States is reported at 92 per 100,000. It is slightly less common in Laotian refugees at 82 per 100,000; it is 59 per 100,000 in Kampuchean (Cambodian) refugees.

Although SUND cannot be predicted, healthy young adults with cardiorespiratory arrest during sleep need to be examined for any underlying cardiorespiratory disorder. A sleep-related disorder, such as OBSTRUCTIVE SLEEP APNEA SYNDROME or REM SLEEP-RELATED SINUS ARREST, may be the cause of the arrest.

SUND   See SUDDEN UNEXPLAINED NOCTURNAL DEATH SYNDROME.

Sunday night insomnia   Difficulty in initiating and maintaining sleep that commonly is seen on Sunday nights. This form of insomnia occurs due to the tendency to go to bed later on Friday and Saturday nights than during the week (because of social events). Typically the awake time on Saturday and Sunday mornings is later than usual, thereby causing the sleep pattern to be slightly delayed on the weekends compared to that of weekdays. Consequently, many people will attempt to fall asleep at an early time on Sunday night in order to achieve an adequate amount of sleep for work or school on Monday. Because the time of going to bed on Sunday night is much earlier than that of the previous two nights, there often can be difficulty in falling asleep, which is characterized by a long period of time spent in bed awake. If the time of falling asleep on Sunday night is similar to the later time of initiating sleep that occurs on the Friday and Saturday nights, then individuals may find that they are sleep deprived upon awakening for work or school on Monday morning. This will lead to a degree of SLEEP DEPRIVATION that is often termed MONDAY MORNING BLUES.

In order to prevent Sunday night insomnia, an individual should maintain a regular time of going to bed seven days a week and not allow the time to be significantly later on Friday or Saturday nights.

sundown syndrome   See DEMENTIA.

suprachiasmatic nucleus (SCN)   Cells that are located at the bottom of the third ventricle in the hypothalamus. This is believed to be the prime central nervous system site that determines endogenous circadian rhythms, the so-called ENDOGENOUS CIRCADIAN PACEMAKER. The suprachiasmatic nucleus (SCN) has connections with the eye by means of the retino-hypothalamic pathway, which is composed of fibers that pass from the optic nerves to the hypothalamus. By means of the retino-hypothalamic tract (RHT), light and dark influence the circadian pacemaker and act as entraining (maintaining a regular 24-hour) stimuli for our circadian rhythms. Other connections pass to local areas of the central nervous system, as well as through the brain stem and up to the pineal gland, causing the release of the hormone MELATONIN in darkness. Destruction of the suprachiasmatic nucleus has produced loss of the circadian rhythmicity of various CIRCADIAN RHYTHMS.

surgery and sleep disorders   Surgery is a primary treatment form considered for patients who have the OBSTRUCTIVE SLEEP APNEA SYNDROME. Patients with this syndrome have UPPER AIRWAY OBSTRUCTION that occurs at the back of the mouth in the region from the nose to the larynx. Surgical procedures that remove excessive tissue or localized lesions in the upper airway have been shown to be effective in the treatment of some patients with this syndrome.

Obstructive sleep apnea may be due to enlarged tonsils or adenoids, craniofacial abnormalities including retrognathia (posterior-positioned lower jaw) or micrognathia (small lower jaw), or generalized soft tissue enlargement, particularly at the level of the soft palate. Various forms of surgery have been devised in order to improve the upper airway so that obstruction during sleep does not occur.

Surgical treatment of obstructive sleep apnea is still widely performed; however, most patients with this disorder are now treated by means of CONTINUOUS POSITIVE AIRWAY PRESSURE (CPAP) devices, a treatment that has very few complications. The CPAP device provides a low pressure of air to the back of the throat, thereby preventing its collapse during sleep. However, some patients do not find this device suitable for use, and surgery may be the only effective treatment available.

The most common form of surgery used in children with obstructive sleep apnea syndrome is tonsillectomy with or without an adenoidectomy (see TONSILLECTOMY AND ADENOIDECTOMY). Enlarged tonsils are a common cause of obstructive sleep apnea in prepubertal children. Children with enlarged tonsils may also have craniofacial abnormalities that contribute to the upper airway obstruction, such as an altered mandibular relationship to the skull with or without retrognathia. In such patients, MANDIBULAR ADVANCEMENT SURGERY can allow the tissues of the tongue to come forward, thereby preventing pharyngeal obstruction. An experimental surgical procedure involves the release of the hyoid muscles. These muscles fasten the base of the tongue to the skull and their release allows the tongue to be moved forward to open up the posterior pharyngeal air space.

Patients who have a long soft palate, an enlarged uvula and narrow pillar of fauces may be suitable for the UVULOPALATOPHARYNGOPLASTY (UPP) operation, which is a soft tissue surgical procedure performed at the back of the mouth. This procedure is effective for patients with either the obstructive sleep apnea syndrome or simple SNORING; however, only 40% to 50% of patients have a successful result by means of this surgery. Two new forms of palatoplasty are LASER UVULOPALATOPLASTY and radiofrequency palatoplasty (see SOMNOPLASTY). Cephalometric radiographs and FIBEROPTIC ENDOSCOPY aid in selecting patients for the uvulopalatopharyngoplasty procedure, thereby leading to improved surgical results. (See also TRACHEOSTOMY.)

sweating   There can be an increase of sweating during sleep; if it is a regular occurrence it is called SLEEP HYPERHIDROSIS. An increase in sweating can be due to febrile illness, specific neurological disorders, such as stroke, or pregnancy. (See also PREGNANCY-RELATED SLEEP DISORDERS.)

synchronized sleep   Term used to denote NON-REM-STAGE SLEEP, particularly in ontogenetic or phylogenetic sleep research. It is derived from the synchronized patterns of EEG (see ELECTROENCEPHALOGRAM) activity that are commonly seen in non-REM sleep, and it reflects the slowing of the EEG. The term is best avoided if other features of non-REM sleep can be determined. A more specific statement of the stage of sleep (see SLEEP STAGES), such as stage two or three sleep, should be given, if possible.

systemic desensitization   Behavioral technique occasionally used to treat INSOMNIA, particularly in patients who have insomnia due to anxiety or negatively-conditioned associations. The patient is required to make a list of various situations that are likely to contribute to the sleep disturbance, and then concentrate upon those items while coupling them with more restful thoughts. The aim of the treatment is to try to turn the unpleasant associations into pleasant ones so they no longer contribute to the disturbed sleep. Systemic desensitization is sometimes used in conjunction with RELAXATION EXERCISES procedures. (See also AUTOGENIC TRAINING, BEHAVIORAL TREATMENT OF INSOMNIA, BIOFEEDBACK, COGNITIVE FOCUSING, PARADOXICAL TECHNIQUES, PROGRESSIVE RELAXATION.)

T

temazepam   See BENZODIAZEPINES.

temperature   Body temperature decreases during sleep and reaches its minimum level before awakening. It reaches its maximum level during the middle of the period of wakefulness that typically occurs during the daytime. A fluctuation of 1.5 degrees Fahrenheit is usually seen between the low point and the highest point during any 24-hour period. The lowest point of body temperature is about three hours before awakening, typically between 3 A.M. and 5 A.M., and then rapidly rises during the time of awakening. Chronobiological studies have demonstrated that normal-sleeping individuals in time isolation will awaken 85% of the time during the rising phase of the body temperature cycle.

There is some evidence to suggest that exercise and WARM BATHS may be beneficial to nighttime sleep by raising the body temperature prior to sleep onset. However, elevation of the temperature of the sleeping environment is generally not helpful to good sleep and can be an environmental stimulus that contributes to INSOMNIA. Persons who sleep in hot tropical areas can sleep well as long as the environmental temperature is constant and the person has adapted to it. A sudden change in the environmental temperature during the sleeping hours can lead to a disturbed night of sleep. (See also CHRONOBIOLOGY, CIRCADIAN RHYTHMS, EXERCISE AND SLEEP, THERMOREGULATION.)

temporal isolation   In 1962, MICHEL SIFFRE spent 59 days in an underground cavern in the French-Italian Alps and discovered that his sleep-wake cycle had a period length of just over 24 hours as a result of being isolated from ENVIRONMENTAL TIME CUES. In 1962, Jules Ashchoff developed a research facility in a German bunker and demonstrated that with isolation from social and temporal cues, many biological rhythms with a 24-hour cycle would free run (see FREE RUNNING) with a period length of just over 24 hours. Internally-generated rhythms were termed CIRCADIAN RHYTHMS by Franz Halberg in 1959. Additional studies on humans were performed by Elliot Weitzman at Montefiore Hospital in New York where healthy subjects were studied in an environment free of time cues for periods of up to six months. From such experiments much was learned about the human circadian timing system and the effect of environmental and time cues in influencing circadian rhythms.

terrifying hypnagogic hallucinations   Terrifying HYPNAGOGIC HALLUCINATIONS, also known as sleep onset nightmares, are terrifying DREAMS that occur at the beginning of sleep. These dreams are similar to NIGHTMARES; however, nightmares usually occur during REM SLEEP, well after sleep onset. The affected person will become drowsy, start to fall asleep, and then see images that become very terrifying. The images cause a sudden awakening, with anxiety and fear; the content of the nightmare can be recalled. Sometimes the associated movement activity in sleep can be very excessive, with calling out and screaming.

Terrifying hypnagogic hallucinations occur in disorders of disturbed REM sleep, such as in NARCOLEPSY, where a SLEEP ONSET REM PERIOD can occur, or following the acute withdrawal of REM-suppressant medications, such as the tricyclic ANTIDEPRESSANTS.

Terrifying hypnagogic hallucinations need to be differentiated from other forms of hallucinatory behavior, such as that seen in more typical hypnagogic hallucinations where the dream content is not terrifying. SLEEP TERRORS occur during SLOW WAVE SLEEP, well after sleep onset, and the terror episodes are associated with fear and anxiety but little dream recall. Rarely, a mental disorder can produce nocturnal hallucinatory behavior; however, the occurrence only at sleep onset would be atypical.

Treatment of terrifying hypnagogic hallucinations involves treatment of the underlying disorder, either narcolepsy or other causes of sleep onset REM episodes, and may involve the use of REM-suppressant medications, such as the tricyclic antidepressant medications.

theophylline   See RESPIRATORY STIMULANTS.

thermoregulation   The body's ability to control body TEMPERATURE within a narrow range. Changes in body temperature and environmental temperature can have important effects upon sleep. The body maintains body temperature within a close range and usually varies it by no more than 1.5 degrees throughout the day. Body temperature falls during sleep, reaching a low point approximately three hours before the time of awakening. Even sleep during the daytime can cause body temperature to fall slightly. Therefore, sleep and circadian factors are important in the control of body temperature.

During sleep, there are specific effects of the sleep state upon the control of body temperature, which is under the control of the preoptic and anterior hypothalamic nuclei (POAH). Thermoregulation changes reduce body temperature during NON-REM-STAGE SLEEP in association with the reduction in the metabolic rate. During REM SLEEP, body temperature in humans increases slightly; however, studies in animals have tended to show that the metabolic rate and body temperature typically are reduced in REM sleep. The slight increase in humans may be related to the increased central nervous system activity. Reduced muscle activity is likely to be responsible for the reduction of metabolic rate and body temperature that is seen in animals.

The control of body temperature varies between sleep states so that the control mechanisms are intact during non-REM sleep and are inhibited during REM sleep. Sweating does not occur during REM sleep, and usual body responses to cold, such as shivering, are not seen during REM sleep. The body's temperature is largely under the control of the environment temperature during the REM sleep state.

Changes in the environmental temperature also have an effect on sleep itself. The amount of SLOW WAVE SLEEP and REM sleep is maximal at an environmental temperature of 29 degrees Celsius (84.2 degrees Fahrenheit); as the body temperature changes, the amount of each sleep stage reduces. In addition, there are changes in the quality of sleep with increased arousals and number of awakenings, and an increased sleep latency. However, a person's adaptation to the environmental temperature influences the effects on sleep that are seen.

Artificial changes in body temperature can have an effect on the quality of sleep. An increase in body temperature prior to the major sleep episode will lead to an increase in non-REM sleep (see WARM BATHS).

The control of body temperature may have important effects upon the infant during its development. Because of the prevalence of SUDDEN INFANT DEATH SYNDROME, the possibility has been raised that an abnormality in the control of thermoregulation during sleep stages may predispose an infant to apneic episodes. Hypothermia has been shown to cause laryngeal hyperexcitability, which can lead to UPPER AIRWAY OBSTRUCTION. Body temperature changes are also useful for the determination of circadian rhythmicity, as they are a marker of the phase of the circadian rhythm. Body temperature changes are commonly recorded in the investigation of shift work and jet-lag effects. (See also CIRCADIAN RHYTHMS, EXERCISE AND SLEEP, SHIFT-WORK SLEEP DISORDER, SLEEP LATENCY, TIME ZONE CHANGE (JET LAG) SYNDROME.)

theta activity   EEG (ELECTROENCEPHALOGRAM) activity with a frequency of 4 to 8 Hz that is generally maximal over the central and temporal areas. Theta activity is commonly seen in lighter stages of NON-REM-STAGE SLEEP but also is present in REM SLEEP. A specific form of theta activity called SAWTOOTH WAVES is characteristic of REM sleep.

tidal volume   The amount of air usually taken into the lungs during a normal breath at rest. It is typically 500 cubic centimeters of air.

time zone change (jet lag) syndrome   Syndrome associated with complaints of difficulty in maintaining sleep and EXCESSIVE SLEEPINESS; typically associated with rapid travel across multiple time zones. The sleep-wake pattern has to be temporarily shifted to another time, the difference in time depending upon the number of time zones crossed. In addition to disturbance of the sleep-wake pattern, there are changes in alertness and performance and general feelings of malaise. The severity and duration of these symptoms is dependent upon not only the number of time zones crossed but also the direction of travel. Adaptation to time zone change is usually quicker following westward travel, where the onset of a new sleep episode is delayed in relation to the prior sleep episode. The tendency for improved adaptation after westward travel is thought to be due to the natural tendency to delay the onset of the sleep episode, the same tendency seen if one is placed in an environment free of time cues.

Once the individual is in the new time zone, adaptation occurs rapidly, with the symptoms of sleep disturbance diminishing with each day in the new environment. Typically, the sleep episode in the new time zone is of shorter duration and may be of lesser quality than that prior to the travel, and this produces a tendency to SLEEP DEPRIVATION and consequent excessive sleepiness. As there is a greater ability to delay our sleep onset than to advance the sleep onset, travel to the east, where sleep is scheduled to occur at a time earlier than the prior sleep onset time, is associated with a greater SLEEP ONSET difficulty.

The disruption in the sleep episode and excessive sleepiness produced by time zone change may induce reduced work performance and interfere with social and occupational activities, but the sleep disturbance usually rapidly abates upon adaptation in the new environment. However, for business persons who frequently travel and have limited time to adapt to the time zone changes, chronic sleep disturbance and impaired work performance may be of particular concern. Airline crews are particularly susceptible to the effects of time zone change.

Polysomnographic studies following time zone change have shown a greater number of arousals and increased stages of lighter sleep with a consequent reduction in SLEEP EFFICIENCY. SLOW WAVE SLEEP generally occurs in normal amounts but there may be reduced REM sleep.

Time zone change sleep disorder can occur in individuals of any age; however, the elderly are believed to be more likely to suffer from symptoms due to their difficulty in maintaining a regular and highly efficient sleep-wake cycle.

JET LAG may be exacerbated by the use of HYPNOTICS. Treatment is directed toward maintaining a regular pattern of sleep in the new environment. A regular sleep onset time and wake time is recommended, with an appropriate sleep duration. An attempt to adapt to the new environmental time is preferable for individuals who plan to be in the new time zone for episodes of one or more weeks. However, if staying in the new time zone for only a few days, maintenance of the prior sleep-wake pattern, even though it is not coordinated with the new environmental time, is preferable.

If a delay in the sleep episode is to be expected in the new environment, attempts to adapt may involve initiating a gradual delay in the original environment prior to travel so the sleep episode is partially adapted.

Daytime flights are said to be preferable to nighttime flights, so the night sleep can occur in a more acceptable environment. Studies have shown that hypnotics use can be beneficial for the first one or two nights in the new time zone in order to enhance the efficiency of the sleep episode. (See also ARGONNE ANTI-JET-LAG DIET, CIRCADIAN RHYTHM SLEEP DISORDERS, ENVIRON-MENTAL TIME CUES, PHASE ADVANCE, PHASE DELAY.)

Tofranil   See ANTIDEPRESSANTS.

tongue retaining device (TRD)   Dental appliance designed to hold the tongue forward to prevent SNORING. The mouthpiece, which is inserted into the mouth and fitted over the upper and lower teeth, contains a compartment that holds the tongue in a forward position by suction. The tongue retaining device works on the principle that the position of the tongue contributes to UPPER AIRWAY OBSTRUCTION, thereby adding to snoring. It is particularly effective for patients who snore while lying in a supine position.

Polysomnographic studies have demonstrated that the TRD can be useful for treating mild OBSTRUCTIVE SLEEP APNEA SYNDROME, especially in patients who are unable either to use a nasal CONTINUOUS POSITIVE AIRWAY PRESSURE (CPAP) device or undergo UVULOPALATOPHARYNGOPLASTY. However, many patients find the device uncomfortable and are unable to tolerate it for more than 50% of the night. In addition, the device appears to be less successful in patients who are more than 50% overweight. (See also ORAL APPLIANCES.)

tonsillectomy and adenoidectomy   Tonsillectomy, with or without an adenoidectomy, is a surgical procedure that is performed for the relief of the OBSTRUCTIVE SLEEP APNEA SYNDROME. This procedure is most commonly performed in children because tonsil enlargement is common in the pre-pubertal age group. However, some adults can also have very enlarged tonsils, or enlarged adenoids, which contribute to UPPER AIRWAY OBSTRUC-TION and therefore may need to undergo this surgery. Many patients treated by a UVULOPALATOPHARYNGOPLASTY (UPP) operation also have removal of tonsils or adenoids if they are enlarged at the time of the UPP surgery.

Tonsillectomy involves removal of the enlarged lymphoid tissue situated between the anterior and posterior pillar of fauces. This tissue is involved in the immune response to infections in childhood but gradually regresses and is of little functional importance in adulthood. Removal of the tonsils is a simple procedure in children, but it assumes greater likelihood of complications, such as excessive bleeding, in adults.

In the majority of children with enlarged tonsils and obstructive sleep apnea, tonsillectomy entirely relieves the obstructive sleep apnea. However, some patients who have craniofacial abnormalities may continue to have obstructive sleep apnea following removal of the tonsils or adenoids. Post-operative polysomnographic monitoring for obstructive sleep apnea is required for patients with severe obstructive sleep apnea who appear to be symptomatic following surgery. Other surgical procedures, for example, MANDIBULAR ADVANCEMENT SURGERY, may be required, or the use of a CONTINUOUS POSITIVE AIRWAY PRESSURE (CPAP) device. (See also SURGERY AND SLEEP DISORDERS, TRACHEOSTOMY.)

total recording time (TRT)   The duration of time from sleep onset (lights out) to the end of the final awakening. The total recording time comprises the TOTAL SLEEP TIME, including stages non-REM and REM sleep, and episodes of wakefulness and movement time that occur until the lights are on; arousal time; or ARISE TIME.

total sleep episode   The duration of the major sleep episode, which usually occurs at night. This is the total amount of time available for sleep, and typically it is approximately eight hours in duration. The total sleep episode includes REM SLEEP and NON-REM-STAGE SLEEP, as well as periods of WAKEFULNESS that occur during the time available for sleep. (See also TOTAL RECORDING TIME, TOTAL SLEEP TIME.)

total sleep time (TST)   The amount of actual sleep that occurs during a sleep episode; consists of\ the sum of the total amount of non-REM plus REM sleep. The total sleep time varies according to age, being greatest in infancy with a gradual reduction as one gets older. (See also SLEEP DURATION, TOTAL RECORDING TIME, TOTAL SLEEP EPISODE.)

toxin-induced sleep disorder   A sleep disorder characterized by either INSOMNIA or EXCESSIVE SLEEPINESS; produced by the ingestion of toxic agents such as heavy metals or organic toxins. The poisoning due to the repeated ingestion of these agents produces central nervous system effects, such as stimulation and agitation, and can also produce depression-causing sleepiness and even COMA. Other symptoms such as cardiac stimulation, respiratory depression, and gastrointestinal upset can occur with the ingestion of the toxic agents. Liver, renal and cardiac poisoning can occur.

This type of sleep disorder is most commonly seen in industrial workers who are exposed to toxic chemicals. It can also be seen in children, who may ingest lead in paint or be excessively exposed to the exhaust fumes of leaded gasoline.

The treatment of the sleep disturbance involves removal of exposure to the offending agent as well as providing good SLEEP HYGIENE measures in order to prevent continuation of the sleep disturbance.

tracheostomy   Regarded as the most effective surgical treatment for OBSTRUCTIVE SLEEP APNEA SYNDROME; involves placing a hole in the trachea and inserting a tube so that the upper airway is bypassed when the individual breathes. The tracheostomy typically is closed during the daytime and open at night so that sleep-related UPPER AIRWAY OBSTRUCTION does not occur.

Tracheostomy is reserved for patients with severe sleep apnea syndrome who are unable to be treated effectively by medical and nonsurgical means. The most effective alternative nonsurgical treatment is by means of a CONTINUOUS POSITIVE AIRWAY PRESSURE (CPAP) device. Some patients, for varying reasons, are unable to use such a system, and tracheostomy is considered if their obstructive sleep apnea is severe enough.

Immediately following the placement of the tracheostomy, patients with severe obstructive sleep apnea notice a dramatic improvement in terms of the quality of sleep at night and relief of daytime sleepiness. There are improved objective clinical features, such as improved oxygen saturation during sleep, reduced cardiac ARRHYTHMIAS, improved quality of sleep and objective evidence of improved daytime alertness.

The complications of tracheostomy are primarily the social difficulties of having a hole at the base of the neck. (Patients are unable to swim or go into small boats where they might fall into the water.) The complications of tracheostomy include recurrent infections, development of granulation tissue at the site of the tracheostomy, and recurrent irritation or cough. More severe problems, such as tracheomalacia (a weakness of the tracheal cartilage) may rarely occur. However, despite the potential complications, tracheostomy can be a dramatically effective and lifesaving treatment for many patients. (See also MANDIBULAR ADVANCEMENT SURGERY, UVULOPALATOPHARYNGOPLASTY, SURGERY AND SLEEP DISORDERS.)

tranquilizers Term introduced in the early 1950s to characterize the calming effect of the medication reserpine. The tranquilizers are often divided into two groups, the major and the minor tranquilizers.

The major tranquilizers include medications, such as phenothiazines, that are often used to treat the major psychiatric disorders. The minor tranquilizers are those that have lesser mind-altering effects and are primarily used for reducing anxiety, such as the BENZODIAZEPINE antianxiety agents. As the term *tranquilizer* can apply to agents with very marked effects on mood and thought, or can apply to agents with very mild effects, the term is best avoided. The terms *antipsychotic* and *antianxiety* medications are preferred. (See also ANXIETY DISORDERS, HYPNOTICS, PSYCHIATRIC DISORDERS.)

transient insomnia Insomnia that is differentiated from SHORT-TERM and LONG-TERM INSOMNIA. The term is synonymous with ADJUSTMENT SLEEP DISORDER and situational insomnia.

triazolam See BENZODIAZEPINES.

triclofos   See HYPNOTICS.

tricyclic antidepressants   See ANTIDEPRESSANTS.

Tripp, Peter   A 32-year-old New York City radio disc jockey who stayed awake for eight consecutive days as a fund-raising event for the March of Dimes birth defects organization. Each day he performed his regular three-hour broadcasts, but he went without any sleep. By the fifth day, Tripp began hallucinating and became increasingly paranoid. At the end of his ordeal, Tripp slept for 13 consecutive hours. Although his psychotic-like thinking cleared up after he slept, Tripp was slightly depressed for several months, possibly linked to his SLEEP DEPRIVATION ordeal. (See also SLEEP NEED.)

TRT   See TOTAL RECORDING TIME.

tryptophan   See HYPNOTICS.

TST   See TOTAL SLEEP TIME.

tumescence   Term used for the engorgement of the penis that occurs in relationship to sexual excitement or REM SLEEP at night. A measure of the ability of the penis to obtain adequate tumescence is used for a better understanding of the cause of IMPOTENCE. (See also IMPAIRED SLEEP-RELATED PENILE ERECTIONS, NOCTURNAL PENILE TUMESCENCE TEST, SLEEP-RELATED PAINFUL ERECTIONS, SLEEP-RELATED PENILE ERECTIONS.)

twitch   A very small body movement such as a foot or finger jerk. A body twitch during sleep is not usually associated with an arousal but is consistently detected either visually or by electromyographic recordings. Body twitches are common during normal sleep, particularly of infants. These movements are often myoclonic jerks, and when they occur in great frequency in neonates the disorder BENIGN NEONATAL SLEEP MYOCLONUS may be present. In adults, twitches can occur at sleep onset and are then termed SLEEP STARTS, particularly if they are associated with a whole body movement.

U

ulcer   See PEPTIC ULCER DISEASE.

ultradian rhythm   Rhythms that have a cycle length of less than 24 hours in duration. The term is used for biological rhythms that occur with a higher frequency than the 24-hour sleep-wake cycle, such as respiratory or cardiac rhythms. Biological rhythms that have a period length greater than 24 hours (such as the MENSTRUAL CYCLE) are known as *infradian rhythms*. (See also CHRONOBIOLOGY, CIRCADIAN RHYTHMS.)

unconsciousness   A mental state in which there is loss of responsiveness to sensory stimuli. States of unconsciousness can be produced by metabolic, pharmacologic or intracerebral lesions. Patients who are unconscious are usually in COMA; however, impaired levels of consciousness may be present with intact sleep-wake cycling and retention of some responses to stimuli.

The term "clouding of consciousness" is often applied to reduced states of wakefulness and awareness in which the patient may be responsive to external stimuli but has a variation in the level of attention, with hyperexcitability and irritability, that alternates with episodes of drowsiness. More advanced degrees of clouding of consciousness can produce a confusional state in which there is difficulty in following commands. A state of DELIRIUM is characterized by disorientation, fear, irritability and a misperception of stimuli. Such patients frequently will have visual hallucinations that can alternate with periods when the mental state appears intact.

The term *obtundation* often applies to an impairment of full consciousness where the individual has some reduction in level of alertness, with decreased awareness of the environment. Such patients may have EXCESSIVE SLEEPINESS or DROWSINESS.

The term STUPOR is often applied to a loss of responsiveness in which the individual can be aroused only by very strong and vigorous stimuli. The patient may be in deep sleep with slow wave activity from which it is difficult to be aroused. After arousal, such subjects typically will lapse back into the unresponsive state. This condition is often associated with organic cerebral dysfunction; however, severe schizophrenia or DEPRESSION can lead to a similar state. (See also DEMENTIA, PSYCHIATRIC DISORDERS.)

upper airway obstruction   Term applied to obstruction that typically occurs during sleep and is associated with the OBSTRUCTIVE SLEEP APNEA SYNDROME. Obstruction can occur anywhere from the nose to the larynx and may not be evident during wakefulness. Causes of such obstruction include a very narrow nasal airway, enlarged adenoids or tonsils, an elongated soft palate, and obstruction at the base of the tongue by tongue tissues, including the lingual tonsil (tonsil sometimes found at the base of the tongue). Predisposing conditions to upper airway obstruction include skeletal abnormalities such as a posterior-placed lower jaw (retrognathia).

Surgery or appliances, such as a CONTINUOUS POSITIVE AIRWAY PRESSURE (CPAP) device, can relieve the upper airway obstruction during sleep and resolve the clinical features associated with the obstructive sleep apnea syndrome. (See also MANDIBULAR ADVANCEMENT SURGERY, ORAL APPLIANCES, SURGERY AND SLEEP DISORDERS, TONSILLECTOMY AND ADENOIDECTOMY, TRACHEOSTOMY, UVULOPALATOPHARYNGOPLASTY.)

upper airway resistance syndrome (UARS)   A disorder consisting of an increased effort of breathing during sleep which produces an arousal that results in sleep fragmentation and subsequent daytime sleepiness. These arousals occur in the absence of APNEAS, HYPOPNEAS and oxygen desaturation. The presence of frequent arousals in a patient complaining of EXCESSIVE SLEEPINESS who does not have apneas and hypopneas should raise suspicion that upper airway resistance syndrome is present.

The best way to document the pressure change is by esophageal pressure monitoring. However, in the absence of pressure monitoring an increased number of arousals (more than 10 per hour) during sleep is typically associated with this syndrome. Approximately 10% of all breaths have negative intrathoracic pressures (less than -10 centimeters of water). Ten percent of all breaths involve an increased effort that is greater than two standard deviations of the value monitored during quiet relaxed breathing. (See also OBSTRUCTIVE SLEEP APNEA SYNDROME.)

upper airway sleep apnea   See OBSTRUCTIVE SLEEP APNEA SYNDROME.

uvulopalatopharyngoplasty (UPP)   A surgical procedure that was developed by Tanenosuke Ikematsu in 1964. This surgical procedure was first used in Japan for the treatment of SNORING and was introduced into the United States by Shiro Fujita in 1979 as an alternative to TRACHEOSTOMY for the treatment of the OBSTRUCTIVE SLEEP APNEA SYNDROME. The surgical procedure for uvulopalatopharyngoplasty involves the removal of redundant and excessive tissue from the pharynx in order to prevent UPPER AIRWAY OBSTRUCTION during sleep. This surgical procedure shortens the soft palate and removes the uvula and the anterior and posterior pillar of fauces that attach to the soft palate. The tonsils, if present, are usually removed.

UPP is a widely used procedure for the treatment of snoring and the obstructive sleep apnea syndrome. However, studies have demonstrated that only 40% to 50% of an unselected group of patients with obstructive sleep apnea syndrome will respond to this procedure. Patients who have been screened by means of upper airway studies have an increased operative success; however, the procedure is ideal for only 20% to 30% of all patients who are evaluated for the obstructive sleep apnea syndrome.

Potential complications of the surgical procedure include insufficiency of the palate closure so that fluids being swallowed may be regurgitated into the nose. (But this complication rarely occurs if the patient is well screened beforehand and an excessive amount of tissue is not removed.) Other complications of uvulopalatopharyngoplasty are those related to anesthesia and other nonspecific surgical complications. Two new forms of palatoplasty have been developed: LASER UVULOPALATOPLASTY and radiofrequency palatoplasty (see SOMNOPLASTY). These procedures have the advantage of being able to be performed in a physician's office without the need for general anesthesia. (See also MANDIBULAR ADVANCEMENT SURGERY, SURGERY AND SLEEP DISORDERS, TONSILLECTOMY AND ADENOIDECTOMY, TRACHEOSTOMY.)

V

Valium   See BENZODIAZEPINES.

ventilation   Movement of air in and out of the lungs. Ventilation can be impaired by a number of disorders that affect the central nervous system, and the nerves and muscles involved in the chest mechanics. Several SLEEP-RELATED BREATHING DISORDERS, such as OBSTRUCTIVE SLEEP APNEA SYNDROME, CENTRAL SLEEP APNEA SYNDROME, CAHS (CENTRAL ALVEOLAR HYPOVENTILATION SYNDROME) and CHRONIC OBSTRUCTIVE PULMONARY DISEASE, can affect ventilation. Ventilation abnormalities during sleep can lead to ALVEOLAR HYPOVENTILATION (abnormal arterial blood gases during the daytime, with HYPOXEMIA and hypercapnia). Relief of the sleep-related breathing disorder can lead to resolution of these daytime blood gas impairments. Other disorders, such as KYPHOSCOLIOSIS and intrinsic lung disease, can also have impaired ventilation during sleep.

Treatment of sleep-related breathing disorders may involve weight reduction (see OBESITY), assisted ventilatory devices, such as a positive pressure ventilator or CONTINUOUS POSITIVE AIRWAY PRESSURE (CPAP) device, or upper airway surgery, such as TRACHEOSTOMY or UVULOPALATOPHARYNGO-PLASTY. (See also SURGERY AND SLEEP DISORDERS.)

vigilance testing   Tests of vigilance to assess the level of alertness during the period of wakefulness as applied in clinical or research settings. Tests may be subjective, by rating scales such as the STANFORD SLEEPINESS SCALE or the visual analogue scale. However, most vigilance testing involves some physiological measure, such as the determination of pupil diameter by PUPILLOMETRY. (The pupil is very sensitive to changes in ALERTNESS and becomes smaller as the level of alertness decreases.)

Other tests involve reaction time tests, such as flicker fusion (rapid alternating pattern of light flashes) studies and letter sorting tasks. These tests determine the ability to concentrate and adequately perform the task at hand.

Other electrophysical means of determining alertness include MULTIPLE SLEEP LATENCY TESTING (MSLT) and MAINTENANCE OF WAKEFULNESS TESTING (MWT), which involve five nap opportunities and measure SLEEP LATENCY on each nap.

Vivactil   See ANTIDEPRESSANTS.

W

wakefulness   A brain state that occurs in the absence of sleep in an otherwise healthy individual. It is the state of being awake that is characterized by EEG wave patterns dominated by ALPHA RHYTHM, or electrocortical activity, between 8 Hz and 13 Hz. This alpha activity is most pronounced when the eyes are closed and the subject is relaxed. Infants tend to have a slower rhythm of about 4 Hz at four months of age, and this increases in frequency with age. The wakefulness rhythm is about 6 Hz at about 12 months of age, 8 Hz at three years of age, and reaches 10 Hz to 13 Hz at 10 years of age. The alpha rhythm remains stable in adults; however, there is often a decline in the elderly, particularly in those with some degree of cerebral pathology. The amplitude varies from person to person, but most often amplitudes of 20 to 60 microvolts are found (rarely, amplitudes above 100 microvolts can be seen). This wakefulness rhythm is thought to be of cortical origin.

In addition to the characteristic alpha activity of wakefulness, there are also BETA RHYTHMS, which occur particularly with increased ALERTNESS, motor activity and in response to environmental stimuli. Wakefulness is often subdivided into quiet wakefulness, where an individual is resting in a relaxed condition, compared with a period of active wakefulness, when the individual is more alert and may be engaged in talking or other motor activities.

wake time   The total time that is scored as wakefulness during a polysomnographic recording. This period of wakefulness usually occurs between SLEEP ONSET and the final wake-up time.

warm baths   Taking a warm bath just before sleep may improve sleep, according to some scientific studies. The beneficial effect of a warm bath is attributed to raising both the core body TEMPERATURE and the more peripheral skin temperature.

weight   Weight plays an important part in exacerbating some sleep disorders. OBSTRUCTIVE SLEEP APNEA SYNDROME more commonly occurs in persons who are overweight, and weight reduction can be associated with an improvement in the symptoms of the syndrome. However, the amount of weight loss required for improvement varies greatly. Some individuals may lose 100 pounds without there being any significant effect, whereas in others, five or 10 pounds of weight loss may produce improvement.

The NOCTURNAL EATING (DRINKING) SYNDROME is a sleep disorder often associated with increasing body weight. People with this disorder will awaken during the night with a compulsion to eat or drink; most of the day's caloric intake may be taken during the hours of sleep. Those with the disorder often seek help in preventing the awakenings to eat in the hope that this will lead to a reduction of body weight. (See also CAHS [CENTRAL ALVEOLAR HYPOVENTILATION SYNDROME], DIET AND SLEEP, OBESITY, OBESITY HYPOVENTILATION SYNDROME, SLEEP-RELATED BREATHING DISORDERS.)

wet dream   See NOCTURNAL EMISSION.

Wilkinson auditory vigilance testing   Proven to be one of the most sensitive performance tests in documenting ALERTNESS and EXCESSIVE SLEEPINESS during the day. In this test, the subject listens through headphones to a recording of a repetitive series of timed pips. These pips of sound are 500 milliseconds in duration, have a regular stimulus interval of 1.5 seconds, and occur on a background of "gray" noise. Occasionally, at unpredictable intervals, one of the tone pips is slightly shorter in duration than the rest (approximately 400 milliseconds). The subject has the task of detecting the shorter signals and indicating their presence by pressing a button. The test continues for 30 minutes and is analyzed in terms of the signals correctly detected, the number of erroneously pushed buttons, and the reaction time from the presentation of the stimulus to the response.

This test is mainly used for research purposes to determine levels of alertness and has little clinical applicability.

World Federation of Sleep Research Societies   Founded in 1989 by the European Sleep Research Society, the Japanese Sleep Research Society, the Latin American Sleep Research Society, and the Sleep Research Society (of the United States). International meetings are held every two years. The first congress was held in 1991. For further information visit the federation's web site at: www.wfsrs.org.

X–Y–Z

Xanax   See BENZODIAZEPINES.

xanthines   See RESPIRATORY STIMULANTS.

yawning   An involuntary movement of the mouth that occurs in humans as well as in such animals as dogs, cats, crocodiles, snakes, birds, and even some fish. A yawn begins with a slow inhalation of air followed by a quicker expiration. Yawns may signify sleepiness as well as stress or boredom.

zaleplon (Sonata)   See HYPNOTICS.

zeitgeber   See ENVIRONMENTAL TIME CUES.

zolpidem   See HYPNOTICS.

zopiclone   See HYPNOTICS.

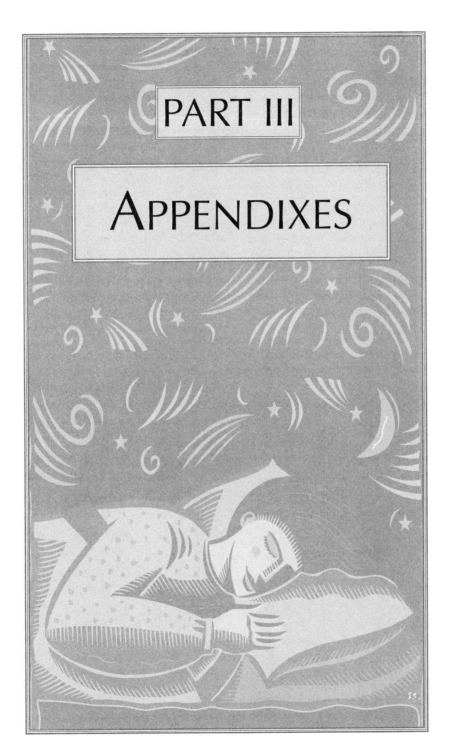

PART III

APPENDIXES

APPENDIX 1
BETTER SLEEP COUNCIL'S GUIDELINES ON HOW TO SELECT A MATTRESS*

By Andrea Herman, Director of the Better Sleep Council

1. Since comfort is a very subjective consideration, the person who is going to use the mattress should test the mattress. If it is a couple, both should be present. Wear comfortable clothes to go shopping for a mattress.
2. There's absolutely no substitute for lying down on a mattress to test it out. (Sitting will not give you as much information since that is not how you will ultimately use it.) Lie down on your back on the mattress.
3. Now close your eyes and try to sense along the length of your body how the mattress is conforming to meet you. The mattress should cradle your body. It should support you along all your curves. It should be comfortable.
4. Turn into the position in which you usually sleep and try it out that way.
5. Take your time even though you may be uncomfortable with the process and want to get through the purchase quickly. You're going to be spending an awful lot of time on that mattress.
6. You and the mattress must be a good match. By the process of elimination, you discover ones you like and ones you don't like.
7. Always find out store policies regarding purchases and exchanges if you get home and find, after several nights, you don't like it.
8. Some states have laws that require the labeling of mattresses so you know if you are getting a new or used mattress.

Better Sleep Council's Guidelines on Mattress Care*

1. Use a washable mattress pad.
2. Vacuum the mattress.
3. If it gets a stain, use light soap and water and dab at it. Never soak a mattress, because it's porous and you will never be able to get it dry.

*This information is based on an interview with Andrea Herman conducted by Jan Yager, Ph.D.

APPENDIX 2
SOURCES OF INFORMATION ON SLEEP INCLUDING SLEEP WEBSITES*

AMERICAN ACADEMY OF SLEEP MEDICINE (AASM)
6301 Bandel Road NW, Suite 101
Rochester, MN 55901
http://www.aasmnet.org

AMERICAN SLEEP APNEA ASSOCIATION (ASAA)
1424 K Street NW, Suite 302
Washington, DC 20005
e-mail:asaa@sleepapnea.org
http://www.sleepapnea.org

AMERICAN SLEEP DISORDERS ASSOCIATION (ASDA)
See American Academy of Sleep Medicine (AASM).

ASSOCIATION FOR THE STUDY OF DREAMS (ASD)
P.O. Box 1166
Orinda, CA 94563
e-mail: asdreamsaol.com
http://www.asdreams.org

BETTER SLEEP COUNCIL
(of the National Association of Bedding Manufacturers) (BSC)
501 Wythe Street
Alexandria, VA 22314
http://www.bettersleep.org

BOOKS FOR SLEEPLESS NIGHTS
http://www.sleephomepages.
  org/books

CENTER FOR SLEEP RESEARCH
Clinical Development Research Centre
The Queen Elizabeth Hospital
Woodville Road
Woodville, South Australia 5011
Australia
http://www.unisa.edu.au/sleep

GOOD SLEEP and CIRCADIAN LEARNING CENTER
Circadian Information, Inc.
125 Cambridge Park Drive
Cambridge, MA 02140
e-mail: info@circadian.com
http://www.circadian.com
http://goodsleep.com

DREAMS
The D.R.E.A.M.S. Foundation
Box 513 Snowdon
Montreal, Quebec
Canada H3X 3T7
http://www.dreams.ca

INTERNATIONAL DIRECTORY OF SLEEP EXPERTS
http://www.websciences.org

NAPPING
The Napping Company, Inc.
26 Orchard Park Drive
Reading, MA 01867
http://www.napping.com

*Since associations and organizations may change their name, address or website information, or even cease to operate, the accuracy of any of the listings in this section cannot be guaranteed. The listings in this section are provided for information only. Inclusion does not necessarily imply endorsement, nor should omission of any sources or resources have any implications. Although a personal reply is not guaranteed, we welcome learning about new potential listings, as well as any corrections that might be considered in the current listings. Suggestions, comments or corrections should be sent to Jan Yager, Ph.D., P.O. Box 8038, Stamford, CT 06905-8038.

NARCOLEPSY INSTITUTE
Sleep-Wake Disorders Center
Montefiore Medical Center
111 East 210th Street
Bronx, NY 10467

NARCOLEPSY NETWORK
10921 Reed Hartman Highway
Cincinnati, OH 45242
e-mail: narnet@aol.com
http://www.narcolpesynetwork.
  org

**NARCOLEPSY AND SLEEP
DISORDERS NEWSLETTER**
http://www.narcolepsy.com

**NATIONAL CENTER FOR SLEEP
DISORDERS RESEARCH**
National Institutes of Health
(Part of the National Heart, Lung, and
  Blood Institute)
NHLB1, Building 31, Room 4A11
9000 Rockville Pike
Bethesda, MD 20892
http://www.nhlbi.nih.gov/about/
  ncsdr/index.htm

**NATIONAL SLEEP FOUNDATION
(NSF)**
1522 K Street NW
Suite 500
Washington, DC 20005
http://www.sleepfoundation.org

**POLYSOMNOGRAPHIC
TECHNOLOGISTS**
Association of Polysomnographic
Technologists (APT)
P.O. Box 14861
Lenexa, KS 66285-4861
http://www.aptweb.org

RESTLESS LEGS SYNDROME
Restless Legs Syndrome Foundation,
Inc.
P.O. Box 7050
Department CP
Rochester, MN 55903-7050
http://www.rls.org

SANDMAN'S SLEEP MALL
http://www.sleepnet.com

SHIFTWORK

The Night Shift Initiative (NSI)
c/o Voron Communications
8001 Castor Avenue
PMB 119
Philadelphia, PA 19152
http://www.nightshift.com

SLEEP APNEA
See listing for American Sleep Apnea
Association.

SLEEP DISORDER CENTERS
http://www.aasmnet.org

SLEEP HOME PAGE
http://www.sleephomepages.org

SLEEP MEDICINE HOME PAGE
http://www.users.cloud9.net/
  ~thorpy

SLEEP RESEARCH ONLINE
c/o WebSciences
10911 Weyburn Avenue
Suite 348
Los Angeles, CA 90024
http://www.sro.org

SLEEP RESEARCH SOCIETY
6301 Bandel Road NW
Suite 101
Rochester, MN 55901
http://www.srssleep.org

THE SLEEP WELL
http://www.stanford.edu/
  ~dement/
See also the related website:
http://www.SleepQuest.com

SLEEPMULTIMEDIA
Sleep Multimedia Inc.
P.O. Box 329-H
Scarsdale, NY 10583

**SLEEP-WAKE DISORDERS
CENTER**
Montefiore Medical Center
111 East 210th Street
Bronx, New York 10467

**SOCIETY FOR LIGHT TREAT-
MENT AND BIOLOGICAL
RHYTHMS**
P.O. Box 591687,
174 Cook Street
San Francisco, CA 94159-1687
http://www.sltbr.org

TALK ABOUT SLEEP.COM

Talk about Sleep, Inc.
P.O. Box 382276
Germantown, TN 38183

(901) 482-2025
http://www.talkaboutsleep.com

TEEN PERSPECTIVE ON SLEEP

SLEEP FROM A TO ZZZZ
http://www.library.thinkquest.
  org/25553

APPENDIX 3
BIBLIOGRAPHY

Encyclopedias on Sleep

Carskadon, Mary, ed. *The Encyclopedia of Sleep and Dreams*. New York: Macmillan, 1993.
Thorpy, Michael J., and Yager, Jan. *The Encyclopedia of Sleep and Sleep Disorders*. 2d ed. New York: Facts On File, Inc., 2001.

Popular and Professional Books and Articles on Sleep in General

Albert, Katherine A. *Get a Good Night's Sleep*. New York: Simon & Schuster, 1996.
Anch, A. Michael, Browman, Carl P., Mitler, Merrill M. and Walsh, James K. *Sleep: A Scientific Perspective*. Englewood Cliff, N.J.: Prentice-Hall, 1988.
Aserinsky, Eugene, and Kleitman, Nathaniel. "Regularly Occurring Periods of Eye Motility and Concomitant Phenomena during Sleep," *Science* 118 (1953): 273–274.
Barnes, C., and Orem J. *Physiology in Sleep*. New York: Academic Press, 1980.
Borbely, Alexander. *Secrets of Sleep*. New York: Basic Books, 1986.
Chopra, Deepak. *Restful Sleep*. New York: Harmony Books, 1994.
Coren, Stanley. *Sleep Thieves: An Eye-opening Exploration into the Science and Mysteries of Sleep*. New York: The Free Press, 1996.
Dement, William C. *Some Must Watch While Some Must Sleep*. New York: Norton, 1976.
———, and Vaughan, Christopher. *The Promise of Sleep*. New York: Delacorte Press, 1999.
Goldberg, Philip, and Kaufman, Daniel. *Everybody's Guide to Natural Sleep*. Los Angeles: Jeremy P. Tarcher, Inc., 1990.
Hales, Diane. *The Complete Book of Sleep*. Reading, Mass.: Addison-Wesley, 1981.
Hauri, Peter. *Current Concepts: The Sleep Disorders*. Kalamazoo, Mich.: The Upjohn Company, 1982.
Hobson, Allan J. *Sleep*. New York: Freeman, 1989.
Horne, James. *Why We Sleep*. Oxford: Oxford University Press, 1988.
Kleitman, Nathaniel. *Sleep and Wakefulness*. Chicago: University of Chicago Press, 1939; revised, 1963.
Lamberg, Lynne. *The American Medical Association Guide to Better Sleep*. New York: Random House, 1984.
Luce, Gay, and Segal, Julius. *Sleep*. New York: Lancer, 1966.
Maas, James B. *Power Sleep*. New York: Harper Perennial, 1999.
Manaceine, Marie de. *Sleep: Its Physiology, Pathology, Hygiene and Psychology*. London: Walter Scott, 1897.
McGinty, D., Drucker-Colin, R., Morrison, A., and Parmeggiani, P. *Brain Mechanisms of Sleep*. New York: Raven Press, 1984.
Mendelson, W. B. *Human Sleep: Research and Clinical Care*. New York: Plenum Press, 1987.
Mitler, Elizabeth A., and Mitler, Merrill M. *101 Questions About Sleep and Dreams*. Del Mar, Calif.: Wakefulness-Sleep Education and Research Foundation, 1996.
Moore-Ede, Martin, and Le Vert, Suzanne. *The Complete Idiot's Guide to Getting Good Night's Sleep*. New York: Macmillan, 1998.
Morton, Leslie T. *A Medical Bibliography*. 4th ed. London: Gower, 1983.
National Sleep Foundation. *2000 Omnibus Sleep in America Poll*. Washington, D.C.: National Sleep Foundation, 2000. http://www.sleepfoundation.org/publications/2000poll.html.

Parkes, J. D. *Sleep and Its Disorders.* London: W.B. Saunders, 1985.

Walsleben, Joyce A., and Baron-Faust, Rita. *A Woman's Guide to Sleep.* New York: Crown, 2000.

Webb, Wilse B. *Sleep: The Gentle Tyrant.* Englewood Cliffs, N.J.: Prentice-Hall, 1975.

BY TOPIC

Adolescence

Carskadon, M. A., "Patterns of sleep and sleepiness in adolescents." *Pediatrician* 17 (1990): 5–12.

Carskadon, M. A., Labyak, S. E. Acebo, C., and Seifer, R., "Intrinsic Circadian Period of Adolescent Humans Measured in Conditions of Forced Desynchrony," *Neuroscience Letters* 260 (1999): 129–132.

————, Wolfson, A. R., Acebo, C., Tzischinsky, O., and Seifer, R., "Adolescent Sleep Patterns, Circadian Timing, and Sleepiness at a Transition to Early School Days," *Sleep* 21 (1998): 871–881.

Thorpy, Michael J., Korman, E., Spielman, Arthur, and Glovinsky, P. B., "Delayed Sleep Phase Syndrome in Adolescents," *Journal of Adolescent Health Care* 9 (1988): 22–27.

Aging and Sleep

Asplund, R. "Sleep Disorders in the Elderly." *Drugs and Aging* 14, no. 2 (1999): 91–103.

Carskadon, M. A., *Brown, E. D., and Dement, W. C. "Sleep Fragmentation in the Elderly: Relationships to Daytime Sleep Tendency,"* Neurology of Aging 3 (1982): 321–327.

Hartmann, Ernest. *The Sleep Book: Understanding and Preventing Sleep Problems in People over 50.* Washington, D.C.: American Association of Retired Persons, 1987.

Morgan, Kevin. *Sleep and Aging: A Research-Based Guide to Sleep in Later Life.* Baltimore, Md.: Johns Hopkins University Press, 1987.

Vitiello, M. V., and Prinz, P. N. "Aging and Sleep Disorders," in R. L. Williams, I. Karacan, and C. A. Moore, eds. *Sleep Disorders.* New York: Wiley, 1988, pp. 293–314.

Weitzman, E. D. "Sleep and Aging" in Katzman, R. and Terry, R. D., eds. *The Neurology of Aging.* Philadelphia: F. A. Davis, 1983, pp. 167–188.

Bedwetting (sleep enuresis)

Cendron, M., "Primary Noctural Enuresis: Current Concepts," *American Family Physician* 59, no. 5 (1999): 1205–1214, 1219–1220.

Ferber, R., "Sleep-Associated Enuresis in the Child," in Kryger, Roth, and Dement, eds., *Principles and Practices of Sleep Disorders Medicine.* Philadelphia: Saunders, 1989, pp. 643–664.

Forsythe, W. F., and Redmond, A., "Enuresis and Spontaneous Cure Rate: Study of 1129 Enuretics," *Archives of Disease in Childhood* 49 (1974): 259–263.

Mikkelsen, E. J., and Rappoport, J. L., "Enuresis: Psychopathology, Sleep Stage, and Drug Response," *Neurological Clinics of North America* 7 (1980): 361–377.

Benefits of Sleep

Blakeslee, Sandra. "Experts Explore Deep Sleep and the Making of Memories." *The New York Times,* November 14, 2000, page F2.

Lipman, Lisa (Associated Press), "Study: Sleep Helps Improve Memory." *The Advocate, November, 2000, page A11.*

Children (see infants and children)

Chronobiology

Halberg, Franz, "Chronobiology," *Annual Review of Physiology* 31 (1969): 675–725.

Kripke, D. F., Gillin, J. C., Mullaney, D. J., Risch, S. D., and Janowsku, D. S. "Treatment of Major Depressive Disorders by Bright White Light for 5 Days" in *Chronobiology and Psychiatric Disorders.* New York: Elsevier Sciences Publishing Company, 1987, pp. 207–218.

Circadian Rhythm Disorders and Body Clocks
(see also adolescence)

Czeisler, C. A., Duffy, J.F., Shanahan, T.L., et. al. "Stability, Precision, and Near 24-Hour Period of the Human Circadian Pacemaker." *Science* 284 (1999): 2177–81.

Czeisler, C. A., Witzman, E. D., Moore-Ede, M. C., Zimmerman, J. C., and Knauer, R. S., "Human Sleep: Its Duration and Organization Depend on Its Circadian Phase," *Science* 210 (1980): 1264–1267.

Kamei, R., Hughes, L., Miles, L., and Dement, W. "Advanced Sleep Phase Syndrome Studied in a Time Isolation Facility," *Chronobiologia* 6 (1979): 115.

Smolensky, Michael, and Lamberg, Lynne. *The Body Clock Guide to Better Health.* New York: Henry Holt, 2000.

Daytime Sleepiness (see excessive daytime sleepiness)

Dreams and Nightmares

Diamond, Edwin. *The Science of Dreams.* Garden City, N.Y.: Doubleday, 1962.

Empson, Jacob. *Sleep and Dreaming.* London: Faber and Faber, 1989.

Fischer, C. J., Byrne, J., Edwards, T., and Kahn, E., "A Psychophysiological Study of Nightmares," *Journal of the American Psychoanalytic Association* 18 (1970): 747–782.

Freud, Sigmund. *The Interpretation of Dreams.* Trans. Joyce Crick. Ed. Ritchie Robertson. New York: Oxford University Press, 2000.

Garfield, Patricia. *Creative Dreaming.* New York: Ballantine, 1974.

Hall, Calvin. *The Meaning of Dreams.* New York: Harper, 1953.

———, "What People Dream About," *Scientific American* 184 (1951): 60–63.

Hartmann, Ernest. *The Nightmare.* New York: Basic Books, 1984.

Hobson, Allan J. *The Dreaming Brain.* New York: Basic Books, 1988.

Jung, C. G., *Dreams.* Trans. R. F. C. Hull. Princeton, N.J.: Princeton University Press, 1974.

Pagel, J. F. "Nightmares and Disorders of Dreaming." *American Family Physician* 2000 Apr 1; 61(7): 2037–2042, 2044. Review.

Drowsy Driving

Brody, Jane E. "Personal Health: Why Drivers Fall Asleep, and How to Avoid Becoming a Traffic Statistic." *The New York Times,* July 5, 1990, page B7.

Findley, L. J., et al. *Driving Performance and Automobile Accidents in Patients with Sleep Apnea."* Clinics of Chest Medicine 13, no. 3 (Sept. 1992): 427–35. Review.

Horne, J., and Reyner, L. "Vehicle Accidents Related to Sleep: A Review." *Occupational and Environmental Medicine.* 56, no. 5 (May 1999): 289–94, Review.

Mitler, M. M. "Sleepiness and Human Behavior." *Current Opinion in Pulmonary Medicine* 2, no. 6 (November 1996): 488–91. Review.

National Sleep Foundation, *2000 Omnibus Sleep in America Poll.* "Drowsy Driving." Washington, D.C.: National Sleep Foundation, 2000.

———. *2001 Sleep in America Poll.* "Drowsy Driving." Washington, DC: National Sleep Foundation, 2001.

Excessive Daytime Sleepiness

Guilleminault, C. "Disorders of Excessive Daytime Sleepiness." *Annals of Clinical Research* 17 (1985): 209–219.

Mahowald, Mark. "Assessing Excessive Daytime Sleepiness: A Complaint to be Taken Seriously," *Sleep Medicine Alert.* Washington, D.C.: National Sleep Foundation, summer 1999.

Roehrs, Timothy, et al., "Excessive Daytime Sleepiness Associated with Insufficient Sleep," *Sleep* 6 (1983): 319–325.

Rosen, Gerald. "EDS in Children." *Sleep Medicine Alert.* Washington, D.C.: National Sleep Foundation, summer 1999.

Roth, T., et al., "Daytime Sleepiness and Alertness," in Kryger, M., Roth, Thomas, and Dement, W., eds. *The Principles and Practices of Sleep Disorders Medicine.* Philadelphia; W. B. Saunders, 1989, pp. 14–23.

History of Sleep

De Marian, Jean-Jacques, "Observation Botanique," in *Histoire de L'Academie Royale des Sciences* (1729): 35–36.

Haymaker, Webb. *The Founders of Neurology.* Springfield, Ill.: Charles C. Thomas, 1953.

Lyons, Albert S. *Medicine: An Illustrated History.* New York: Abradale Press, 1978.

Moruzzi, Giuseppe. "The Historical Development of the Differentiation Hypothesis of Sleep." *Proceedings of the American Philosophical Society* 108 (1964): 19–28.

McHenry, Lawrence C., Jr. *Garrison's History of Neurology.* Springfield, Ill.: Charles C. Thomas, 1969.

Rosner, Fred. *Julius Preuss' Biblical and Talmudic Medicine.* New York: Sanhedrin Press, 1978.

Siegel, Rudolph E. *Galen on the Affected Parts, from the Greek, with explanatory notes.* London: S. Karger, 1976.

Infants and Children

Cuthbertson, Joan, and Schevill, Susie. *Helping Your Child Sleep Through the Night.* Garden City, N.Y.: Doubleday, 1985.

Dickinson, Amy. "Eyes Wide Shut (Sleep-deprived parents of newborns get advice from two camps. Listen to only one at your peril.) *Time,* November 13, 2000.

Durand, M., et al. "Ventilatory Control and Carbon Dioxide Response in Preterm Infants with Idiopathic Apnea." *American Disease of Childhood* 139 (1985): 717–720.

Ferber, Richard. *Solve Your Child's Sleep Problems.* New York: Simon and Schuster, 1985.

Ferber, Richard, and Kryger, Meir. *Principles and Practices of Sleep Medicine in the Child.* New York: Saunders, 1995.

Guilleminault, C., ed. *Sleep and its Disorder in Children.* New York: Raven Press, 1987.

Kahn, A., et al., "Insomnia in Cow's Milk Allergy in Infants," *Pediatrics* 76 (1985): 880–884.

Kahn, A., et al., "Normal Sleep Architecture in Infants and Children." *Journal of Clinical Neurophysiology* 13, no. 3 (May 1996): 184–97. Review.

Konner, Melvin, "Where Should Baby Sleep?" *New York Times Sunday Magazine,* January 8, 1989, pp. 39–40.

Lugaresi, E., et al., "Fatal Familial Insomnia and Dysautonomia with Selective Degeneration of Thalmic Nuclei," *New England Journal of Medicine* 315 (1986): 997–1003.

Rae-Dupress, Janet. "It's tricky getting a baby to sleep like one." *U.S. News & World Report,* October 16, 2000, page 70.

Sheldon, Stephen, Riter, S., and Detrojan, M. *Atlas of Sleep Medicine in Infants and Children.* Armonk, N.Y.: Futura, 1999.

Sperling, Dan, "Sleep Disorders of the Kiddie Kind," *USA Today,* June 22, 1989, page 5D.

Thach, B., "Sleep Apnea in Infancy and Childhood," *Medical Clinics of North America* 69 (1985): 1289–1315.

Insomnia

Ancoli-Israel S. "Insomnia in the Elderly: A Review for the Primary Care Practitioner." *Sleep* 23 (February 2000) Suppl. 1:S23–30.

Bootzin, R., and Nicassio, P. M. "Behavioral Treatment for Insomnia," in M. Hersen, R.M. Eissler, P.M. Miller, eds. *Progress in Behavior Modification*. New York: Academic Press, 1978, pp. 1–45.

Hauri, Peter, "Primary Insomnia," in Kryger, M., Roth, Thomas, and Dement, W., eds, *The Principles and Practices of Sleep Disorders Medicine*. Philadelphia; W. B. Saunders, 1989.

Hawi, Peter, and Linde, Shirley. *No More Sleepless Nights*. 2d ed. New York: Wiley, 1996.

Kales, Anthony, and Kales, Joyce D. *Evaluation and Treatment of Insomnia*. New York: Oxford University Press, 1984.

Kales, A., et al. "Personality Patterns in Insomnia," *Archives of General Psychiatry* 33 (1976): 1128–1134.

Morin, C. M. *Insomnia: Psychological Assessment and Management*. New York: Guilford, 1993.

Morin, E. M., et al., "Nonpharmacological Treatment of Late-Life Insomnia," *Journal of Psychosomatic Research* 42, no. 2 (1999): 103–116.

"New Insomnia Drug: Are There any Medications to Treat Insomnia That Won't Leave Me Feeling Groggy the Next day?" *Johns Hopkins Medical Letter Health After 50* 12, no. 1 (March 2000) 8.

Roth, T. "New Trends in Insomnia Management." *Journal of Psychopharmacology* 13, no. 4 (1999) Suppl. 1: S37–40. Review.

Seidel, W. F., and Dement, W. C. "Sleepiness in Insomnia: Evaluation and Treatment," *Sleep* 5 (1982): S182–S190.

Shapiro, Colin M. *Conquering Insomnia*. Hamilton, Ont.: Empowering Press, 1994.

Spielman, Arthur J., "Assessment of Insomnia," *Clinical Psychology Review* 6 (1986): 11–25.

Spielman, Arthur J., Caruso, L., and Glovinsky, P., *A Behavioral Perspective on Insomnia Treatment*," Psychiatric Clinics of North America 10 (1987): 541–553.

Spielman, Arthur J., Saskin, Paul, and Thorpy, Michael J. "Treatment of Chronic Insomnia by Restriction of Time in Bed," *Sleep* 10 (1987): 45–56.

Zisapel, N., "The Use of Melatonin for the Treatment of Insomnia," *Biological Signals and Receptors* 8, nos. 1–2 (1999): 84–89.

Jet Lag

Ehret, Charles F., and Lynne Waller Scanlon. *Overcoming Jet Lag*. New York: Berkley, 1983.

Ayes, Kathleen. *Beat Jet Lag*. London: Thorsons, 1991.

Oren, Dan A., et al. *How to Beat Jet Lag*. New York: Holt, 1993.

Stone, B. M., et al., "Promoting Sleep in Shiftworkers and Intercontinental Travelers," *Chronobiology International* 14, no. 2 (1977): 133–143.

Napping

Anthony, William A. *The Art of Napping*. Burdett, N.Y.: Larson Publications, 1997.

Dinges, David F., and Broughton, Roger J., eds. *Sleep and Alertness: Chronobiological, Behavioral, and Medical Aspects of Napping*. New York: Raven Press, 1989.

Leonhardt, D. "More bosses encourage napping on the job." *The New York Times,* October 13, 1999.

Riley, T. L., ed. *Clinical Aspects, Sleep and Nap Disturbance*. London: Butterworth, 1985.

Rohrlich, Marianne. "Restful Destinations for the Nap-Inclined." *The New York Times,* January 20, 2000, page F10.

Stern, Gary M. "Naps Help Boost Energy, Reduce Stress." *Investor's Business Daily,* February 1, 2000, page 1.

Narcolepsy

Altrich, M. S., "Diagnostic Aspects of Narcolepsy," *Neurology* 50, no. 2, Suppl. 1 (1998): S2–S7.

Bassetti, C., and Aldrich, M. S. "Narcolepsy." *Neurologic Clinics* 14, no. 3 (August 1996): 545–71. Review.

Faraco, J., et al., "Genetic Studies in Narcolepsy, a Disorder Affecting REM Sleep," *Journal of Heredity* 90, no. 1 (1999): 129–132.

Green, P. M., and Stillman, M. J. "Narcolepsy: Signs, Symptoms, Differential Diagnosis, and Management." *Archives of Family Medicine* 7, no. 5 (September–October 1998): 472–478. Review.

Guilleminault, C., Passouant, P., and Dement, W. C. *Narcolepsy.* New York: Spectrum, 1976.

Roth, Bedrich. *Narcolepsy and Hypersomnia.* Basel: Karger, 1980.

Thorpy, Michael J., et al., "Objective Assessment of Narcolepsy," *Archives of Neurology* 40 (1983): 126–127.

Utley, Marguerite J. *Narcolepsy.* DeSoto, Tx.: M. J. Utley, 1995.

Wise, M. S., "Childhood Narcolepsy," *Neurology* 50, no. 2 Suppl. 1 (1998): S37–S42.

Restless Legs Syndrome

Ekbom, K. A., "Restless Leg Syndrome," *Neurology* 10 (1960): 867–873.

Silber, M. H., "Restless Leg Syndrome," *Mayo Clinic Proceedings* 72, no. 3 (1997): 261–264.

Psychology and Sleep

Aikman, Walter, and Ann. *Stress.* New York: Bantam, 1974.

American Psychiatric Association. *Diagnostic and Statistical Manual of Mental Disorders,* 4th ed. Washington, D.C.: American Psychiatric Association, 1994.

Beck, A. T., Rush, A. J., Shaw, B. F., and Emery, G. *Cognitive Therapy of Depression.* New York: Guilford Press, 1979.

Gillin, J. C., "Are Sleep Disturbances Risk Factors for Anxiety, Depressive and Addictive Disorders?" *Acta Psychiatrica Scandinavica Supplement* 393 (1998): 39–43.

Johnson, L. C. "Psychological and Physiological Changes Following Total Sleep Deprivation" in Kales, A., ed., *Sleep: Physiology and Pathology.* Philadelphia: Lippincott, 1969.

Mamelak, M., "Neurodegeneration, Sleep, and Cerebral Energy Metabolism: A Testable Hypothesis," *Journal of Geriatric Psychiatry and Neurology* 10, no. 1 (1997): 29–32.

Reite, M., "Sleep Disorders Presenting as Psychiatric Disorders." *Psychiatric Clinics of North America* 21, no. 3 (1998): 591–607.

Rosa, R. R., Bonnett, M. M., and Kramer, M., "The Relationships of Sleep and Anxiety in Anxious Subjects." *Biological Psychology* 16 (1983): 119–126.

Sussman, N. "Anxiety Disorders." *Psychiatric Annals* 18 (1988): 134–189.

Thase, M. E. "Depression, Sleep, and Antidepressants," *Journal of Clinical Psychiatry* 59, no. 4 (1998): 55–65.

Zarcone, V. P., "Sleep and Schizophrenia," in Williams, R. L., et al., *Sleep Disorders.* New York: Wiley, 1988, pp. 175–188.

Seasonal Disorders and Light Therapy

Chesson, A. L., Jr. Littner, M., Davila, D., Anderson, W. M., Grigg-Damberger, M., Hartse, K., Johnson, S., and Wise, M. "Practice Parameters for the Use of Light Therapy in the Treatment of Sleep Disorders." *Sleep* 1999 Aug 1; 22 (5): 641–60.

Terman, M., et al. "Light Treatment for Sleep Disorders: Consensus Report. Sleep Phase and Duration Disturbances." *Journal of Biological Rhythms* 10 (1995): 135–147.

Yager, Jan. "Living Through January." *Newsday.* January 5, 1988, page 39.

Shift Work

Coleman, Richard M. *Wide Awake at 3:00 A.M.* New York: Freeman, 1986.

Dotto, Lydi. *Losing Sleep.* New York: Morrow, 1990.

Moore-Ede, Martin. *The Twenty-four-Hour Society.* Reading, Mass.: Addison-Wesley, 1993.

Van Reeth, O., "Sleep and Circadian Disturbances in Shift Work: Strategies for Their Management," *Hormone Research* 49, nos. 3–4 (1998): 158–162.

Sleep Apnea

Dickens, Charles. *The Posthumous Papers of the Pickwick Club.* London: Chapman and Hall, published in serial form, 1836–37.

Fairbanks, D. N. F., et al., eds. *Snoring and Obstructive Sleep Apnea.* New York: Raven Press, 1987.

Guilleminault, C., "Sleep Apnea Syndromes; Impact of Sleep and Sleep States," *Sleep* (1980): 227–246.

Guilleminault, C., and Dement, William C., eds., *Sleep Apnea Syndromes.* New York: Alan R. Liss, 1978.

Guilleminault, C., and Kowall, J., "Central Sleep Apnea in Adults," in Thorpy, Michael J., ed., *Handbook of Sleep Disorders.* New York: Dekker, 1990.

Kryger, M., "Fat, Sleep, and Charles Dickens: Literary and Medical Contributions to the Understanding of Sleep Apnea," *Clinics of Chest Medicine* 6 (1985); 555–562.

Leech, Judith A. *Falling Asleep in the Middle of Life.* Ogensburg, N.Y.: AYD Medical Services, 1999.

Pascualy, Ralph A., and Soest, Sally Warren. *Snoring and Sleep Apnea: Personal and Family Guide to Diagnosis and Treatment.* New York: Raven Press, 1994.

Shepard, J. W., Jr. "Hypertension, Cardiac Arrhythmias, Myocardial Infarction, and Stroke in Relation to Obstructive Sleep Apnea." *Clinics of Chest Medicine* 13, no. 3 (Sept 1992): 437–1958. Review.

Sullivan, C. E., et al., "Reversal of Obstructive Sleep Apnea by Continuous Positive Airway Pressure Applied Through the Nares," *Lancet* (1981): 862–865.

Thalhofer, S., et al., "Central Sleep Apnea." *Respiration* 64, no. 1 (1997): 2–9.

Woodson, B. T. "Surgical Approaches to Obstructive Sleep Apnea." *Current Opinion in Pulmonary Medicine* 4, no. 6 (November 1998): 344–350. Review.

Young, T., et al. "The Occurrence of Sleep-disordered Breathing Among Middle-aged Adults." *New England Journal of Medicine* 328, no. 17 (April 29, 1993): 1230–1235.

Sleep Deprivation

Allmon, Stephanie. "Wake-up Call Sounded on Need for More Sleep." *The Washington Times,* April 26, 2000, page A2.

Brink, Susan. "Sleepless Society." *U.S. News & World Report,* October 16, 2000, pages 62–71.

Horne, J. A., "Sleep Function; with Particular Reference to Sleep Deprivations," *Annals of Clinical Research* 17 (1985): 199–208.

Howerton, Michael. "Sleepless in Stamford? Earlier School Starting Times Worry Some Parents, Officials." *The Advocate,* August 6, 2000, page 1, A7.

Johns, M. W. "A new model for measuring daytime sleepiness: The Epworth Sleepiness Scale." *Sleep* 14 (1991): 540.

Murphy, Kate. "Sleep: Health & Fitness: An 'Epidemic' of Sleeplessness." *Business Week,* May 8, 2000, page 161.

Rechtschaffen, A., et al., "Sleep Deprivation in the Rat: X. Integration and Discussion of the Findings," *Sleep* 12 (1989): 68–87.

Sleep Disorders and Sleep Disorders Medicine

Aldrich, Michael S. *Sleep Medicine*. New York: Oxford University Press, 1999.

American Sleep Disorders Association. *ICSD—International classification of sleep disorders. Revised: Diagnostic and coding manual*. Rochester, Minn.: American Sleep Disorders Association, 1997.

Billiard, M., Guilleminault, C., and Dement, W. C., "Menstruation-Linked Periodic Hypersomnia," *Neurology* 25 (1976): 436–443.

Borbely, A. A. "A Two-process Model of Sleep Regulation." *Human Neurobiology* 1, 195–204.

Broughton, R., "Sleep Disorders: Disorders of Arousal?" *Science* 159 (1968): 1070–1087.

Coleman, Richard, "Periodic Movements in Sleep (Nocturnal Myoclonus) and Restless Leg Syndrome" in Guilleminault, C., ed. *Sleeping and Waking Disorders: Indications and Techniques*. Menlo Park, Calif.: Addison-Wesley, 1982, pp. 265–295.

Driver, H. S. "Sleep in Women." *Journal of Psychosomatic Research* 40, no. 3 (March 1966): 227–30. Review.

Ferini-Strambi, L., and Zucconi, M. "REM Sleep Behavior Disorder." *Clinical Neurophysiology* 111, Suppl. 2 (September 2000): S136–140.

Fritz, Roger. *Sleep Disorders*. Naperville, Ill.: National Sleep Alert, Inc., 1993.

Giraudoux, Jean. *Ondine*, Adapted by Maurice Valency. *New York: Random House, 1954.*

Kamei, R., Hughes, L., Miles, L., and Dement, W. C., "Advanced Sleep Phase Syndrome Studied in a Time Isolation Facility," *Chronobiologia* 6 (1979): 115.

Kryger, M., Roth, Thomas, and Dement, William C., eds. *The Principles and Practices of Sleep Disorders Medicine*. 3rd ed. Philadelphia: W. B. Saunders, 2000.

Lavie, Peretz. *The Enchanted World of Sleep*. New Haven, Conn.: Yale University Press, 1996.

Moruzzi, G., and Magoun, H. W. "Brain Stem Reticular Formation and Activation of the EEG," *Electroencephalography and Clinical Neurology* 7 (1949): 455–473.

Parkes, J. D. *Sleep and Its Disorders*. London: W. B. Saunders, 1985.

Shaver, J. L. and Zenk, S. N. "Sleep Disturbance in Menopause." *Journal of Women's Health and Gender-Based Medicine* 9, no. 2 (March 2000): 109–118.

Shepard, John W., Jr., ed. *Atlas of Sleep Medicine*. Armonk, N.Y.: Futura, 1991.

Shneereson, John. *Handbook of Sleep Medicine*. Oxford, England: Blackwell Science Ltd., 2000.

Thorpy, Michael J., ed. "International Classification of Sleep Disorders." American Sleep Disorders Association, 1990.

———. *Handbook of Sleep Disorders (Neurological Disease and Therapy* series, W. Koller, series editor). New York: Marcel Dekker, 1990.

Thorpy, Michael J., and Glovinsky, Paul B. "Parasomnias," *Psychiatric Clinics of North America* 10 (1987): 623–639.

Vgontzas, A. N., and Kales A. "Sleep and its Disorders." *Annual Review of Medicine* 50 (1999): 387–400. Review.

Weitzman, E. D., Czeisler, C. A., Coleman, R. M., et al. "Delayed Sleep Phase Syndrome," *Archives of General Psychiatry* 38 (1981): 731–746.

Williams, R. L., Karacan, I., and Moore, C., eds. *Sleep Disorders: Diagnosis and Treatment*. 2nd edition. New York: Wiley, 1988.

Yager, Joel. "Nocturnal Eating Syndromes: To Sleep, Perchance to Eat." *Journal of the American Medical Association 283, no. 7 (1999).*

Sleep Hygiene

Baekaland, F., and Lasky, R. "Exercise and Sleep Patterns in College Athletes." *Perceptual and Motor Skills* 23 (1966): 1203–1207.

Fidell, S., Perasons, K., Tabachnick, B. G., and Howe, R. "Effects on Sleep Disturbance of Changes in Aircraft Noise Near Three Airports." *Journal of the Acoustical Society of America* 107, no. 5, pt. 1 (May 2000): 2535–2547.

Hicks, R. A. and Youmans, K. "The Sleep-promoting Behaviors of Habitual Short- and Longer-sleeping Adults." *Perceptual and Motor Skills* 69, no. 1 (August 1989): 145–146.

Lukas, J. S., "Noise and Sleep: A Literature Review and a Proposed Criteria for Assessing Effects," *Journal of the Acoustical Society of America* 58 (1975): 1232–1242.

Okamato, K., Nakabayashi, K., Mizuno, K., Okudaira, N. "Effects of Truss Mattress Upon Sleep and Bed Climate," *Applied Human Science* 17, no. 6 (November 1998): 233–237.

Reimao, R., Souza, J. C., Gaudioso, C. E., Guerra, H. D., Alves, A. D., Oliveira, J. C., Gnobie, N. C., and Silverio, D. C. "Nocturnal Sleep Pattern in Native Brazilian Terena Adults." *Arquivos De Neuropsiquiatria* 58, no. 2A (June 2000): 233–8.

Tiffin, R., Ashton, H., Marsh, R., and Kamali, F. "Pharmacokinetic and Pharmacodynamic Responses to Caffeine in Poor and Normal Sleepers." *Psychopharmacology* (Berlin) 121, no. 4 (October 1995) (4): 494–502.

Williams, R. L., et al. "EEG of Human Sleep." *Sleep: Clinical Applications,* New York: Wiley, 1974.

Sleep Medications and Related Topics (alcohol, caffeine, nicotine)

Dobkin, Bruce H. "Sleep pills," *New York Times Sunday Magazine,* February 5, 1989, page 39.

Curatolo, P. W. and Robertson, D., "The Health Consequences of Caffeine," *Annals of Internal Medicine* 98 (1983): 641–653.

Hughes, Rod J. "Clinical Applications of Melatonin in Sleep Medicine." *Sleep Medicine Alert.* Washington, D.C.: National Sleep Foundation, spring 1999.

Kales, Anthony, et. al., "Chronic Hypnotic Drug Use: Ineffectiveness, Drug Withdrawal Insomnia and Dependence," *Journal of American Medical Association* 227 (1974): 511–517.

Kripke, D. F., Simons, R. N., Garfinkel, L., and Hammond, E. C. "Short and Long Sleep and Sleeping Pills: Is Increased Mortality Associated?" *Archives of General Psychiatry* 3 (1979): 103–116.

Nicholson, A. N., "Hypnotics: Clinical Pharmacology and Therapeutics," in Kryger, M. H., Roth, T., and Dement, W. C., eds. *Principles and Practices of Sleep Medicine.* Philadelphia: Saunders: 1989, pp. 219–227.

O'Brien, Robert, and Chafetz, Morris. *The Encyclopedia of Alcoholism.* New York: Facts On File, Inc., 1982.

O'Brien, Robert, and Cohen, Sidney. *The Encyclopedia of Drug Abuse.* New York: Facts On File, 1984.

Tinsley, J. A. and Watkins, D. D., "Over-the-Counter Stimulants: Abuse and Addiction," *Mayo Clinic Proceedings* 73, no. 10 (1998): 977–982.

United States Surgeon General. *The Health Consequences of Smoking.* Washington, D.C.: U.S. Government Printing Office, 1981.

Sleep Paralysis

Goode, G. B., "Sleep Paralysis," *Archives of Neurology* 6 (1962): 228–234.

Hishikawa, Y., "Sleep Paralysis," in Guilleminault, C., Dement, W. C., and Passouant, P., eds. *Narcolepsy.* Vol. 2. *Advances in Sleep Research.* New York: Spectrum, 1976, pp. 97–124.

McKecknie, J., "Incidence and Diagnosis of Sleep Paralysis," *Nursing Times* 94, no. 22 (1988): 50–51.

Roth, B., Bruhova, S., and Berkova, L., "Familial Sleep Paralysis," *Archives Suisses Neurological Neurochir Psychiatry* 102 (1968): 321–330.

Sleep-Related Asthma

D'Ambrosio, C. M., et al. "Sleep in Asthma," *Clinics of Sleep Medicine* 19, no. 1 (1998): 127–137.

Martin, R. J., "Nocturnal Asthma and the Use of Theophylline," *Clinical & Experimental Allergy* 28, Suppl. 3 (1998): 64–70.

———, "Nocturnal Asthma" in Martin, R. J., ed., *Cardiorespiratory Disorders During Sleep.* New York: Futura, 1984, pp. 119–146.

Snoring

Hausfeld, Jeffrey N., with Alice E. Fugate. *Don't Snore Anymore.* New York: Three Rivers Press, 1999.

Sudden Infant Death Syndrome (SIDS)

American Academy of Pediatrics. Task Force on Infant Sleep Position and Sudden Infant Death Syndrome. "Changing Concepts of Sudden Infant Death Syndrome: Implications for Infant Sleeping Environment and Sleep Position." *Pediatrics* 105, no. 3, pt. 1 (March 2000): 650–656. Review.

Naeye, R. L., "Sudden Infant Death," *Scientific American* 242 (1980): 42–56.

Hoppenbrouwers, T. and Hodgman, J. E., "Sudden Infant Death Syndrome (SIDS)," *Public Health Reviews* 11 (1938): 363–390.

Scragg, R. K., et al., "Side Sleeping Position and Bed Sharing in the Sudden Infant Death Syndrome," *Annals of Medicine* 30, no. 4 (1998): 345–349.

Willinger, Marian. "Back to Sleep Program Significant in Reducing SIDS." *Sleep Medicine Alert.* Washington, D.C.: National Sleep Foundation, winter, 1999.

Time Management (see also circadian rhythm)

Barkas, J. L. (a/k/a Jan Yager) *Creative Time Management.* Englewood Cliffs, N.J.: Prentice Hall, 1984.

Croft, Chris. *Time Management.* London: International Thomson Business Press, 1996.

Hall, Edward T. *The Dance of Life: The Other Dimension of Time.* Garden City, N.Y.: Doubleday, 1983.

Yager, Jan. *Creative Time Management for the New Millenium.* Stamford, Conn.: Hannacroix Creek Books, 1999.

Zerubavel, Eviatar. *Hidden Rhythms: Schedules and Calendars in Social Life.* Chicago: University of Chicago Press, 1981.

ABOUT THE AUTHORS

MICHAEL J. THORPY, M.D.

Michael Thorpy, M.D., board certified in sleep disorders medicine, is director of the Sleep-Wake Disorders Center at Montefiore Medical Center, Bronx, New York. Both a clinician and a well-published researcher, Dr. Thorpy serves as associate professor of neurology at Albert Einstein College of Medicine and is the chairman of the Sleep Section of the American Academy of Neurology. In addition, Dr. Thorpy is the past secretary of the National Sleep Foundation (NSF) and directs the NSF's National Narcolepsy Registry, which is located at Montefiore.

Dr. Thorpy was born in New Zealand and earned his medical degree from the University of Otago in 1973. He has published extensively on narcolepsy, insomnia and sleep disorders. His seven books include *The Encyclopedia of Sleep Disorders.* His curriculum vitae lists more than 50 articles, including peer-reviewed publications in journals such as *The New England Journal of Medicine.* Dr. Thorpy's Sleep Medicine Home Page is one of the major sleep websites on the Internet, and his computerized textbook of sleep, *SleepMultiMedia* (on CD-ROM), is the only one of its kind. In 1993, he was awarded one of the sleep field's highest honors: The Nathaniel Kleitman Award from the American Sleep Disorders Association.

Dr. Thorpy is frequently quoted in the media, including *The New York Times, The Washington Post* and *Good Housekeeping.* He has been interviewed on TV and radio including appearances on *The Today Show* and *20/20.*

JAN YAGER, Ph.D.

Dr. Yager has a Ph.D. in sociology from the Graduate Center of the City University of New York (1983) where she had a National Science Foundation predoctoral fellowship in medical sociology through a joint program of Mt. Sinai Medical School and the Graduate Center of the City University of New York. Previously, she did a year of graduate work in psychiatric art therapy at Hahnemann Medical College.

An award-winning and prolific author, Dr. Yager's 15 books include *Creative Time Management for the New Millennium, Friendshifts ®: The Power of Friendship and How It Shapes Our Lives* and *The Help Book* and dozens of magazine, newspaper, and website articles in *Parade, McCall's, Woman's Day, Redbook, The New York Times, Harper's,* and others. She is the coauthor, with Michael J. Thorpy, M.D., of *The Encyclopedia of Sleep and Sleep Disorders.*

Dr. Yager, the former J. L. Barkas, is a member of the American Sociological Association and the National Speakers Association. A speaker and workshop leader, Dr. Yager has been interviewed on numerous TV and radio shows, such as *The Today Show, The Oprah Winfrey Show, The View* and ABC radio, and has also been quoted or featured in *The Wall Street Journal, USA Today,* The Associated Press, *The New Yorker, People* and *The New York Times.* Her website is: http://www.JanYager.com

INDEX

Page numbers followed by the letter *f* indicate figures. **Boldface** page numbers indicate the primary entry on a topic.

continuous positive air-
way pressure (CPAP)
116–117
alcohol ingestion
and 86
automatic 38–39
bilevel 38
limitations of
116–117
mechanism of 116
nasal 33, 38,
116–117
nasal congestion
and 197
for sleep apnea 33,
38–39
convulsions **117**
cortisol **117**
asthma caused by
269
depression and 72
functions of 117
secretion of 72,
117, 148
cosleeping 62
cot death **117** *See also*
sudden infant death
syndrome
coughing **117–118**
causes of 117
treatment of
117–118
CPAP *See* continuous
positive airway pres-
sure
cramps **118**
nocturnal leg **205**
Creative Dreaming
(Garfield) 132
creativity
dreams and **132**
sleep and 73
Creutzfeldt-Jakob dis-
ease 143
crib death **118** *See also*
sudden infant death
syndrome
Crick, Francis 264
Critchley, Michael 175
CSS *See* Clinical Sleep
Society
cyclothymia 189
Cylert *See* pemoline
Czeisler, Charles 53,
111, 120

D

Daly, Dan 295
Darwin, Charles 100
daydreaming **119**
daytime sleepiness *See*
excessive sleepiness
death during sleep **119**
death rates, sleep dura-
tion and 7, 119, 252
deep sleep **120**
delayed sleep phase
120

delayed sleep phase
syndrome **120–122**
causes of 121
diagnosis of 121,
122
prevalence of 121
symptoms of 58,
64–65, 120–121
treatment of 53,
59, 65, 111, 122
delta sleep **122** *See
also* slow wave sleep
delta waves 9*f*, 11,
122, 135, 279
Dement, William C. 7,
8, 16, 24, 77–78, 91,
122, 147, 175, 241,
256, 278
dementia **123**
causes of 123
diagnosis of 123
vs. fatal familial
insomnia 143
symptoms of 68,
123
treatment of 123
depression **123–124**
and delayed sleep
phase 121
diagnosis of 190
and insomnia
30–31
and sleep stages
71–72, 189
symptoms of
123–124, 189,
231
treatment of 92,
124, 188
deprivation, sleep
256–257
depression and 72
effects of 7,
256–257
questionnaire on 6
REM **241**
Descartes, René 224
desensitization, sys-
temic **301**
Dewan, Edmond M.
129
dextroamphetamine
sulfate (Dexedrine)
294
diary, sleep 5, 6*f*, 263
Dickens, Charles 33,
100, 209, 210–211,
224
diet **124–125**
Argonne anti-jet-
lag 95–96, 125
effects of 18, 124
and weight reduc-
tion 210
DIMS *See* disorders of
initiating and main-
taining sleep

Dinges, David 7
disorders of excessive
somnolence (DOES)
125–126
disorders of initiating
and maintaining
sleep (DIMS)
126–127
disorders of the sleep-
wake schedule *See*
circadian rhythm
sleep disorders
diurnal 127
DOES *See* disorders of
excessive somno-
lence
Doll, Erich 33
L-dopa **178**
dopamine **127–128**
effects of 127
in narcolepsy 128
prolactin and 148,
230
dream(s) **128–132**
brain activity dur-
ing 130–131
content of **128,**
129–130, 146
and creativity **132**
effects of 78
functions of 69,
128, 129, 171
gender and 128,
130
interpretation of
146, **171**
lucid 131, **181**
REM rebound and
239
REM sleep and
77–78, 129, **241**
sleep atonia and
254
sleep mentation in
263–264
study of 128–129
visual component
of 129–130
dream anxiety attacks
128
drowsiness **132–133**
drowsy driving **133**
drugs 183–185 *See also*
specific types
drunkenness, sleep
259 *See also* confu-
sional arousals
duration, sleep
259–261
age and 259–260
definition of 259
factors affecting
259–261
in infants 5,
60–61, 162, 259
and mortality rates
7, 119, 252

dustman 248
dyspnea, nocturnal
203, 220, 270
dyssomnia **133**
dystonia, nocturnal
paroxysmal 63,
205–206

E

early morning arousal
134
ear plugs 207
eating (drinking) syn-
drome, nocturnal
51–52, 125,
203–204, 315
Economo, Constantin
von 156
EDS (excessive daytime
sleepiness) *See*
excessive sleepiness
EEG *See* electroen-
cephalogram
efficiency, sleep **261**
Egan, P. 248
Ehret, Charles 95
Ekbom, Karl A. 47,
244
Elavil *See* amitriptyline
elderly sleep 67–68
advanced sleep
phase in 58, 59
need for 5
electrical status epilep-
ticus of sleep (ESES)
134–135
diagnosis of 135
symptoms of
134–135
treatment of 135
electroencephalogram
(EEG) **135–136**
history of 104
procedure for
135–136, 225
electromyogram (EMG)
136, 225
electro-oculogram
(EOG) **136,** 226
electrosleep 283–284
EMG *See* electromyo-
gram
emission, nocturnal
131, **204–205**
endogenous circadian
pacemaker **137,**
217, 300
endoscopy **137**
fiberoptic 137,
143
enuresis, sleep **261**
causes of 63
definition of 63
features of 97
treatment of
63–64
environment, sleep,
history of 4

effects of 19, 88,
183–184, 294
respiratory **244**
therapeutic uses for
293–294
types of 293
stimulus control therapy 32, **296–297**
Stokes, William 109
strain gauge **297**
stress 17, **297**
stupor **297, 310**
subclinical electrical
status epilepticus of
sleep (SESE) 135
sudden infant death
syndrome (SIDS)
297–298
cause of 61–62,
297
risk factors for
61–62, 163, 298
sudden unexplained
nocturnal death syndrome (SUND) 97,
298–299
Sullivan, Colin 33, 116
SUND *See* sudden
unexplained nocturnal death syndrome
Sunday night insomnia
102, **299**
sundown syndrome
See dementia
suprachiasmatic nucleus (SCN) **300**
and circadian
rhythms 105,
137, 156–157,
217, 300
and melatonin
secretion 185
surgery, for sleep disorders **300–301** *See
also specific types*
swallowing syndrome,
sleep-related abnormal **268**
sweating **301**
sweats, night 262–263
SWS *See* slow wave
sleep
Symonds, Charles 205
synchronized sleep
301
systemic desensitization
301

T

tachypnea, sleep-related neurogenic **275**

talking, sleep **282**
Tartini, Guiseppe 132
temperature
body **302,**
303–304
environmental
302, 304
temporal isolation **302**
terrifying hypnagogic
hallucinations
302–303
terrors *See* sleep terrors
thermoregulation
303–304
theta activity 10, 11,
135, 248, **304**
theta coma 114
Thornby, Michael J.
22
Thorpy, Michael 171,
197
thyroid hormone 152,
157
thyroid-stimulating
hormone 157
tidal volume 107, **304**
time zone change syndrome *See* jet lag
timing of sleep, insomnia associated with
168
TMN *See* tubero-mammillary nucleus
tongue retaining device
(TRD) **306**
tonsillectomy 34, 39,
300, **306–307**
total recording time
(TRT) **307**
total sleep episode
307
total sleep time (TST)
307
toxin-induced sleep
disorder **307**
tracheostomy 40, 117,
209, **307–308**
tracheotomy 33
tranquilizers **308**
transient insomnia 83,
308
transition disorders,
sleep-wake **284**
TRD *See* tongue retaining device
tricyclic antidepressants
31
for depression 92
side effects of 31,

45
Tripp, Peter 256, **309**
TRT *See* total recording
time
L-tryptophan 124,
125, 250
TST *See* total sleep
time
tubero-mammillary
nucleus (TMN) 187
tumescence **309**
twitch **309**
L-tyrosine 128

U

UARS *See* upper airway resistance syndrome
ulcer disease, peptic
220
ultradian rhythm 247,
310
unconsciousness **310**
UPP *See* uvulopalatopharyngoplasty
upper airway obstruction **310–311**
causes of 310–311
early descriptions
of 33
and snoring 34
treatment of 311
upper airway resistance
syndrome (UARS)
35, **311**
upper airway sleep
apnea *See* obstructive sleep apnea syndrome
uvulopalatopharyngoplasty (UPP)
311–312
complications of
312
effectiveness of
117, 311–312
procedure for 311
for sleep apnea 33,
39, 117, 301,
311
for snoring 33,
289–290, 301,
311
submucous resection with 197
uvulopalatoplasty
laser 39, **178,** 290,
312
radiofrequency 39,
290, 312

V

vegetative state 113
ventilation **313**
vertex sharp waves
175
vigilance testing **313**
Wilkinson auditory
315
vitamin A deficiency
199
Vivarin 107

W

Wadd, William 33
wakefulness 98, **314**
wake time **314**
walking, sleep *See*
sleepwalking
warm baths **314**
weight **314–315**
ideal 209
reduction of 210
and sleep apnea
17, 37, 209,
314–315
Weitzman, Elliot 53,
120, 151, 302
Wells, William Hughes
33
Westphal, Carl
Friedrich Otto 42
wet dreams *See* nocturnal emission
Wilkinson auditory vigilance testing **315**
women
dream content in
128, 130
sleep disturbances
in 14, 66–67
World Federation of
Sleep Research
Societies **315**
Wyzinski, Peter W.
236–237

Y

yawning **316**
Yoss, Robert 295

Z

zaleplon (Sonata) 20,
30
Zappert, Julius 149,
174
zeitgeber *See* environmental time cues
zolpidem (Ambien)
20, 30
Zwilling, George 251